Sexual Cultures in East Asia

This book is the first to examine the social construction of sexual identity and the social stigma attached to the HIV/AIDS epidemic in East Asia. By studying sex work in the context of socio-economic change, the contributors persuasively argue that a discourse of sexuality forms a central point from which examinations of broader social and political relationships can take place. In an area where the discussion of sexuality is still largely a taboo subject, *Sexual Cultures in East Asia* provides a unique collection of case studies that highlight the difference between sexual attitudes within East Asia, and also the relationship between seemingly 'new' behaviour and traditional ideologies.

Specific issues discussed in relation to the AIDS epidemic and the social construction of sexual risk and sexual identity include:

- how sexual identity is formed and/or transformed
- networks which can channel or condition selection of sexual partners
- the complex relationship between traditional filial duty and prostitution
- gendered relations of power
- the relationship between kinship, sex education, marriage, NGOs and sex

By using a multidisciplinary approach, which includes sociological, medical and historical perspectives, Micollier highlights how East Asian sexual identity is most definitely a social construction. Designed specifically for social scientists and those involved in AIDS development programs, this book will appeal to anyone interested in sexuality and Asian cultures.

Evelyne Micollier is an Affiliated Research Fellow of the International Institute of Asian Studies, The Netherlands.

RoutledgeCurzon-IIAS Asian Studies Series

Series Co-ordinator: Dick van der Meij
Institute Director: Wim A.L. Stokhof

The International Institute for Asian Studies (IIAS) is a postdoctoral research centre based in Leiden and Amsterdam, The Netherlands. Its main objective is to encourage Asian Studies in the Humanities and the Social Sciences and to promote national and international co-operation in these fields. The Institute was established in 1993 on the initiative of the Royal Netherlands Academy of Arts and Sciences, Leiden University, Universiteit van Amsterdam and Vrije Universiteit Amsterdam. It is mainly financed by The Netherlands Ministry of Education, Culture, and Sciences. IIAS has played an active role in co-ordinating and disseminating information on Asian Studies throughout the world. The Institute acts as an international mediator, bringing together various entities for the enhancement of Asian Studies both within and outside The Netherlands. The RoutledgeCurzon-IIAS Asian Studies series reflects the scope of the Institute. The Editorial Board consists of Erik Zürcher, Wang Gungwu, Om Prakash, Dru Gladney, Amiya K. Bagchi, James C. Scott, Jean-Luc Domenach and Frits Staal.

Images of the 'Modern Woman' in Asia
Edited by Shoma Munshi

Nomads in the Sedentary World
Edited by Anatoly M. Khazanov and Andre Wink

Reading Asia
Edited by Frans Husken and Dick van der Meij

Tourism, Heritage and National Culture in Java
Heidi Dahles

Asian-European Perspectives
Edited by Wim Stokhof and Paul van der Velde

Law and Development in East and Southeast Asia
Edited by Christoph Antons

The Indian Ocean Rim
Edited by Gwyn Campbell

Rethinking Chinese Transnational Enterprises
Edited by Leo Douw, Cen Huang and David Ip

Indonesian Sea Nomads
Cynthia Chou

Diasporas and Interculturalism in Asian Performing Arts
Edited by Hae-Kyung Um

Reading East Asian Writing
Edited by Michel Hockx and Ivo Smits

Sexual Cultures in East Asia
Edited by Evelyn Micollier

Hinduism in Modern Indonesia
Edited by Martin Ramstedt

Sexual Cultures in East Asia

The social construction of sexuality and sexual risk in a time of AIDS

Edited by Evelyne Micollier

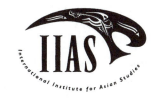

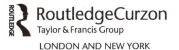

LONDON AND NEW YORK

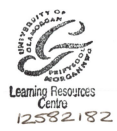

Learning Resources
Centre
12582182

First published 2004
by RoutledgeCurzon
11 New Fetter Lane, London EC4P 4EE

Simultaneously published in the USA and Canada
by RoutledgeCurzon
29 West 35th Street, New York, NY 10001

RoutledgeCurzon is an imprint of the Taylor & Francis Group

Printed and bound in Great Britain by MPG Books Ltd, Bodmin

British Library Cataloguing in Publication Data
A catalogue record for this book is available from the British Library

Library of Congress Cataloging in Publication Data
A catalog record for this book has been requested

ISBN 0-415-30871-2

Contents

ACKNOWLEDGEMENTS

This volume is a product of a research project focusing on AIDS, sexuality, and civil society in East Asia and in China in particular (1998–2001). The book was prepared during an International Conference on July 6–7, 2000 in Amsterdam organized by the International Institute for Asian Studies. The editor acknowledges the competent support of the IIAS staff during the book production's process. I am particularly grateful to Dr Rogier Busser, Dr Dick van der Meij and Rosemary Robson (BA Hons.) for copy-editing the manuscript, and for the lay-out.

I am also very thankful to all the participants in the workshop including those whose presentations are not part of this volume, but who contributed positively to the discussions, namely Dr Han ten Brummelhuis, University of Amsterdam, Dr Liao Susu, Beijing Union Medical College, Dr Zhao Pengfei, Shanghai Family Planning Research Institute, and Dr Lily Ling, The Hague Institute of Social Sciences.

My sincere gratitude goes to the referees for their constructive comments, which have been a source of reflection for the editor and the contributors in this book. I thank all the contributors – those who have been conscientiously revising their conference papers and those who have joined us in the publishing phase. The final works appearing in the volume, however, remain their personal views and responsibility. Indeed, views expressed throughout the papers may not be shared by the editor, and to some extent, the contents developed remain the responsibility of the authors also.

I thank the European Science Foundation for its consistent financial support for the research project and the conference and the NWO (Dutch Foundation for Scientific Research) for the funding provided for the conference. Finally, I am indebted to IIAS support for my research activities as a European Science Foundation research fellow attached with IIAS (1998–2000) and as a long-term affiliated fellow (2001–2002).

NOTES ON CONTRIBUTORS

MARIE-EVE BLANC is currently an Associated Research Fellow at IRSEA (Institute for Research on South-East Asia) of the CNRS (French National Center for Scientific Research) in Marseilles, and a Research Project Manager with ANRS funding (National Agency for AIDS Research, France). She holds a PhD in Sociology from the University of Provence (France). Her current project is about sexual behaviours, knowledge and management of HIV/AIDS risk among young urban Vietnamese men, and is carried out with POPCON (Population Consultants) in Hanoi. She has been working with ANRS since 1999. She presented papers at conferences and published a number of articles on gender and health issues in the context of Vietnamese culture. She co-edited *Asian Societies Confronted by AIDS*, Paris: L'Harmattan, 2000 (in French).

ANNUSKA DERKS is a PhD Candidate in Anthropology at the University of Nijmegen, The Netherlands, and currently holds a teaching position at the Institute of Anthropology, University of Bern, Switzerland. She has worked since 1995 as a research officer for the Center for Advanced Study in Phnom Penh and as a consultant for international organizations working on trafficking and sex work in Cambodia. Among her publications are papers on trafficking in Cambodia and Southeast Asia. Her forthcoming PhD *Moving Women, Moving Selves* focuses on the complex interplay of migration, gender, and identity in Cambodia.

CHRISTIAN HENRIOT (PhD) is Professor of Modern History at Lumière-Lyon 2 University and Director of the Institut d'Asie Orientale. His research interests cover Chinese urban history, women's history and the Sino-Japanese war. His major publications in English are: *Shanghai 1927–1937: Municipal Power, Locality, and Modernization*, Berkeley, The University of California Press, 1993; Prostitution and Sexuality in Shanghai: A Social History, 1849–1949, New York/Cambridge, Cambridge University Press, 2000; *New Frontiers: Imperialism's New Communities in East Asia, 1842–1952*, with Robert Bickers (eds.), Manchester, Manchester University Press, 2000.

MEI-LING HSU (PhD) is currently a Professor of Journalism at the National Chengchi University in Taipei, Taiwan. She has recently published a Chinese book entitled *AIDS and the Media*, Taipei, Chuliu Publisher, 2001; also 'Pattern of responses to HIV transmission questions: Rethinking HIV knowledge and its relevant to AIDS prejudice,' *AIDS Care,* 14(4), (2002, co-authored with C-Y Lew-Ting), and 'An exploration of AIDS prejudice: Fear of infection and moral devaluation' in *Public Health in Taiwan* (forthcoming, also co-authored with C-Y Lew-Ting). Her research projects in Taiwan include a review of health communication research and education, a textual analysis of news discourses of sex workers, foreign labour and HIV/AIDS, evaluations of health campaigns of HIV/AIDS, TB and enterovirus infection, respectively, and an interdisciplinary effort in increasing health literacy via the mass media.

PAULA-FRANCES KELLY is currently a PhD candidate in Confucian Philosophy and its implications on gender and the AIDS epidemic. She holds a degree in Education and Graduate Diplomas in Sociology (Research and Evaluation) and in Community Development and a Masters of Arts degree (Criminology). She directs the non-government development organization, PKA(Asia)Inc and consults for international NGOs, UN agencies, private development companies and bilateral agencies. She has lived in Vietnam for over ten years but has worked in the Southeast Asian Region for more than thirty years. Her work entails development programme identification, implementation, monitoring, and evaluation. This requires research: economic, contextual, social, gender, and cultural. Her overriding research interest is that of cultural values and attitude perpetuation, and how these impact on behaviours (individual and institutional). For many years she has researched religion and cultures in the region and used her findings in programme development for health – predominantly for HIV/AIDS/STI reduction – for women's empowerment, environment, community development, trafficking migration, and training.

WEN-CHI LIN is currently a doctoral student at the Department of Journalism, National Cheng-Chi University, Taipei, Taiwan. She has written her master's thesis, *The Rhetoric of AIDS as Constructed In News Discourse: An Analysis of China Times and United Daily*, in 1996. She has also translated two books into Chinese, including *Communication: An Introduction*, Taipei, Weber Publisher, 2000, authored by Karl Rosengren, and *Identity and Difference*, Taipei, Weber Publisher, 2002, edited by Kathryn Woodward. Her research interests include rhetorical criticism, discourse analysis, and culture research. She has been working with Dr Mei-Ling Hsu in a textual analysis of news discourses of sex workers, foreign labour and HIV/AIDS, as well as evaluations of health campaigns of HIV/AIDS, TB and enterovirus infection in Taiwan.

WIM LUNSING was a Temporary Lecturer in Social Anthropology at Oxford Brookes University, an Associate Research Professor in Japanese Studies at the University of Copenhagen, and a Research Fellow at the University of Tokyo. He has a BA (1985) and MA (1988) in Japanese Studies from the University of Leiden and a PhD in Social Anthropology (1995) from Oxford Brookes University. He has presented papers at numerous conferences in Europe, North America, and Asia and has given lectures at various universities in Europe and Japan. Apart from his book: *Beyond common sense: sexuality and gender in contemporary Japan*, London, New York, and Bahrain, Kegan Paul International, 2001, he has published various papers on lesbian and gays issues, on fieldwork methods and ethical issues, and on sex culture and sex work in contemporary Japan.

EVELYNE MICOLLIER was a long-term research fellow at IIAS (International Institute for Asian Studies, Leiden) (1998–2002), and is currently an Associated Research Fellow at IRSEA (Institute for Research on South-East Asia) of the CNRS (French National Centre for Scientific Research) in Marseilles. She was a visiting scholar at the Institute of Ethnology of the Academia Sinica in Taipei (1995–1996). She holds an MA (1988) in Chinese Studies and a PhD in Medical Anthropology from the University of Provence (France). She has both presented papers at international conferences and published a number of articles on health and religious issues in the context of Chinese culture. She co-edited *Asian Societies confronted by AIDS*, Paris: L'Harmattan, 2000 (in French).

PAN SUIMING is Professor of Sociology and Director of the Institute for Research on Gender and Sexuality at the Beijing Renmin (People's) University of China. He is also an expert in AIDS prevention at the China Health Ministry, an expert on Marriage and Family at the China Civil Affairs Ministry, a pornography prevention expert at the China News and Publishing Ministry, and vice-chair of the China AIDS Network. He has published a number of papers in international journals on sexuality, sex education, AIDS prevention and awareness, gender, and sex work in PR China (in English), and presented his works at international conferences. He has also published nine books in Chinese between 1988 and 2002 about sexuality, sexology, the sex industry, sexual behaviours and relationships in China today. He has recently published (in Chinese): *Study of Three 'Red Light Districts' in Southeastern China*, 2002; *Nation-wide Sampling Survey of Chinese Sexual Behavior and Relationships*, 2001; *Case-study of a Chinese 'Red Light District'*, 2000.

ANKE VAN DER KWAAK is an anthropologist working at the Health, Care and Culture Section of the VU University Medical Centre. She teaches courses on culture and health, reproductive health, and qualitative research design. Currently, she is working on a research project on female circumcision and the Somali Community in the Netherlands. Her recent publications are: Edien Bartels, Anke van der Kwaak en Han Bartels, 'Meisjesbesnijdenis in justitieel perspectief' (Female circumcision from a legal perspective) *Proces. Tijdschrift voor berechting en reclassering.* 'Cultuur in de strafrechts-praktijk', maart/april, 2002, nr.3/4, pp. 49–53. M. van Dijk, J. Visschedijk en A.H. van der Kwaak, 'Client satisfaction – Guidelines for assessing the quality of leprosy services from the clients perspective' (*Leprosy Review*, forthcoming).

IAN WALTERS (PhD) is Senior Lecturer in Anthropology at Northern Territory University, Australia. He has been researching in Vietnam for nearly a decade, working mainly in material culture studies and Vietnamese pasts. More recently he has begun to research Vietnam's sex industries, with an interest in the relations between policy, culture, and commercial sexuality. He is the author of *Dasher Wheatley and Australia in Vietnam* (1998) and co-editor of *Altered States: Material Culture Transformations in the Arafura Region* (2001). He is currently working on a book manuscript called *Social Evil: Prostitution Policy and Culture in Vietnam.*

IVAN WOLFFERS is a Professor at the VU University Medical Center, section of Health Care and Culture. He holds an MD and a PhD. He is the Editor of *Research for Sex Work,* a yearly Newsletter. He provides technical support and capacity building to the network 'CARAM Asia' (Co-ordination of Action Research on AIDS and Migration). The Secretariat is located in Kuala Lumpur/Malaysia.

TSUI-SUNG WU is currently a doctoral student at the Department of Journalism, National Cheng-Chi University, Taipei, Taiwan. With her research interest in sexuality and sex agenda, she wrote her master's thesis, *The homosexuals in newspapers: A discourse analysis of homosexuality reports in Taiwan*, in 1998, which was later published as a book chapter in C.R. Ho (ed.) *A Study of Homosexuality*, Taipei, Chiulu Publisher, 2001. She has also conducted an in-depth analysis of male prostitutions in Taiwan, which was presented at the Fifth International Conference On Sexuality Education, Sexology, Trans/Gender Studies and LesBigay Studies, and is under being prepared as a book chapter. She has been working with Dr Mei-Ling Hsu in a textual analysis of news discourses of sex workers, foreign labour, and HIV/AIDS in Taiwan.

INTRODUCTION

EVELYNE MICOLLIER

Plural discourses on sex, components and methods of workings of sexual cultures in Asia need to be explored in more depth, and this book should be taken as one brick added to the edifice of this specific body of knowledge. The main focus of our book is the study of sexual cultures and commercial sex work in East Asian societies. Most chapters have been revised from papers presented at the IIAS Conference 'Health, Sexuality, and Civil Society in East Asia', which took place in Amsterdam on July 6–7 2000, while a few contributors have joined us in the publication process (Henriot, Kelly, Walters). The book is organized in two parts: (1) 'Sexual cultures: caught between traditions and transitions' and (2) 'The social construction of sexuality and sexual risk in the light of STDs/AIDS control'. Topics discussed may, of course, overlap in the two parts. The first part deals with issues related to sexual cultures such as the role of commercial sex work, the kinship system, matrimonial strategies, gender roles in the family, gendered power relations in society and in the building of these cultures in transition. A dialectical relation between traditional and new elements in the ideological and behavioural configuration of sexual cultures is underlined throughout the papers. The second part examines specific issues related to the HIV/AIDS epidemic and the social construction of sexual risk. As Parker (1995:362) put it, 'The social construction of sexual excitement and desire, ways in which sexual identities are formed and transformed, the relations of power and domination that may shape and structure sexual interactions, and the social/sexual networks that channel and condition the selections of potential sexual partners may all be salient issues that must be taken into account in developing more effective strategies for AIDS prevention.'

As many scholars have shown since Foucault (1976), sexuality is a dense nodal point for competing power relations and discourses of sexuality play a crucial role in efforts both to regulate and reform the political, economic, and social orders (Bristow 1997; Di Leonardo and Lancaster 1997). The complexity of the subject and the multi-layered social phenomena to be examined suggested that the perspective of the book should be multidisciplinary. Indeed, the contributors are sociologists (Blanc, Pan), anthropologists (Derks, Lunsing, Micollier, Walters), a historian (Henriot), communication specialists (Hsu, Lin, Wu), a development expert

(Kelly), medical doctors and/or medical anthropologists (Wolffers, Van der Kwaak).

East Asian societies are usually labelled family-oriented 'Confucianized societies' and are, roughly speaking, characterized by hierarchical human and social relations, authoritarian political organizations, a high level of social codification, and gender inequality. They share a common cluster of values, a cultural feature relevant to be used as a working hypothesis for the study of the intimate side of the Self such as sexual behaviours, meanings, and ideas. The relevance of a cultural constraint in the social construction of sexuality is discussed in a number of papers (Blanc, Derks, Kelly, Micollier, Wolffers). In our understanding, East Asia includes the Chinese world (P.R.China, Hong Kong, Taiwan, Singapore and the Chinese diasporas), Vietnam, Korea and Japan. The comparative perspective is trans-Asian and is thus a proximity comparison – a tentative endeavour to draw comparative lines between East Asian countries, and in a broader perspective between East and Southeast Asia. A few papers document the situation in Mainland Southeast Asia (Vietnam, Cambodia, Thailand) and Insular Southeast Asia (Indonesia). Vietnam is the most obvious and significant link between East and Southeast Asia, a fact explaining the number of papers (3) focusing on Vietnam in the book (Blanc, Kelly, Walters). Throughout these papers, there is a remarkable contrast in the description of Vietnamese attitudes towards sexuality although it should be noted simultaneously that there is an ambivalence towards sex workers in most East and Southeast Asian societies.

SEXUAL CULTURES: GENDER AND SEXUALITY

In our understanding, the concept of sexual culture is borrowed from Herdt (1997:10): 'A "sexual culture" is a consensual model of cultural ideas about sexual behaviour in a group. Such a cognitive model involves a world-view of norms, values, beliefs, and meaning regarding the nature and purpose of sexual encounters. It also involves an affective model of emotional states and moral guidelines to institutionalize what is felt to be "normal, natural, necessary, or approved" in a community of actors.'

Societies differ greatly in their normative codes of sexual conduct and the expression of desires, needs, and sexuality may change drastically in the course of life (Mead 1961). Most academic works stress the differences between Asian and Western sexual cultures focusing on the comparison between a much mythicized 'East' and 'West', along the lines of an Orientalist intellectual tradition, and by doing so falling into the research bias of 'exoticizing' the Other and considering Asian culture as one to be opposed to the West. Moreover, most of the discussion on sexuality in Asia takes place in Western academic arenas pursued by either Western scholars or Asian scholars based in the West. This work will diverge from this common perspective in discussing differences within Asia, mainly by drawing a few comparative lines between sexuality in East Asia and Southeast Asia, and in bringing together Western scholars and Asian scholars from Asia in our collective editorial project.

Even though sexuality is an important aspect of life, it remains a difficult subject for scholarly research. In Western societies, the sexual liberation and the feminist movement from the 1960s favoured the rise of plural discourses on sex. It allowed people to live experiences questioning traditional normalization and regulation of sexual relations. However, even contemporary anthropological research, with every tool of fieldwork and all imaginable theoretical sophistication, has difficulties in obtaining reliable information about these recent changes in sexual behaviour and meanings in Western societies. The *mise en discours* of sexuality in Europe in relation to power and control has been extensively researched by Foucault (1976). He argued that the regulation of sexuality in Europe was a political tool for both the state and the church in their agonistic strive for power and control over the people. In Asian societies, sex is far less an object of discourses and studies than in the Christian and republican traditions. The social significance of sexuality in various contexts, namely marital, extramarital, commercial, is different in Asia as compared to Western societies. In general, it is even more difficult to study sexuality in Asia than it is in the West. Despite these problems, Dikötter (1995) has shown in a pioneering work that a similar state discourse regulating and monitoring closely sexual behaviours and meanings did prevail in modern China and, to some extent, still exists in contemporary China. In contrast to China, there is almost no state discourse on sex in most Southeast Asian countries.

The papers further contribute to explaining how and why sexuality is not a primordial acquisition or comprehensible in terms of totalizing or essentializing theories but is definitely a social construct within an open, dynamic and contingent set of social, political, and economic relations.[1] These theories were challenged by social scientists who demonstrated that sexual conduct was socially and culturally constructed (among them, Gagnon, and Simon 1973; Gagnon 1977; Weeks 1985). As soon as the theory of natural gender difference is rejected, a structural social inequality between men and women, thus the power of gender, becomes obvious; gendered power relations appear then as an important factor to explain the differences between the sexual lives of men and women (Gagnon and Parker 1995:14). The local discourse on sexuality, its incorporation into people's worldviews, disciplinary efforts to normalize it, and divergent critical voices highlight the modern tendency for sexuality to become a central point in contesting broader issues of identity politics and gender relations. Representations of gender and sexuality are far more than before created through a whole range of forms from the commercialized images of the female eroticized body to those of the supportive and self-sacrificing wife. For instance, in China, the views of medical experts, agents of the state, as well as commercial bodies interested in responding to consumer demand come together in transmitting such images: 'Indeed, the explosion of sexually explicit material since the 1980s and the transformation of sexual practices among urban young people denote the emergence of what could be called a new sexual culture in China's urban centers.' (Evans 1995:387; 389). However, ideas and practices rooted in the traditional system can still be remodelled and re-emerge in new conditions through a process of cultural revivalism, men and women being agents both complying with and resisting competing constructions of sexuality: for instance, there is an implicit gender code prescribing for the middle-class Chinese woman the respect of Confucian family values and of the status quo (Maclaren 1998:196).

COMMERCIAL SEX WORK AND MARRIAGE

This book mainly documents female sex work. However, one has to keep in mind that male prostitutes do constitute about one third of the total number of sex workers on an international scale even though all figures and estimates about prostitution should be taken cautiously (Davis 1993). Commercial sex work should be analysed as a complex social phenomenon closely related to drastic socio-economic changes occurring in Asia and to cultural traditions as well. Identifying social, cultural, economic and environmental factors of commercial sex work[2] are at the core of most papers (Derks, Kelly, Lunsing, Micollier, Pan, Walters, Wolffers). These factors are, of course, related to sex roles in the family and in society. Some forms of prostitution have their roots in traditional forms of debt bondage, which was a well-established social institution in Southeast Asia, the Indian Subcontinent, and China (Testart 2000).

Female prostitution in East and Southeast Asia is mainly meant for native men. Even in Thailand, where international sex tourism is fully developed and where sex tours are so common, prostitution for foreigners constitutes only about twenty per cent of all commercial sex exchanges. Forms of prostitution range on a continuum from slavery to free operation by girls and free choice about engaging in the sex industry. There is a high turnover among sex workers; prostitution is not a fixed career. For a woman, involvement in sex work during a period of her life may generate a long-term stigma or an improvement in her living conditions, if she uses the money earned to develop other lucrative activities. The agency of prostitutes is an important issue to be raised in the analysis of prostitution. Sex workers may make impressive careers or slowly improve their position: the origin of Thai women's economic activities in Europe took place at some point in the sphere of sex work. For instance, they have managed to open Thai restaurants, and the very existence of Thai communities in Germany, Holland, and Scandinavia is evidence of the agency of sex workers. Their agency is related to women's position in the kinship system (Brummelhuis 1997; 2000). The Thai situation offers the greatest contrast to India where women are strictly bound to male agnatic families. As for China, even though traditional kinship systems are agnatic, socialist ideas and practices have influenced other rules of behaviour, and deep changes in gender roles within marriage. In the context of East and Southeast Asia, some similarities can be pointed out. The common Western idea that sex for money can be clearly distinguished from a love or a marriage relationship does not exist in Asia, where economic factors are always essential in the building up of social and/or intimate relationships. In such a context, prostitution and marriage are closely interrelated institutions so much so that any discussion about prostitution should extend to the issue of marriage for several reasons. Firstly, they both combine sex and money according to positions in the kinship system. Second, a man tends to make a division between the woman he will marry and the person(s) to whom he is sexually attracted. The married woman will be the mother of his children and have access to the family economic resources. Sex roles within marriage tend to suppress any sexual agency or subjectivity of the wives, who are supposed to be 'good women'. A 'good woman' is per definition not a 'whore' and should not take any sexual initiatives. Asian women are trained to look for a husband and they know at a very early stage that it behoves them to look for a husband in the future. In that context, the fact that women use their bodies strategically, their youth and their beauty, to get money is consistent with their education in society and in the family, and not even in contradiction with a 'globalizing' context.[3]

As Derks shows in her paper about sex work in Cambodia, 'researching sex work gives of a picture of the contradictions that exist between oppression and exploitation on the one hand side and power and freedom on the other hand side.' Lunsing offers an anthropological perspective on sex work in Japan with the question about the agency of prostitutes at the core of his analysis. He shows that 'the economic aspects of sex have become more explicit than they have been for some time' and that 'there is an actual increase of sex being traded for money' in Japan, which is not the result of any 'globalizing' process but is rather related to a traditional sexual permissiveness. Pan's paper is composed of selected extracts from his pioneering book about the underground sex industry in China recently published in Chinese (Pan 1999). His book is the first ever published on the subject based on sociological first-hand data. For that reason, it provides a new valuable source for an overall understanding of the development of a sex industry in China. The emergence, patterns, and methods of working of a red light district can be drawn from his work based on three case-studies conducted in three different towns in South China (provinces of Guangdong, Guangxi, and Guizhou). Pan, from the 'Sociological Research Institute on Gender and Sexuality' (*Xing shehuixue yanjiusuo*) at the China People's University (*Zhongguo renmin daxue*, Beijing), and his research associates did field research about sex work in 1998 and 1999. The results were unveiled in two books (Pan 1999; 2000) which provide a deep insight into actual and contextualized working and living conditions of sex workers, and a record of their voices kept silent until now. Their long-term project research is still underway: another field research was done in 2001. The institute directed by Pan is the first of its kind in P.R.China. Its aim is to document different aspects of sexuality such as sex work, sexual identity and homosexuality by using methodological tools of sociology and anthropology rather than those of biomedical sciences, epidemiology and public health as is usually the case in China. In her paper about sex work and sexual culture in China, with a few references to Vietnam and Korea, Micollier uses some of Pan's findings in addition to her own fieldwork data, and discusses the role of sex work in the social construction of sexuality. She argues that a whole range of cultural, social, and economic factors tend to shape a sexual culture in which sex work plays the main role because of marriage rules and women's traditional roles in the Confucian family. Sexuality is thus approached through the dialectical relation between marital and extra-marital sexual life. Two papers in the book emphasize the structural relations between prostitution and marriage (Derks, Micollier). The study of sex work at international and national levels shows that movements of the population are closely interrelated with the flourishing of a sex industry (Herdt 1997; Blanc 1998, Husson 1998, Micollier 1998). One explanatory factor of its rapid expansion in developing Asian countries is linked to an economic development, which stimulates the mobility of the labour force. Besides, sex work is a way for women to climb the social ladder in society, and that social factor is a recurrent motive for engaging into prostitution (Brummelhuis 1997). Through such social mobility, poor women can support their families and middle-class women involved in occasional high-class prostitution may alleviate economic dependency on parents or husbands to satisfy consumerist and individualist aspirations. As

Derks subtly notes, mobility in the context of sex work is an aspect to be studied in more depth as a multi-layered process involving changes of settings and changes of behaviour as well. Wolffers, Kelly and Van der Kwaak go further in their analysis by talking about 'shifting identities' when they refer to drastic changes of conduct of sex workers at home or in work settings. They distinguish self-defined identities and identities defined by others, and underline that sex workers commonly keep their different identities well-separated from each other, an attitude mainly attributable to societal disapproval and legal prohibition. Their paper documents the situation in Vietnam, Thailand, and Indonesia, drawing a few comparative lines between East and Southeast Asian countries. Walters focuses on the economic factors underlying the development of a sex industry in Vietnam, and identifies some cultural factors as well: he explains for instance that female prostitutes support their families and that, by doing so, fulfil their filial duties: 'Those involved in the sex industries see themselves as making sensible and filial contributions to family, employer, and the country.' One should recall here that filial piety was among the most important Confucian values, if not the most important, in traditional China, Vietnam, and Korea, and still is to some extent. Kelly analyses gender and sexuality as social constructs in the context of the Vietnamese society with a feminist perspective. On the basis of her experience as a development expert, she chooses to use a number of research reports focusing on implications for intervention, which are usually more scarcely referred to in academic works.

Sexuality and Sexual Risk in a Times of AIDS

Sex education, State/NGOs relations are approached through the analysis of local STDs/AIDS campaigns (Blanc, Micollier Part Two, Wolffers *et al.*). Throughout all the papers, it is constantly reiterated that sexuality may generate and stimulate a debate in society involving the State and diverse actors of civil society through the issue of controlling communicable diseases as STDs, including the HIV/AIDS epidemic. News analysis of discourses about the AIDS epidemic sheds light on the social construction of disease as a social stigma (Hsu *et al.*). Henriot's paper offers a historical study on STD control and prostitution during the Republican period in Shanghai (1912–49). Henriot concludes: 'While no direct parallel with the Republican period can be traced, the dominant mode of intervention by the Chinese authorities has been stigmatization and repression. As in the past, the approach to the problem of prostitution and STDs – a problem made more sensitive with HIV and AIDS – is derived from prejudiced views rather than a genuine attempt to confront the social dynamics that run below prostitution and from a deliberate policy of imposing a blackout on these issues, especially the extent of HIV in China, both internally and externally.' His research appears as complementary to anthropological and sociological studies conducted in contemporary China (Pan 1999, 2000; Micollier 1999; Jeffreys 1997). The issue of *Chinese Sociology and Anthropology* edited by Jeffreys (1997) aims at clarifying the nature and the effects of government regulations of prostitution in China today, offering a specific reading of the relationship between State and society. It is a contribution to the understanding of the particular forms of knowledge and institutional practices explaining how prostitution could be conceptualized as an object of political concern and as a target for corrective intervention: translated materials from Chinese reveal the highly differentiated and organized nature of prostitution in China today, and detailed various responses to this social problem.

Whether we can or cannot talk about an 'emerging civil society' or a 'civil society' really needs to be asked through the lens of public health issues related to sexuality (Blanc, Hsu *et al.*, Micollier part II). For instance, in China, although the State is still trying to regulate sexual life and attitudes towards sex (Dikötter 2000), people are being submitted to diverging influences. They tend to act and think away from prescriptions coming either from traditional family ideology or from State discourses. A public health issue can both reveal and fuel social change. In her paper about sex education in Vietnam, Blanc shows how sex education programmes are implemented at school and out of school, and which tensions and negotiations are at work in the process. She emphasizes the tensions engendered by cultural taboos, which fuel the resistance of the teachers and the families as well. These tensions have to be negotiated between all the actors involved, namely the official bodies ruling the educational and the health-care system, the educational and health personnel, the families, and the local NGOs, which have been developing in the context of a emerging civil society during the 1990s.

DISCUSSION: SELECTED POINTS

In addition to the points mentioned earlier, the following issues were raised during the discussion at the 2000 IIAS Conference designed to be a research workshop:

At this stage of the current research on gender and sexuality, as Brummelhuis noticed, the existence of transgender is no longer considered a curious, marginal phenomenon but appears as a very interesting topic for further study about the relationships between sexuality and gender. Gender is not a strictly dichotomic concept but rather a bipolar one usually stretching out on a 'male–female' continuum. Ethnographic studies conducted in Latin America have inspired a new idea showing that gender and sexual identities can be drawn on a bipolar 'male–non male' continuum rather than a 'male–female' one, referring to the famous Latin 'macho' figure (Balderston and Guy 1997). Moreover, there is a prevalence of more fluid constructions of sexual identities questioning a strict homosexual–heterosexual polarity (Green and Babb 2002). In Asia, transgender people (third gender) have been known for a very long time in some countries such as India, Thailand, Burma, Indonesia, and the Philippines. Locally, there is a plurality of discourses on them emanating from the modern health-care sphere (sexologists and health workers), the popular sphere or the 'globalizing' sphere.

What does openness towards sexuality mean? Openness is again a social construct and if we begin the analysis with Western concepts, most Asian people may appear prudish and silent about sexuality. Indeed, as Brummelhuis and Herdt (1995:16) explain, 'it is necessary to spell out for certain societies the distinctions between prudery, sex-positivity, openness and repression in specific – public and private – cultural contexts (Parker 1995). Actually, the Western case might be extreme and atypical, due to its high tolerance for sex in public discourse, compared to the face of its elaborate ideologies and practices of repression (Foucault 1976).' For instance, the attitude of men towards sex work is significant: while it is very difficult for most Western men to admit visiting prostitutes, it is quite easy for most Asian men to do so. A simple reason is that a Western man who visits prostitutes, is perceived by others and perceives himself as a loser because it seems to spell out that he could not find a girlfriend. In contrast, visiting prostitutes is a mark of status and of masculinity for an Asian man. This example shows differences in values toward sex work, which have implications in the social construction of masculinity.

Why is it so easy to sell people's bodies? There seems to be no normative constraints to the treating people's bodies, to the commodification of the bodies of one's children and women. As Lunsing put it, love and sex may be considered commodities 'whether it takes place in marriage, love relationships, or in the context of prostitution.' Bodies have become a vehicle to getting cash. In the Chinese context, pre-revolutionary conditions, the communist ideology, and the international 'globalizing' model seem to have created an ideal ideological and behavioural configuration for the expansion of prostitution. A simple reason may be that poverty is more shameful than prostitution. Taking the risk to adopt a reductionist view, one may observe that 'local' bodies are now unavoidably bounded to financial 'international' flows. As Pan pointed out in the discussion, the officer class in China still buy beauty rather than sex as it is the tradition mainly to invigorate the process of traditional social networking (*guangxi* system of social relations). He argues that this feature has nothing to do with any 'globalizing' process. Through the surveys of his long-term research, it appears that most male clients ideally want to have a wife, a girlfriend, and a prostitute to serve and accompany them.

Although sexuality is a difficult subject for social science research to tackle as mentioned earlier, it has to be investigated in order to evaluate sexual risk and to design appropriate AIDS prevention programmes, as well as for a better understanding of human beings and of human life in the context of culture. Public health and educational purposes are obvious. Furthermore, the study of sexual risk in the Era of AIDS and its culture-bound factors are a pressing issue as the AIDS epidemic is spreading at an alarming rate in the most populated countries of the world – China and India, and is currently gaining ground in Asian countries. East and Southeast Asian societies share several factors which make the implementation of appropriate STDs/AIDS programmes more difficult, namely a sharp increase in 'indirect' sexual services,[4] the volatility and diversity of entertainment settings, and a high turnover of prostitutes. Other aspects of sexual cultures and sexual risk in times of epidemics also need to be explored further, and in this book, a few topics among many were selected. The relationship between sexuality and identity remains to be documented in the context of East Asian cultures: indeed, structural factors of gender, class, and age underlie the social construction of identity at different levels – individual, familial, local, national, and even 'globalized'.[5] The question of sexual identities and the erasing of boundaries needs to be addressed: queer, gay, lesbian, and transgender cultures are emerging or are being re-shaped, caught between traditional beliefs and practices, between the visible and invisible aspects of attitudes and discourses, redesigned to cope with the transitions undergone in societies. Even though first hand data used by most contributors were collected using a methodology designed to understand public discourses – official, popular, and traditional – about sexuality, they were also intended to listen to the actual voices of sex workers and sexual minorities as well, addressing the problem of the social stigmas associated with them and the discourses on them may have raised difficulties and consequently silenced some voices. These voices still need to be heard to deepen our knowledge of the social construction of sexuality, and to help in the building up of more appropriate anti-AIDS strategies in the context of East Asian 'civil societies.'

NOTES

1 See Manderson and Jolly (eds), a work which also apprehends sexualities as social constructs in the Asian context; for an insightful theoretical approach and a well-documented state of the field of sex research, see Parker and Gagnon (eds) (1995), and their introduction in particular (pp. 3–16).
2 I will use 'commercial sex work' rather than 'sex work' on the grounds that we should consider some forms of sex work as non-commercial exchanges (sex work performed in such conditions that it becomes slavery, and forced sex in marital life).
3 Some ideas in this paragraph were inspired by the paper presented by H.T. Brummelhuis (2000).
4 Epidemiologists usually distinguish 'direct' prostitution from 'indirect' prostitution. In East and Southeast Asia, the distinction is not very useful because commercial sex work takes so many different forms and takes place in a whole range of settings.
5 For an interesting discussion on the paradoxes of identities and on how 'sexuality is woven into the web of all our identities,' (p. 36), see Weeks (1995).

REFERENCES

Balderston, D. and D.J. Guy (eds) (1997) *Sex and Sexuality in Latin America*. New York: New York University Press.

Blanc, M.E. (1998) 'De la ville à la campagne: itinéraire de l'épidémie du VIH/Sida au Vietnam,' in: 'Migrations et Sida,' special issue of *Migrations et Santé* 94–5, pp. 11–29.

Bristow, J. (1997) *Sexuality*. London: Routledge.

Brummelhuis, H.T. and G. Herdt (eds) (1995) *Culture and Sexual Risk. Anthropological Perspectives on AIDS*. Amsterdam: Gordon and Breach Publishers.

– (1997) 'Mobility, Marriage, and Prostitution: Sexual Risk among Thai in the Netherlands,' in: G. Herdt (ed.) *Sexual Cultures and Migration in the Era of AIDS. Anthropological and Demographic Perspectives*. Oxford: Clarendon Press, pp. 167–84.

– (2000) 'Sexualities: Tentative Comparisons Between Southeast Asia and East Asia,' paper presented at the IIAS Conference on 'Health, Sexuality, and Civil Society in East Asia', Amsterdam, July 6–7.

Davis, N.J. (1993) *Prostitution: An International handbook on Trends, Problems, and Policies*. Westport, Connecticut: Greenwood Press.

Dikötter, F. (1995) *Sex, Culture and Modernity in China. Medical Science and the Construction of Sexual Identities in the Early Republican Period.* London: Hurst Co.

– (2000) 'La sexualité et les maladies sexuellement transmissibles en Chine: discours médical et représentations sociales,' in: M.E. Blanc, L. Husson et E. Micollier (eds) *Sociétés asiatiques face au sida.* Paris: L'Harmattan, pp. 23–40.

Di Leonardo M. and R.N. Lancaster (eds) (1997) *The Gender/Sexuality Reader: Culture, History, Political Economy.* New York: Routledge.

Evans, H. 1995 'Defining Difference: The Scientific Construction of Sexuality and Gender in the People's Republic of China,' *Signs. Journal of Women in Culture and Society* 20(2), pp. 357–94.

Foucault, M. (1976) *Histoire de la sexualité I. La volonté de savoir.* Paris: Gallimard.

Gagnon, J.H. (1977) *Human Sexualities.* Glenview, IL: Scott Foresman.

Gagnon J.H. and R.G. Parker (1995) 'Introduction: Conceiving Sexuality,' in: R.G. Parker and J.H. Gagnon (eds) *Conceiving Sexuality. Approaches to Sex Research in a Postmodern World.* New York and London: Routledge, pp. 3–16.

Gagnon J.H. and W. Simon (1973) *Sexual Conduct: The Social Sources of Human Sexuality.* Chicago: Aldine.

Green J.N. and F. Babb (eds) (2002) 'Gender and Homosexuality,' *Latin American Perspectives*, forthcoming.

Herdt, G. (1997) 'Sexual Cultures and Population Movement : Implications for AIDS/STDs,' in: G. Herdt (ed.) *Sexual Cultures and Migration in the Era of AIDS. Anthropological and Demographic Perspectives.* Oxford: Clarendon Press, pp. 3–22.

Husson, L. (1998) 'Le VIH en Indonésie: un virus de "bord de route", fortement lié aux migrations,' in: 'Migrations et Sida,' special issue of *Migrations et Santé* 94–5, pp. 31–54.

Jeffreys, E. (ed.) (1997) 'Prostitution in Contemporary China,' *Chinese Sociology and Anthropology*, fall 30(1).

Maclaren, A. 1998 'Chinese Cultural Revivalism: Changing Gender Constructions in the Yangtze River Delta,' in: K. Sen and M. Stivens (eds) *Gender and Power in Affluent Asia.* London, Routledge, pp. 195-221.

Manderson L. and M. Jolly (eds) 1997 *Sites of Desire, Economies of Pleasure. Sexualities in Asia and the Pacific.* Chicago and London: The University of Chicago Press.

Mead, M. (1961) 'Cultural Determinants of Sexual Behavior,' in: W.C. Young (ed.) *Sex and Internal Secretions.* Baltimore, MD: Williams and Wilkins, pp. 1433–79.

Micollier, E. (1998) 'Mobilité, marché du sexe et de la drogue dans le contexte du VIH/Sida en Chine du Sud,' in: 'Migrations et Sida,' special issue of *Migrations et Santé* 94–5, pp. 55–82.

– (1999) 'L'Autre: porteur originel et/ou vecteur privilégié du VIH/SIDA (Chine populaire-Taiwan)' in: C. Fay (ed.) 'Le sida des autres : constructions locales et internationales de la maladie,' *Autrepart* (Cahiers des sciences humaines), IRD-L'Aube 12, pp. 73-86.

Pan, Suiming (1999) *Zhongguo dixia 'xing changye' kaocha* (Investigation on China's underground sex industry). Beijing: Qunyan chubanshe.

– (2000) *Shengcun yu tiyan. You zhei yang yi ge 'hongdeng qu'* (Existence and experience: There is this kind of 'Red Light District'). Beijing: Zhongguo renmin daxue, Xing shehui xue yanjiusuo (China People's University, Institute for Research on Gender and Sexuality).

Parker, R.G. (1995) 'The Social and Cultural Construction of Sexual Risk, or how to Have (Sex) Research in an Epidemic,' in: H.T. Brummelhuis and G. Herdt (eds) (1995) *Culture and Sexual Risk. Anthropological Perspectives on AIDS*. Amsterdam: Gordon and Breach Publishers, pp. 257–70.

Parker R.G. and J.H. Gagnon (eds) (1995) *Conceiving Sexuality. Approaches to Sex Research in a Postmodern World*. New York and London: Routledge.

Testart, A. (2000) 'L'esclavage pour dettes en Asie orientale,' *Moussons. Recherche en sciences humaines sur l'Asie du Sud-Est* 2, pp. 3–29.

Weeks, J. (1985) *Sexuality and its Discontents: Meanings, Myths, and Modern Sexualities*. London: Routledge and Kegan Paul.

– (1995) 'History, Desire, and Identities,' in: R.G. Parker and J.H. Gagnon (eds) *Conceiving Sexuality. Approaches to Sex Research in a Postmodern World*. New York and London: Routledge, pp. 33-50.

Part One
Sexual Cultures – Caught between Traditions and Transitions

CHAPTER 1

SOCIAL SIGNIFICANCE OF COMMERCIAL SEX WORK: IMPLICITLY SHAPING A SEXUAL CULTURE?

EVELYNE MICOLLIER

This chapter discusses the role of sex work in the social construction of sexuality, mainly in the context of Chinese culture as well as a few examples from the Vietnamese or the Korean context. In our approach to sex work, one of the main working hypotheses is the relevance of cultural constraints such as the Confucian ideas or the Taoist lore on the analysis of sexual cultures. Cogently, the aim is not to overestimate cultural factors at the expense of social and economic factors, but to identify the different factors involved in the social construction of sexuality. All these factors are closely interrelated to shape a sexual culture where sex work lies at the core of the ideological and behavioural configuration – sex work thus becoming part of an 'unspoken' set of sexual norms and values paralleling the 'straight' set (heterosexuality, connubiality, intimacy, and reproduction over pleasure). One should bear in mind that a culture undergoes a continuous process of interpretation, and is not therefore a fixed system giving a ready reference to all the beliefs and behaviour of the people in society. Indeed, at the present, sexual cultures are in transition and produced within a complex nexus of divergent forces, including traditional sexual mores, modern medical discourse, women's movements, patriarchal imperatives, consumerism, and corporate globalization. In this context, representations of sexuality and sexual behaviours are embedded in a social world structured by and saturated with power relations of gender and class. Sexuality therefore provides a consistent site for exploring the various aspects of the social sphere. Our approach explicitly diverges from those relying perhaps too easily on the notion of 'structure' to define culture and comprehend tradition.

SEX WORK: PAST AND PRESENT IN THE CONTEXT OF CHINESE CULTURE

A dialectical relationship bridges past and present, tradition and modernity in the context of contemporary societies. To speak of traditions and heritage does not mean that the world was a static entity prior to the modern era, but implies that 'tradition and past customs provide questions and characterizations that confront every generation anew' (Gutmann 1996:15). Gutmann develops the idea of 'contradictory consciousness' in order to explain that people share both a 'consciousness inherited from the past – and from the experts – that is largely and uncritically accepted, and another, implicit consciousness that unites individuals with others in the practical transformation of the world.' This notion is useful to explain that, when contradictions, tensions between social and cultural values and norms, arise, they are negotiated rather than suppressed in specific and unpredictable ways. In the context of Chinese sexual culture, this process is always in the making as it is well known that, for instance, behaviours and ideas towards premarital sex and marriage of young people have changed but traditional values and norms confronted with these changes, always have to be negotiated by the same actors at the individual and social levels. Commercial sex work as part of the sexual culture appears less contradictory and easier to negotiate for the actors as it is part of tradition as well as part of contemporary consumerist life.

Although references to prostitution in ancient history are vague, we can trace the institution of government-run prostitution taking the form of either government-owned markets or recruited female army camp followers back to at least the Western Han dynasty (second century BC). This state institution reached its peak in the Tang (seventh-ninth century AD) and in the Song dynasties (tenth-thirteenth century AD), two historical periods known for their economic prosperity and the development of art, science, and culture in China. In the Tang dynasty, some prostitutes were connected with local governments, and their lives and business activities were almost totally controlled by local officials. A higher class of prostitutes, living in a special district of the capital and conducting their business with a relative freedom, was under the control of the Imperial government.

The courtesan institution
In ancient and medieval China, most women had no opportunity to have an education and were expected to avoid formal contact with men; to fill a social gap, the category of courtesans emerged as a part of society, their role being primarily to entertain a man and be his friend. Married officials, artists, or merchants, were all accompanied in their public life by courtesans skilled in literature, dance, or music whose primary role was not sexual. These women eventually became famous historical figures.

Another kind of prostitution – private and commercial prostitution – developed during the Ming and Qing, the two last Chinese dynasties acknowledged for allowing the development of trade and a merchant class especially in South China. These formed a new elite either in competition or collaborating with the traditional Confucian gentry elite. The southern cities of Guangzhou, Shanghai, Suzhou, Hangzhou (well known for tea, and silk trade), and in the north, Nanjing, Tianjin, and Beijing, were very famous for their flourishing trade in prostitution (Ruan 1991:69–70). Significantly, these cities were all centres of economic and political power, as well as cultural development.

The prostitutes working in privately owned brothels provided mainly sexual services. From the Song to the Ming dynasties, both forms of prostitution – government and privately owned – coexisted. During the seventeenth century, the early Qing dynasty (the Mandchu, non-Chinese dynasty), local and imperial government-controlled prostitution was abolished. Consequently, this activity became mainly private. Again for most of the Republican period (1912–1949) and up till now in Taiwan, both forms of prostitution coexist: State-run registered legal prostitution and illegal prostitution.

The situation in Mainland China ineluctably changed after 1949: all commercial sex activity was banned by the implementation of a whole set of repressive measures. Communism, a European Judaeo-Christian-born ideology, attributes prostitution to socio-economic factors. Applying this idea to Chinese society, the revolutionaries wanted to relieve the peasants of their debts and from the exorbitant rents and taxes that had forced them to sell their daughters into prostitution. Finally, all the repressive measures which were designed to suppress prostitution never worked, although it became quite invisible for sometime. Although this may have been only through a tightly controlled propaganda. A recent event, which took place during the 1990s in Taiwan, is worth recalling here: Chen Suibian, the newly elected president of Taiwan, who was then the mayor of Taipei, decided to abolish registered prostitution declaring it an illegal activity in the capital city. Needless to say, businesses simply moved to the outskirts of the city where they were still allowed. The newly outlawed registered prostitutes organized street gathering standing up for their rights to work. They cogently argued that they could not change their occupation for lower paid work as most of their relatives were used to living on their high income.

This brief and rather simplistic historical overview shows that tolerance and even the official promotion of prostitution in China has a long history. Courtesans, their biographies and activities, are described in many historical sources, but one cannot say that this social phenomenon is well documented in the sense that it was considered as a very normative aspect of the male elite life. Therefore it was not very interesting to report much about it. We do have more details about a few courtesans because they had developed special skills, either artistic or sexual, or had a specific influence on elite circles. In contrast, almost no information is available on lower class prostitutes and their clients, as the popular daily life history of the general population has still to be written. That is why in this brief historical overview, I have tried to make it clear that most of the literature about the institution of the courtesan refers to the life of upper classes in spaces and times characterized foremost by economic prosperity in the context of political power, expansion of trade, and the development of art.

Prostitution was a well-organized business and the female managers of some brothels had detailed manuals for the training of prostitutes. A manual used in the cities of Suzhou, Yangzhou, and Shanghai in the 1920s, registered accounts of the accumulated experiences of many prostitutes, and listed the requirements needed for a woman to be a successful prostitute (Ruan 1991:74- 5). In Beijing and Tianjin, the female managers preferred to use the *Sunu jing* (Classic of the Virgin). This book takes the form of a conversation between a virgin and *Huangdi*, the mythical Yellow Emperor and god of medicine. The implication is that the acquisition of skills in sexual techniques was more important than refined manners. This classic describes Taoist sexual practices which include sexual positions, movements during intercourse, and breathing exercises, even though the *Sunu jing* is not classified as part of the *Daozang* (Taoist canon).

A traditional cultural feature inescapably relevant to the study of sexuality is the Taoist sexual theory. Taoism is considered to be one of the three pillars of the classical Chinese tradition, the other two being Confucianism and Buddhism. Written primary sources on Taoist ideas about sexuality and sexual techniques are numerous as are secondary Chinese sources and more recently Western literature.[1] Sexual practice is part of the broader category of health or corporal practices including, for instance, meditation techniques which are themselves an integral part of religious practice. Each component of the sexual lore, which is considered to be one element in a global system, is related to all the others. The key concepts organizing this system are those of *yin-yang* and *qi*, the vital dynamic element circulating in the human body as well as in the cosmos. The following categories of belief still have an influence on contemporary sexual behaviour: health, longevity and/or immortality can be reached by sexual activity. Intercourse with virgins, preferably young virgins, contributes to men's health. Youth is currently more valued than beauty, and a virgin has not yet had her Yin depleted. Multiplicity of sexual partners is recommended. The notion of *Cai Yin pu Yang* means to take the Yin to nourish the Yang, and conversely *Cai Yang pu Yin* means to take the Yang to nourish the Yin. These notions are commonly used in health practices as Qigong, Taijiquan, martial arts, various sorts of meditation, and so forth.

The *jing* seminal essence is precious and by extension the essence of everything, an idea also used in meditation techniques for the purpose of transforming *qi* into *jing*. The seminal essence can return to the brain and nourish it. Preventing or interrupting ejaculation by pressing a vital point in the perineal area is highly valued. The best sexual satisfaction is associated with coitus without ejaculation (Ruan 1991:54–5).

In the context of prostitution, these ideas can still explain the preference for virgins and very young girls for the acquisition of health, and the fear of wasting seminal essence through frequent ejaculations. It is worth noting that the women described in erotic novels, and in medical or philosophical treatises on sex are often courtesans.

According to Pan (2000), nowadays, prostitutes perform no special sexual techniques and are no longer trained using old Taoist manuals, as it was the case in ancient and even modern China. In this sense, a tradition is now lost. Most prostitutes surveyed are no different in their sexual behaviour and ideas from other Chinese women. Their work comes closer to international patterns of prostitution.

The works of Henriot (1997) and Hershatter (1997) account for the only extensive historical research done about prostitution in Modern China. The authors have both focused on sex work in modernizing Shanghai. Making use of the accounts of reform programmes for prostitutes in the early 1950s, Hershatter emphasizes the resistance of the sex workers to change, and their affective links to their madams and their offspring. These emotional attachments have to be connected to the Confucian family ideology, the filial piety of children towards their parents being a central value of the ideological configuration. A dutiful prostitute will show filial piety towards her madam. Her madam can be accounted a symbolic substitute for her mother, a psychological process reinforced by the fact that she has often been sold by her family, and that she is a migrant worker far away from home.

There were morally good or bad courtesans according to common stereotypes prevailing in Modern China. The bad courtesans came from low class families, from rural areas, and were lascivious; the good ones came from good or elite families who had financial problems and were forced to sell their daughter. She sent the money back to her family showing her strong filial piety. Such women acquired virtue through their display of filial piety and thus were morally good. The presumption was that they did not enjoy sex much.

Hershatter's findings tend to demonstrate the inanity of post-1949 government policies towards prostitution, of which the aim was to eradicate the phenomenon. Pertinently, recent discourses tend to hint that prostitutes are more like autonomous bread-winners than miserable victims of a social system: 'If the subaltern voices of prostitutes could be heard more clearly outside of detention centres, it is possible that they would give more prominence to a labour framework than the people who regulate and study them do' (Hershatter 1997:392). The author adopts a feminist perspective: the accounts she registers of pre-1949 prostitution suggest that the prostitute was essentially a victim of a gendered power society characterized by male domination; in contrast, through her reports on contemporary prostitution, sex workers seem to enjoy a certain degree of agency.

Henriot is more concerned with the question of modernity, urbanization, and sexuality in China. His main point is related to the sexualization of the services provided: he explains how in the courtesan institution, the process of seduction matters more than sexual intercourse. The transforming of the institution into commercialized sex in modernizing Shanghai supposes a change in sexual behaviour (Leung 2000:185). This may be wide of the mark. As Leung suggests, 'commercialized sex' involving popular prostitutes seems to have been as wide-spread as the courtesan system in urban centres since at least the Song dynasty. The modern experience of Shanghai might not be so different from earlier history. Perhaps when the old literati culture was dying out in the twentieth century, the demand for the kind of non-sexual services that courtesans provided may have decreased.

In contemporary societies, recent research carried out in Taiwan (Hwang 1996), in Korea, and in China (Pan 1999) and Vietnam (Nguyen-vo 1997), where middle-class cultures have emerged more recently, show that male political and business elites adopt a kind of behaviour reminiscent of that of the traditional literati, as they like to discuss and settle business deals in expensive *jiujia* (wine houses) seeking the services of hostesses. This attitude is part of a tacit middle-class social code involving a public re-affirmation of gender, status, and class.

The following example is cited by Leung (2000:185–6):

> In Taipei, a client admits in an interview that it always takes him some time to get to know his preferred hostess well enough to have sex with her. He explains: 'If a man desire a female, he only needs to go to a brothel, and it is not expensive. But he is not interested ... Men these days have high standards ... the more (women) tantalize you, the more you desire them, and you don't want the vulgar and the cheap.' Similarly, interviewed professional *jiujia* hostesses, who reject being called 'prostitute' *jinü*, detest men asking for sex at first encounter whom they have the right to refuse.

Such relationships are not so different from those of the nineteenth century courtesan system described by Henriot.

In Vietnam, there is a process of commodification of sexual pleasure for domestic consumption integral to liberalizing economic practices (Nguyen-vo 1997). The buying of sexual pleasure in the business and political milieu has become an important means of facilitating clientele connections to gain access to the means of production and exchange. The activity of consuming pleasure has become the mark of this entrepreneur class. Borrowing from Butler's concept of 'performative gender' (1990), Nguyen-vo argues that the forms of consumption and commodification of pleasure constitute performances of class and nation, predicated on a gender difference. Consuming women and their bodies allows men to construct themselves not just as men, but as Vietnamese men of a certain class.

The process of establishing personal connections primarily takes the form of the offer and consumption of sexual pleasure, and usually takes place in *bia om* (literally 'hug beer') that provides food, drinks, and a range of semi-sexual or entertainment services such as hugging, kissing, and fondling the men, and strip-tease. Sexual intercourse could eventually occur in these places but that is not the most common service they provide.

As Leung (2000:186) pointed out, 'first, the modernization of the economy does not necessarily wipe out the courtesan institution or reduce the courtesans to 'simple objects' of consumption, though it might well have modified the institution as social needs of the elites changed. Indeed they are quite a few examples of ex-hostesses being married to rich businessmen in Taiwan and other East Asian countries. Second, it was perhaps a myth that sex was only secondary in the courtesan institution. Courtesans, after all, are sexual objects that cannot simply be defined quantitatively by the frequency of sexual intercourse with their clients.'

WOMEN'S TRADITIONAL ROLES:
TENSIONS IN THE CONFUCIAN FAMILY

Confucian principles governing family relations have built up a gender hierarchy to such an extent that tensions between women in the family context have become structural. This is because any benefit for any woman has to be gained at the expense of another one. An actual adherence to Confucian rules was probably heavily dependent on social class and status of the family. Women's lives and conditions in peasant families are virtually undocumented. Even though they were bound to hard work in difficult conditions, peasant women enjoyed a relative autonomy and had less conflicting relations with the other women (Freedman 1979). As Sievers (1999:170) explains,

Generally speaking, the higher the status, the more Confucian the family appears as a probable hypothesis. In gentry's families, women needed more than wisdom and assertiveness to survive; resilience, toughness, and an ability in what Margery Wolf has called 'uterine politics' (1972) were required. In Wolf's analysis, women manipulated two institutions ranged against them – property and Confucian values – in a way that could bring them power and relative security in old age. By successfully tying sons to her, and assisting them in their efforts to achieve power in the family, a woman might acquire reflected authority, plus a commitment to the claims of filial piety that would bring security and respect, as she grew older. That such a woman was often brought into direct conflict with other family members, especially other women, was axiomatic. The structure of the Confucian family system guaranteed conflict among women as a constant.

The structural reasons for the endless conflicts between mothers-in-law, daughters-in-law, and sisters-in-law were rooted in the regulations of the division of property. Property had to be shared by agnatic males who together owned it jointly as a collective person. The division of property was expected to take place after the death of a senior generation member. However, division could occur earlier for a number of reasons, for instance conflicting fraternal relationships often fostered by sisters-in-law. In such a situation, female in-laws had diverging interests in the early division of property, and they were competing fiercely for the loyalties of male relatives. In a comparative perspective, it is worth noting that in two other Confucianized countries, namely Korea and Japan, the Confucian family model did not play a major role in women's lives until the fifteenth century for Korea and the seventeenth century for Japan. Neither Japanese nor Korean traditions, previous to the import of Confucianism and Buddhism, focused on prescriptive female representations or on women's family duties. The folk religions of both Japan and Korea offered representations of powerful women, and this tendency was not really challenged by the drastic changes experienced in both societies over time (Sievers 1999:171–2).

From the family system described above, who were those daughters who ended up, or down, as concubines or prostitutes? What is the meaning of 'voluntary' sex work in a cultural context in which the pattern of individualism has not yet emerged, and may never become a dominant trend in society? In our understanding, an individualistic pattern of socialization means that an individual, a person, takes a decision for herself, and is consequently responsible for her own actions or is free, namely compelled to choose between several alternatives. In her modern history of Chinese prostitution, Gronewold (1982) argues that the Chinese social system in which women are considered another marketable and replaceable product is the main factor explaining the wide-spread and consensual commodification of women rather than any philosophical and/or religious tradition, whether this be Taoist, Buddhist, or Confucian. However, social systems are produced within philosophical and/or religious systems and world-views in the representational terrain. Symbolic and practical aspects are closely interrelated to create a social system regulating among other relationships – gender power and family relations in society. During times of famine and other economic hardships, the inferior status of women occasionally led to extreme measures, such as the deliberate infanticide of female babies. But even at the best of times female children were undervalued, as indicated by the folk adage 'A boy is worth ten girls.' Whereas male children were rarely sold, a general trade in women developed. They were marketed as adopted daughters, future daughters-in-law, and as servants. The traditional ideal in the Chinese family was to keep sons and daughters at home until they were of marriageable age and then to negotiate favourable unions. Sexual virtue among women was highly valued, but virtue lost its significance in difficult times when a daughter could be a liability. A family might choose among five alternatives for the future of a daughter: 'A socially accepted course was to give her into adoption whereby she became either a daughter or a future daughter-in-law for the adopting family. It was also acceptable to sell her directly into marriage for a small sum. A less desirable but more profitable alternative was to sell her into domestic service. This entailed risk for the girl because her ultimate fate rested with the purchaser, who might arrange a favourable marriage for her or might resell her to someone else, including a brothel owner. A fourth alternative was to sell her as a concubine for a household; the girl would be forced to serve as a maid for a wife and a sexual partner for an aging male. Finally, the least respectable but most lucrative option was the prostitution market'(McCaghy and Hou 1993:281). It is worth noticing that the most respectable choice is the least profitable one. Pre-1949 China has been recognized as having 'one of the largest and more comprehensive markets for exchanges of human beings in the world' (Watson 1980:223). The distinction between slavery and other forms of servitude is based on the existence of a kinship link between master and 'bought' dependent (Watson 1980:243). According to the most common estimates, there was a market involving about two million people in the 1920s: the 'mui-tsai,' or 'mooi-jai,' were mostly young girls sold by parents who surrendered all their rights to her to the buyer, including to right to rename them. Commonly labelled 'small slaves,' they fuelled brothels, were used as concubines or as farm girls. The sale of wives as slaves by their husbands was also not a rare phenomenon. Although these practices were considered illegitimate, by both the Imperial law (at least the Qing code, 1644–1911) and Confucian ethics, both of which sanction the idea of making profit out of relatives, they were probably deeply rooted in the Chinese tradition (Testart 2000:10).

Nowadays, when economic difficulties occur, daughters are still more likely than sons to be sacrificed to aid the family. The practice of putting daughters up for adoption symbolizes both women's social standing and supplements the supply of prostitutes. For instance, until recently in Taiwan up to forty per cent of all daughters were put up for adoptions in future in-law families through the *simpua* social institution.

Up to seventy per cent of the women arrested for prostitution in China admitted that selling their bodies was their main source of income. Many also admitted that their husbands approved of and even encouraged them to do this in order to supplement the family income. Paralleling the current increase in prostitution, bigamy and adultery have become widespread in China, and are raising tensions in family and society (*Criminal Justice International* 1989). The resurgence of prostitution has crossed the Chinese borders to expand into an international network. Vietnamese women are sold in China to become wives, concubines, or prostitutes (*Agence France Presse* 1991); Chinese women are being sold to brothels and massage parlours to work as prostitutes in Thailand (*Shijie ribao* [*World Journal*] 1992) (Xin Ren 1993: 96–7).

Gender and class differentiation in entertainment service activities
A repetitive act of class differentiation is performed by the men who use a hostess service. Women's use of the sex trade for class advancement and upward social mobility does not automatically grant them a clear class identity. The distribution of the cultural signs of class therefore works differently for the men who buy and for the women who sell. Both parties are not partners in this business game, but rather actors in a well defined, hierarchized, and gender-powered social structure shared up by its inherent cultural values.

The social stratification of courtesans paralleled the gentry's model of social distinctions and the so-called 'flower-list' elections (since mid-seventeenth century) paralleled the selection of the exclusively male successful candidates in the imperial civil-service examination (Hershatter 1997:165). Courtesans were addressed with such respectable names as *xiansheng* (sir) or *laoshi* (teacher), a fact that could be interpreted as a mark of valued and recognized social status. However, these views inform us only about the representations of the gentry class about prostitutes and courtesans rather than about historical facts because, they were the ones who would write down the history and, of course, data used by historians are limited to these written sources. Very few data on how courtesans perceived themselves, their clients, and their role and status in society are available: courtesans' voices have quite simply been lost unfortunately, we are compelled to admit that even in contemporary sociological and anthropological studies, the voices of prostitutes still need to be heard. Most social scientists have built up their works from news clips, media voices, and official or regulatory discourses rather than by listening to voices, discourses, and experiences, or observing the work and living conditions of prostitutes. Moreover, the current context of the HIV/AIDS epidemic threat does not help by medicalizing the issue of prostitution, labelling prostitutes' activities high-risk sexual behaviour, although it has encouraged more social research on the widespread phenomenon which is unbounded by time or space.

According to Pan's paper in this volume, sex workers involved in the sex industry in contemporary China can be classified into seven vertical layers, paralleling the social stratification. The first one is the second wife, who offers sexual services instead of the emotional, reproduction services, and co-habitation usually or ideally provided by the first wife and/or concubine. The second layer is the hired prostitute for a business trip or for a longer period but within the context of business activities. The third layer is constituted by escort girls working in three different settings (singing parlours or karaoke bars, dance halls, and restaurants-bars), who provide 'on-the-spot escort,' consisting of titillation sexual services without actual sexual intercourse, and/or 'follow you escort' including sexual intercourse. 'Chink girls' who live in their own room in a hotel on a relatively stable basis, and solicit hotel customers by telephone, are part of the fourth layer. They offer a one-time sexual intercourse service rather than all-night sex. The fifth layer is composed of barbershop or massage girls working at barbershops, sauna centres, and feet-washing rooms: their services consist of washing hair or feet and giving massages. Streetwalkers who find customers in recreational places and offer one-time sexual intercourse service are the sixth layer. The seventh layer are the prostitutes for poor transient peasants or workers called 'women who go to, or live in a shed,' playing the role of public wife who charges for the services she provides.

While the women of the lowest layers strictly provide multiple sexual services, those of the second and third layers are involved in social relationships and lives of their clients. Second wives are involved in a more complete relationship including an eventual co-habitation. Such a typology shows how it may be difficult to draw a clear line between sexual and non-sexual services, as sexual intercourse is not a consistent criterion by which to define sex work in this cultural context. The definition of sexual service should be extended to encompass the whole range of sex workers' social roles and practical activities related or not to sex *stricto-sensu*. Indeed, in the same paper, Pan describes a whole range of sexual services classified in various layers.

IDENTIFICATION OF SOCIAL FACTORS

The rate of illiteracy is high among sex workers, and partly explains why so many women from poor rural areas are willing to participate in the sex trade as a last resort to make money.

There is little doubt that sex work is regarded as a way towards upward social mobility: in my ethnographic research, I found quite a few sex workers who wished to become a concubine or a second wife. More rarely their ultimate goal was to get married, but this hope seemed too unrealistic except if one could find a foreigner, who would be more willing to be involved in a marriage transaction they thought.

Prostitution is also a result of an anomic situation in which a woman might find herself. For instance, failure in a university entrance examination, in particular in an urban, middle-class context, education being so much valued by the family and society in Chinese culture, can drive ashamed young women into prostitution and young men into delinquency. This process can be analysed in terms of a resistance to an oppressive system imposed on the youth.

The rate of female suicide in Chinese rural counties is very high and China is one of the few countries in the world where women commit suicide more frequently than men (Lee and Kleinman 2000). The main culprit was traditionally related to arranged marriage, child marriages, adoptions and abuses by the husband's family, and still is exacerbated by the problem of the generation gap. The parents want a traditional marriage for their daughter and she resists. The suicide of women can be also analysed in terms of resistance to a traditional model which exerts unendurable pressure on women. This pressure is now reinforced psychologically for them, because they know some women can escape from this system. Social change can mean that they find themselves in an anomic situation. Migration and eventually sex work is then seen as a way to escape from an unwanted forced marriage. Away from the coils of their family, they hope that they will be able to manage their own lives.

Sex work has an influence on mobility and vice-versa: temporary migratory movements of the population and sex work are two closely interrelated social phenomena (Liao 2000, Evans 2000, Feingold 2000, Xie 2000). In a case-study on the impact of new economic opportunities on women's status and gender relations in the border region of China and

Vietnam, Xie (2000) admits that sex work among other activities may provide new chances for some women, and that work in the sex industry contributes to the development of both the micro- and macro-economies. From a broader regional perspective, it is now recognized that sex workers from China are involved in a trans-Asian network covering most East and Southeast Asia countries; this trend indicates that they participate in inter-regional mobility among sex workers in Asia (Zi Teng 2000:143).

THEORIES OF PROSTITUTION:
A TRADITIONAL SEXUAL CULTURE STRUCTURED BY COMMERCIAL SEX WORK

In order to understand the roots and characteristics of prostitution in Chinese society, we must revert to the attitude of traditional Confucian philosophy regarding the role of women. A woman's duty, first and foremost, was to continue the family line – that is, to bear her husband's male children. Women were regarded as reproductive mechanisms to continue the family lineage. To maintain social harmony, it was considered necessary to inculcate in women a lack of temptation and a feeling of contamination from enjoying sex. Confucianism appears to be a relevant cultural constraint, first of all because it is an all-encompassing ideology regulating all aspects of social life.

Some components of the Confucian family ideology have deep implications for the social construction of sexual cultures. Marriage is conceived of as a social fusion constituting the elementary unit, the matrix of any social exchange. In the context of matrimonial exchange, sexuality and sexual life are reduced to reproductive behaviour in order to obtain sons. This idea explicitly denies erotic desire, excluding the chance of erotic satisfaction and sexual pleasure through marriage, indeed even considering them as dangerous because they are difficult to control. Erotic desire and sexual pleasure would endanger the harmony of the family, being perceived as an unstable, changing element. Therefore they could forebode eventual disorder which would disturb family order and consequently – social, political and cosmological orders. Indeed, Confucianism regulates all human relationships and at all levels of social organization: a family, a clan or a lineage being the elementary social unit, and produces a social and political model, a specific mode of government. Sexual appeal, desire, and pleasure are strongly related to the human emotions and feelings that had to be silenced in order to secure the reproduction and endurance of the social order. Confucian ideology implicitly admits that sexual drives and desires have to be fulfilled outside marriage. A whole social context encourages the development of 'commercial sex work' and a number of female sex worker's roles. In Western Christian traditions, monogamy was the rule, and extra-marital affairs were considered a transgression. Prostitution was, and still is to some extent, a taboo subject; the prostitute as well as the client were considered to be behaving in a sinful way. Paradoxically, an ambiguity lies in the widely shared idea that sexual performance, seduction, and plurality of partners are criteria which shape the social construction of male identity. If a man aims to refrain from sex, his attitude may be thought to be that of a loser. In most Asian societies, the same attitude is perceived as virtuous because the control of desires and emotions is first of all socially prescribed for social harmony, and secondly shows the path to spiritual achievement for inner-life fulfilment.

In China, any discussion about sexual pleasure was a challenge to Confucian tradition. For centuries, public talk about sex has been and continues to be a taboo in Chinese culture. A number of Ming and Qing dynasty classics, such as The Golden Lotus and The Dream of the Red Chamber, offer elaborated descriptions of the joys of intimacy, romance, and sex. Consequently, generations of emperors banned the works mainly because they contravened Confucian modesty.

Sexual liberation means consumerism. The dominant model for female teenagers as an object of self-identification tends more and more to be an elegant, high-class sex worker: the image of such a sex worker suggests that she is a liberated new woman and an ideal consumer. There is a tolerance towards newly claimed sexual identities through consumerism: the legal marriage (legal as the law do not specify that a marriage has to be contracted between a man and a woman) of a lesbian couple living in Beijing, whom I had the opportunity to interview, is a good example. Both women have a middle-class intellectual and artistic background.

Young, middle-class women, for instance university students, may eventually become occasional high-class sex workers for a few years before getting married without questioning the traditional model. They will do this work to get more money and will spend that money for themselves buying expensive clothes, accessories, and the like. Their behaviour is related to a consumerist and individualist ideology. The emergence of individualism is a noticeable trend among young, educated, urban people. This pattern is already fully developed in Taiwanese and Korean society but in China, it is more surprising. In spite of a recent history offering totally different models for and images of women, images of women as sexual objects are gaining ground at an astonishing speed, so much so that as Wolf (1985) concludes 'The revolution is postponed.' The sexualized model has replaced the strong revolutionary woman in all the media, in advertising, and in the feminine press.

Prostitution is not systematically produced by poverty and the sex worker does not always remit her income to family and relatives in her village. However, in terms of numbers, socio-economic factors still explain the involvement of many women in prostitution in China, as it is the case in most developing countries. Indeed, most prostitutes are migrant workers, have a low level of education, and usually come from poor rural areas. This pattern is dominant in provinces populated by minorities where local cultures are non-Chinese. Two combined factors – the traditional status of women and the capitalist-type exploitation of workers meaning low pay, hard work, no rest, and no respect of international labour laws – explain the choice of women to prostitute themselves.

Discourses and behaviours related to the introduction of Viagra in the context of culture should really be investigated as these have generated interesting debates in society. In Taiwan, medical professionals, politicians, traditional physicians, women and men have all taken part in the societal discussion on the Viagra craze, and debates have been concerned with redefining gender relations and the norms of sexuality. These diverging voices demonstrate at least one thing – that sexuality and gender relations are indeed socially constructed, and always in a process of being deconstructed and reconstructed: they are neither 'given phenomena' nor 'precultural drives anchored inside us, beyond the reach of social influences' (Di Leonardo and Lancaster 1997:1).

A set of sexual norms underlies current discourses, namely hetero-sexuality, connubiality, and the primacy of intimacy over pleasure. These 'straight' norms are subtly reaffirmed and naturalized even when the object of criticism is the masculinist narrative that most commonly animates them – to wit, men are innately promiscuous, male sexuality is inherently profuse and proceeds from men's bodies and physiology, and women desire love more than sex.

My own fieldwork conversations and Festa's (2000:22–3) case-study focused on the Viagra craze in Taiwan indicate that extramarital sex is the preferred context in which non-impotent men use Viagra, challenging the dominant discourses about the impact of Viagra use in the marital sexual context. Ning (1999) and Zhang (1999) suggest that extramarital sex is regularly pursued by most men in Taiwan with some of them being involved in long-term affairs. Moreover, in her study of popular discourse on extramarital affairs Chang (1999:70) notes that the media have labelled affairs a 'new epidemic.' She also provides new data for the study of sexual culture that is – that even wives are increasingly engaged in affairs, leading to the speculation that more Taiwanese women 'construe sexual activity as part of lifestyle and identity rather than an enactment of familial and marital commitments' (Chang 1999:69–72). She shows how extramarital affairs dialectically engage issues of cultural inheritance, modernization, body representations, gender relations, and sexuality. According to both Chang (1999) and Ning (1999), sexual performance is often the paramount concern of extramarital affairs.

Host bars targeting a female clientele are documented in Taiwan, Korea, and Japan. There is evidence that sexual tourism designed for Japanese women is increasing with Indonesia as a common destination. I have myself done fieldwork in a few host bars in Taipei, Seoul, and Kwangju (Southeast Korea) designed for the entertainment of women. The clientele was composed mainly of three categories of women, namely young prostitutes, middle-aged career women, and middle-class housewives. Their motives in seeking male entertainers may also differ from those of men who are looking for female entertainers. A major difference may be that female escort and accompaniment are regarded as a mark of social distinction and status for men, and frequenting prostitutes is seen as an important factor in the social construction of male sexuality and is consequently highly valued in society. Unfortunately, the motives of women who frequent male hosts and the perception of their attitude by different social categories in society are not yet documented as I cannot draw more general lines from my own limited fieldwork data. Further research about these settings will eventually shed a new light on East Asian sexual cultures in transition and on the culturally bound transformation of gender relations. However, the fieldwork data I could gather lead me to speculate about a 'normative' sexual culture developing in the context of pleasure settings designed for men as well as for women. The result is that gender relations or marital rules are reproduced and a social order mainly based on traditional values is preserved in spite of noticeable social changes. Meanwhile, a sexual culture shaped by commercial sex is reinforced by the development of a sex market designed for women. The current trend is in fact to create a both gender model instead of an exclusively male model. If these working hypotheses are confirmed, I will argue that the traditional male model reproduces itself once again along the lines of gender differentiation by adjustment to a social change, which allows women to take a small share in the market economy. Indeed, some middle-class women nowadays have a high level of education, make a career, can become quite wealthy, and can afford to spend money in pleasure settings.

CONCLUDING REMARKS

Subversions of social and familial 'explicit' norms, such as extramarital affairs, betray the tensions at the core of mainstream society and intervene in the shaping of an 'implicit' sexual culture. Most of those affairs take place in the context of prostitution. Creating a sexual culture for both sexes in which commercial sex work plays a major role is a way to negotiate these tensions, creating – because it is far from being a marginal solution to solve the contradictions – a 'normative' implicit sexual culture in which commercial sex work is at the core of the ideological and behavioural configuration. All kinds of extramarital affairs are thus becoming less subversive, tending to be included in a set of unspoken or unspeakable social norms. The sex industry is currently built upon at least two overlapping conceptual and behavioural models – the traditional one and the international 'globalizing' one. These interacting models may explain some of the tensions and contradictions in societies confronted by social change: research on sex work is an original way to shed light on the process of social change through a so-called globalization. I will conclude with a comment by Pan who makes an overall analysis of prostitution in China in terms of the labour market (cited by Hershatter 1996:224): 'A family of three were talking about prostitution. The husband said "One act of prostitute on X city is worth three years of my salary". The wife immediately reacted "Then, never visit a prostitute". The daughter unexpectedly said "I should do this job".'

NOTE

1   See for a list of written sources, Ruan (1991:52–4).

REFERENCES

Agence France Presse (1991) 'Vietnamese Women Sold into Prostitution in China and Cambodia, September.

Butler, J. (1990) *Gender Trouble. Feminism and the Subversion of Identity.* New York: Routledge.

Chang, Jui-Shan (1999) 'Scripting extramarital affairs: marital mores, gender politics, and infidelity in Taiwan,' *Modern China* 25(1), pp. 69–99.

Criminal Justice International (1989) Newsletter editor 'Resurgence of Prostitution in China,' June.

Dikötter, F. (1995) *Sex, Culture and Modernity in China. Medical Science and the Construction of Sexual Identities in the Early Republican Period.* London: Hurst Co.

Di Leonardo M. and R.N. Lancaster (eds) (1997) *The Gender/Sexuality Reader: Culture, History, Political Economy*. New York: Routledge.

Festa, P. (2000) 'The Blue Whirlwind Strikes Below the Belt: Male Sexuality, Gender Politics, and the Viagra Craze in Taiwan,' paper presented at the 6th NATSA Conference, June 16–19, Harvard University, Mass.

Evans, G. (2000) 'Transformation of Jinhong, Xishuangbanna, PRC,' in: Evans, G., C. Hutton and Kuah Khun Eng (eds) *Where China Meets Southeast Asia. Social and Cultural Change in the Border Regions*. Bangkok: White Lotus and Singapore: Institute of Southeast Asian Studies, pp. 162- 82.

Feingold, D.A. (2000) 'The Hell of Good Intentions: Some Preliminary Thoughts on Opium in the Political Ecology of the Trade in Girls and Women,' in: Evans, G., C. Hutton, and Kuah Khun Eng (eds) *Where China Meets Southeast Asia. Social and Cultural Change in the Border Regions*. Bangkok: White Lotus and Singapore: Institute of Southeast Asian Studies, pp. 183–203.

Freedman, M. (1979) *The Study of Chinese Society*. Stanford: Stanford University Press.

Gronewold, S. (1982) 'Beautiful Merchandise: Prostitution in China 1860– 1936 ' *Women & History* 1, Spring, pp. 1–114

Gutmann, M.C. (1996) *The Meanings of Macho: Being a Man in Mexico City*. Berkeley, University of California Press.

Hinsch, B. (1990) *Passions of the Cut Sleeve. The Male Homosexual Tradition in China*. Berkeley: University of California Press.

Henriot, C. (1997) *Belles de Shanghai. Prostitution et sexualité en Chine aux XIXè-XXè siècles*. Paris: CNRS éditions.

Hershatter, G. (1997) *Dangerous Pleasures. Prostitution and Modernity in Twentieth-Century Shanghai*. Berkeley: University of California Press.

Hershatter, G. (1996) 'Chinese Sex Workers in the Reform Period,' in: E.J. Perry (ed.) *Putting Class in its Place. Workers Identities in East Asia*. China Research Monograph 48, Berkeley: The Regents of the University of California, pp. 199–243.

Honig E. and G. Hershatter (1988) *Personal Voices. Chinese Women in the 1980s*. Stanford: Stanford University Press.

Hwang, Shu-Ling (1996) 'Taiwan tezhong hangye funü: shou hai zhe? xingdong zhe? piancha zhe?' (Women in Taiwanese sex industry: Victims, Agents or Deviants?), *Taiwan shehui yanjiu jikan* (Taiwan: a Radical Quarterly in Social Studies) 22, April, pp. 119–20.

Lee S., Kleinman A. (2000) 'Suicide as Resistance in Chinese Society,' in: E.J. Perry and M. Selden (eds) *Chinese Society. Change, Conflict, and Resistance*. London: Routledge.

Leung, A.K. (2000) 'Prostitution in Modern Shanghai: Two Recent Studies,' *Nan Nu. Men, Women and Gender in Early and Imperial China* 2(1), pp. 180–7.

Liao, Susu (2000) 'Sex work in rural communities in Hainan and Guangxi, China: Its Significance in STD/AIDS Prevention and Reproductive Health,' paper presented at the IIAS Workshop 'Health, Sexuality, and Civil Society in East Asia,' Amsterdam, July 6–7.

McCaghy, C.H. and C. Hou (1993) 'Taiwan,' in: N.J. Davis (ed.) *Prostitution. An International Handbook on Trends, Problems, and Policies.* Westport, Conn.: Greenwood Press, pp. 273–99.

Nguyen-vo, Thu-Huong (1997) 'Prostitution in a liberalizing Vietnam: the economy, hierarchy, and geography of pleasure,' paper delivered at the 1997 ASPAC Conference, June 26–29, Asiloma.

Ning, Ying-Bin (1999) 'Wei'ergang lunshu de fenxi: xiandai yongyao yu shenti guanli' (On Viagra: modern drug-use and body management), *Taiwan shehui yanjiu jikan* (Taiwan: a radical quarterly in social studies), 33, pp. 225–52.

Pan, Suiming (1999) *Zhongguo dixia 'xing shangye'* (The underground sex industry in China). Beijing, Qunyan chubanshe.

Pan, Suiming (2000) 'Three "Red Lights Districts" in China,' paper presented at the IIAS Workshop 'Health, Sexuality, and Civil Society in East Asia,' Amsterdam, July 6–7.

Ruan, F.F. (1991) *Sex in China. Studies in Sexology in Chinese Culture.* New York: Plenum Press.

Shijie ribao (World Journal) (1992) 'Chinese communists join Thailand Government to crack down on Prostitution,' July 7, in Chinese.

Sievers, S. (1999) 'Women in China, Japan, and Korea,' in: B.M. Ramusack and S. Sievers (eds) *Women in Asia. Restoring Women to History.* Bloomington and Indianapolis: Indiana University Press, pp. 157–254.

Testart, A. (2000) 'L'esclavage pour dettes en Asie orientale,' *Moussons. Recherche en sciences humaines sur l'Asie du Sud-Est* 2, pp. 3–29.

Van Gulik, R. (1961) *Sexual life in Ancient China.* Leiden: Brill.

Xie, Guangmao (2000) 'Women and Social Change along the Vietnam-Guangxi border,' in: Evans, G., C. Hutton and Kuah Khun Eng (eds) *Where China Meets Southeast Asia. Social and Cultural Change in the Border Regions.* Bangkok: White Lotus and Singapore: Institute of Southeast Asian Studies, pp. 312–27.

Xin, Ren (1993) 'China,' in: N.J. Davis (ed.) *Prostitution. An International Handbook on Trends, Problems, and Policies.* Westport, Conn.: Greenwood Press, pp. 87–107.

Watson, J.L. (1980) 'Transactions in People: the Chinese Market in Slaves, Servants, and Heirs,' in: J.L. Watson (ed.) *Asian and African systems of Slavery*. Berkeley: University of California Press, pp. 223–50.

Wolf, M. (1985) *Revolution Postponed. Women in Contemporary China*. Stanford: Stanford University Press.

Zhang, J.Y. (1992) *Psychoanalysis in China. Literary Transformations (1919–1949)*. Ithaca, New York: Cornell University.

Zhang, Li-Wen (1999) 'Lai yike yeyeye kuang Taiwan lanxing de misi' (Pop one pill and go all night – a Taiwanese male fantasy), *Zhongguo shibao*, March 29, p. 8.

Zi Teng (2000) *Research Report on Mainland Chinese Sex Workers*. Hong Kong: Zi Teng NGO.

CHAPTER 2

THREE 'RED LIGHT DISTRICTS' IN CHINA

PAN SUIMING

Translated by Liu Zhenghong

Nowadays, the definition of a red light district in China is as follows: many prostitutes (not individuals) gathered together within one and the same location. In this demarcated territory, the sex industry is distinctively present on a particular scale and it occupies a primary position. The geographical border of this district should be relatively obvious enough for it to be readily distinguishable from the surrounding area. The sex industry of this area should be widely acknowledged and should confine its operations within the boundaries of the district.

At present, the sex industry operates in almost every city in China, but few locations can be truly rated a red light district. In this paper, I will describe three types of red light district. The first one is located in Town A in the economically highly developed area around the Zhujiang Delta. I classify this delta area as 'Lately Developed and Extroversive,' having recently taken flight because of the introduction of foreign investment. It principally services the people of Hong Kong and Taiwan. The second is Town B, an economic and technological development zone close to an industrial city in the hinterland of Guangxi Province. Its primary function is to provide services for passing drivers and businessmen as well as the nearby urban population, covering a need which appeared with the development of transportation and the establishment of the economic development zone. In view of this I call it 'Roadside By-growth.' The third is Town C lying in a booming gold-mining area on the borders of Hunan and Guizhou Provinces. The emergence of this red light district, which at present serves only for local residents, is entirely based on the opening up of the gold deposits. Therefore it should be categorized as 'local haphazard.'

There were three principal fieldwork methods which I employed in my observations in these red light districts: monitoring at a set location at a set time; making door-by-door visits; and participant observation which required remaining in some of the places for a time, interviewing the owners of recreation centres about their business operations, chatting with the female sex workers and the 'procuresses' as if they had nothing to do with the matter in hand, interviewing those soliciting the prostitutes by pretending to be one of them. This is the appropriate juncture to mention that a certain diffidence generally forces the Chinese to refer to female sex workers obliquely as *xiao jie* (miss).

Today in China, although the sex industry is still illegal, this has not precluded it from forming its own system and operating mechanism. Producing and marketing blue (pornographic) materials is its advertising department. Escort services provide its show case and sales department. The medical treatment of STDs (sexually transmitted diseases) is its after-sales department. Those who directly 'buy sex with money' or 'exchange money for sex' are its core 'production' department. Besides those immediately concerned, there are many affiliated industries, such as the hotel industry, the entertainments industry and so on. If the added output value of those affiliated industries deriving from prostitution and escort services is included, the economic scale of the Chinese sex industry may be expanded many times over.

The results of my long-term research have mainly been published in Chinese in a number of books and articles. This paper gives an idea of the extensive research and monographic work I have carried out on prostitution in China. This work has contributed to the identification of social and economic factors related to sex work: official figures are analysed; the stratification of sex workers and of prostitution, and various layers of sexual services are described and explained in different settings; finally, the attitudes of local people towards sex workers, male control and the economic scale of the sex industry are emphasized.

THE CHARACTERISTICS OF AND ACTUAL CONDITIONS IN ESCORT SERVICES IN CHINA

Escort services refer to people (mostly female) offering services like keeping company to customers (mainly male), while the latter drink, sing or go dancing in public places, in exchange for a direct monetary transaction. There are three inherent key factors in escort services: they occur in public places and the person who offers such a service is not acquainted with the client beforehand. At present, there are few telephone reservations for escort services in China. Secondly, escort service may involve indulging on pornographic activities in various measures, including foreplay. Finally a direct cash deal is carried out at the service spot, the price and scale of which are clear and definite and are approved of by both parties.

There are many other forms of escort service, such as swimming companion, travelling escort, business trip escort, cinema-going companion, and so on. In fact, escort service is an ancient Chinese tradition. Throughout history there have always been courtesans/prostitutes with whom men did no more than drink, sing, dance and eat instead of having sex. Among the upper classes such occasions were regarded as normal social activities. There is no specific charge for providing an escort service in the Chinese Penal Code at present. Until the summer of 1998, as many as forty-three cities had begun to levy individual income tax from the 'Public Misses' (local name of female sex workers). However, in March 1999, legal regulations were proclaimed by the Chinese government that prohibited escort services for profit in any form to be conducted in public places of recreation. If violated, the perpetrators would be fined by the Public Security Bureau. The major reason behind this legislation is that escort service is usually the prelude to prostitution. Following this form of logic, any occupation may be prohibited as long as any hint of intimate relations is thought to be involved. Cogently some policewomen were also found to be engaged in such intimate relations. One is tempted to ask will the government prohibit such an occupation as the police? Taking this prelude logic as a yardstick, any normal service job, as long as it is performed by women, may become the prelude to more intimate relations and thus should be prohibited. Carried to its logical extreme, the government ought to continue prohibiting women from stepping out of their houses.

In recent years, more and more laid-off female workers from the overheated manufacturing industries have been engaging in escort services to earn an income. Their husbands or brothers see them to and from work and even provide covert protection in dance halls. When they demand more than simply companionship from these women, the customers are only asking for trouble. It is a pity that the Chinese government now prohibits such re-employment.

In Beijing, because of the official ban, the price for non-sexual escort services for about three hours has been raised to an all-time high of $25 (equal to seven days wages of a labourer). Nevertheless, in many middle- or small-sized cities, where escort services are not prohibited, the price may be as low as $3.5. In Town A: on spot A, between 19:30 and 23:20, twelve of the sixty-three escort girls secured customers. Simple arithmetic shows that the business rate is less than 20 per cent. On Spot B, between 19:40 and 23:30, forty-three escort girls came in and only eleven of them found customers. Consequently the rate of business was 26 per cent. On Spot C, between 20:10 and 23:45, seventy-six escort girls streamed in and only about eighteen of them found customers, therefore the business rate was 24 per cent. So the business rate of escort girls is a little lower than that of the barbershop girls, a category to which I shall return a little later. A particular feature of Town A is the scarcity of true massage girls or true escort girls.

Any woman undertaking this work is required to know how to give a massage or perform escort services whether or not they are willing to perform sexual services, but such girls are few and far between. Because local prostitution is flourishing, misconceptions and misunderstandings have taken root among the people. Almost all the female sex workers there believed that all the customers who approached them were seeking sexual services and the so-called massage and escort services were just a cover-up.

Therefore, they assume that as long as they are willing to let their sexual services, they do not have to acquire any other specific skills. Likewise, the customers are inhibited by such misconceptions and misunderstandings; they think they have to take a girl to bed if they come. The mutual misunderstanding and the logical consequences of it only deepen the confusion. If a male customer requires only a normal massage or a non-sexual escort service, he will be thought odd by almost all and sundry. In Town C, in the beginning only sexual intercourse pure and simple was on offer. However, such direct prostitution met fierce opposition from the local government. So after a period of unremitting resistance by the government, it disappeared. Some cadres think that it is the strict government prohibition that has forced the owners of recreational premises to adopt a style of business in which they have to sell sex in the guise of an escort service. The owners of recreational premises look at matters differently. It is their belief that the direct prostitution of the past was not the best way to tackle the job because it was too one-sided and the market was not good. Pertinently, simple prostitution does not bring in any extra income even though the investment required in it is not small, and therefore it is not worthwhile economically. So the present escort-first and go-to-bed later style is actually a multi-product operational style that has expanded the market potential. Therefore, even if the government has not pre-empted the attack, most owners of recreational premises would have expanded in this direction, since it seems to be the proper half-way house between the official prostitution prohibition policy and the need for prostitution among the populace. It is also a business price to which some concessions have been made by both parties that may eventually solve the theoretical predicament that China is facing. Thus the government may claim: 'There is no (officially recognized) prostitution in China for the time being, though underground prostitutes still exist' and be absolutely correct. From a social point of view, such a claim means confirmation of the present status quo and even helps to cause it.

THE SCALE OF PROSTITUTION IN CHINA

The number of prostitutes has been officially investigated and gone into even-handedly all over the country. In 1982, China released its first proclamation prohibiting prostitution. According to statistics from the Public Security Department, the number of prostitutes in 1984 was 12,281. This broke the 100,000 barrier in 1989 and rose above 200,000 in 1991. By 1992, it had increased to 250,000 and 246,000 in 1993. If the figure remained at 250,000 from 1994 to 1997, after which it roared to about 2,120,000. A very authoritative book says: the rate was 25 per cent to 30 per cent around 1991, but another expert says it was only 10 per cent. I visited City G, City H and City L at the beginning of 1994. I carried out a survey by questionnaire, which I distributed among the population of the whole city aged between sixteen and seventy using a multi-strata random sampling method. In the above-mentioned three cities, 1.7 per cent of the people admitted to having had sexual relations with persons other than their spouses and having given them money or valuable gifts as well. Of these, 0.7 per cent confessed to receiving money or valuable gifts from the other party. If the floating population is included, this figure must be enlarged at least one time. However, in City G, even if you add the prostitution population to that of the drug addicts, the figure of the persons dealt with accordingly by the Public Security departments was a mere 7000. That is, the arrest rate of City G that year was only 5 per cent of its historical occurrence rate, perhaps even only 2.5 per cent. Of the overall adult population of the above-mentioned three cities, besides those who admitted they had tried sex work, 3.2 per cent admitted to having toyed with the idea of buying sex, while 1.0 per cent admitted having tried. Of these 2.0 per cent admitted with the idea of selling sex while 0.5 per cent admitted actually having done so.

I surveyed all undergraduates in Beijing by mail using multi-strata sampling in 1991 and again in 1995. I repeated this throughout the whole country in 1997. The result was as follows: in 1991, 23.0 per cent of all the undergraduates in Beijing had at least once thought of finding an underground prostitute. The figure was as high as 34.8 per cent in 1995 and reached 46.8 per cent of the undergraduates throughout the whole country in 1997. This has constituted a significant increase in the statistics, while the figure of the persons who admitted having tried prostitution has been kept below 1 per cent. In 1991, 11.3 per cent of the undergraduates in Beijing had at least once thought of selling sex. There was no obvious change in 1995 and it remained at 11.3 per cent. In 1997, the rate increased to 15.4 per cent but this is not a significant statistical difference. In addition, those who confessed they had at least once actually done so remained 0.3 per cent to 0.4 per cent.

The above figures may not indicate an increase in the number of those who had toyed with the idea or had tried, but suggest that those who had had such thoughts or had put such thoughts into action had grown increasingly brave about admitting this. Even so, the figures also demonstrate that the potential market for the sex industry is expanding.

THE STRATIFICATION OF PROSTITUTES: THE GENERAL CIRCUMSTANCES

The Chinese sex industry formed seven vertical layers in 1996. The second wife is at the top of the layers. The substantial difference between concubines, 'girls fed by VIPs' (companion to the rich) or factual marriage and the second wife lies in the fact that the second wife charges on a time basis. What they offer first and foremost is sexual services, instead of emotional services, reproductive services or companionship and so on. Only the unit by which they compute service time is longer than is general with secret prostitutes. They usually collect money monthly.

The second layer is the hired companion who is called a hired prostitute by the Public Security Bureau. They do not cohabit long with their clients, but are simply 'hired' during one business trip or a period of business activities.

The third layer is composed of escort girls who are active in three places (singing parlours, dance halls and restaurants). The services they offer are based on 'on-the-spot escort' (they keep a client company in a particular place,) but they strive for 'follow your escort' (to go out with those who have solicited their escort services).

The fourth layer is comprised of a group known as "chink girls" in local parlance. There is no collective name for them in other places. Sometimes they are called 'lodgers.' They rent their own rooms and tend to live fairly permanently in hotels. They find customers by telephone. If a man shows such an inclination, he will press the doorbell that emits the sound 'chink' and then enters to make the deal on the spot. There are usually more one-time sexual intercourse encounters rather than 'all-night sex' in their service packet.

Barbershop girls or massage girls constitute the fifth layer. They are well known for washing hair, giving massages or 'washing feet.' They work with various barbershops, saunas or 'feet washing' rooms and usually 'get to work on the spot.' They have fewer opportunities for 'follow your escort' or for all-night sex.

Streetwalkers or street girls belong to the sixth layer. They usually pick up customers outside a hotel door, the doors of a cinema or other recreational places and then find other places for one-time sexual intercourse.

The seventh layer consists of 'women who go to or live in a shed.' They mainly make deals with peasant-workers from other places. Some do this work occasionally or as part-time co-work which involves living with a group of peasant workers, like a public wife who charges. They are the 'lowest and the poor peasants' among the prostitutes. Some do it for only a bowl of soup.

Although all seven layers are prostitutes in the strict sense, the goods they offer are different. What the two lowest levels offer is simply the opportunity for one-time sexual intercourse. The fourth and the fifth layers offer multiple sexual behaviour. The second and third layers are involved in a sort of social association, and the first layer indulges in a sort of co-habitation. The aims of the underground prostitutes of the seven layers are definitely different. The objective of the second wife and hired prostitute is to become real concubine one day, perhaps even to become a real wife. They look for formal sexual relationships, so they sometimes ask nothing from or even subsidize their customers when they want to hook big fish by playing them on a long line, though this does not prevent them from haggling over every penny as well. What escort service of the third layer and chink girls are looking for is not only money, they are after a more luxurious life-style that might well be dangling within their reach. So they stubbornly keep and guard that battlefield, even though they may not have customers or may even go hungry. The living and working conditions of those barbershop girls, massage women or street girls of the fifth and the sixth layers almost beggar the belief of ordinary people. The probability of their being exploited and being harmed is also much greater. This is not to say that they are completely without help and, they can still overcome their life-style and survive. For the prostitutes belonging to the seventh layer, who are called 'women who go to or live in shed,' earning money is their dream. Some temporarily organized 'peasant worker teams' take them in. They are housemaids during the day and 'public wife' at night. They usually do not have a fixed price. What the peasant workers give them is material assistance instead of tips. Therefore, the highest and the lowest prostitutes resemble wives, whether they charge or not.

VARIOUS LAYERS OF CHINESE 'SEXUAL SERVICES'

Classical sexual service means sexual intercourse completed by penetration by the client's penis in exchange for money. The difference between 'open fire once' (one-time sexual intercourse) or 'hire for one night' (all-night sex), lies only in the degree of service.

Special sexual service means sexual exchange such as oral intercourse or anal intercourse. The separation of sexual intercourse from sexual exchange and the distinction between the classical sexual services and special ones is not only very important academically, it is also significant to the research on the actual state of sex work. To my knowledge, among the present Chinese underground sex workers, the majority, especially those who were born in the lower social classes, refuse to provide special sexual services, because these are not acceptable in the sexual culture of their class. They think such practices as oral intercourse or anal intercourse very 'dirty,' 'sick,' or 'over the top.' They also consider those who do it as 'abnormal,' 'boring,' and 'bullying.' The upshot is that many prostitutes will not offer such services, no matter how much they are paid since they have a strong physical aversion to and truly feel sickened by such behaviour, even to the point of nausea. That is, they still stubbornly keep to the most traditional sexual practices in their sexual ideas, sexual behaviour and sexual techniques. The only openness they are prepared to reveal is they are ready to exchange the use of their own genitals for money. Nevertheless, they attach two implied conditions: their clients must rent their genitals for 'normal and proper' use. Their mouths and anuses are not for sale. In this respect, they are no different from most other Chinese women.

Fondling service means allowing caressing, but not involving their own genital organs. They do not allow the customers to have sexual intercourse or any other form of sexual exchange, but they do allow the customers to touch the other sexually sensitive parts of their body. Many escort services allow such activities. For instance, in the South, touching a prostitute's breast is called 'fondle ball' (caressing a female breast). Another sexual service is cinema escort, which is divided into 'early half court' and 'later half court' and the prices of which differ greatly. These two words indicate in fact that in the dark cinema, the girls allow the customers to touch the upper and lower halves of their bodies. These are also known as 'accepting caressing services.'

Output caressing sexual services consist of the female sex workers touching the customers' sexually sensitive parts without allowing their customers to touch that same parts of their own bodies. Many heterosexual massages provide this service. In a number of places, there is a massage sexual service called 'anti-aircraft' meaning the massage girls perform masturbation hand jobs for their customers who lie down on a bed, with their penises looking like guns firing at aircraft. A further service is called 'ice and fire,' which is ranked as the 'five clouds' (the fifth level of service), meaning a massage girl sucking the penis of her customer first with ice water in her mouth, then sucking it with hot water in her mouth. The so-called 'nine clouds' (highest heaven) means a girl sucks each sexually sensitive part of her customers' body including anus and stabs that part with her tongue. Of course, this is the most expensive service, equal to twenty to thirty-three days of the labourer's wages. If there is a depression in the sex market, some very traditional girls will learn these skills quickly. Cogently these services are better than sexual intercourse if we are thinking in terms of the prevention of STDs/HIV. The division of the caressing sexual services into 'accepting' and 'output' is significant. Some females would rather be massage girls who give hand jobs than be part of an escort service; they will not let the customers touch their body. They think it is unacceptable to sell the sensitive parts of their body to the customers. So the girls are not naked at this moment, even when giving a hand job. Trade rules state that customers should not touch the body of the massage girls. However, other girls are just the opposite. They think it is passive to be caressed by the customers to whom they are offering companionship. This is understandable because it does not mean they like it themselves. Nevertheless, to give massage and a hand job to the customers is active participation and shows them to be very 'coquettish,' 'low' and very 'dissolute.' Customers' tastes differ greatly too. Some men think it is not enough just to touch the girls during escort service, even after having forked out so much money. They consider it is still far removed from actually having sex. On the other hand, there is yet another group of men who think masturbation is 'metamorphosis' and 'harmful,' so why should they spend money on it? Still others compute and find that it is more satisfactory for them to touch the girls themselves during escort service than to have a hand job in which they do not have the chance to touch the girls with their own hands, no matter how good the hand job is.

Female sex workers may also offer naked dances, strip-teases, or bisexual shows and sexual intercourse shows. Today, the performance of sexual services is very limited for two reasons. First, some local prostitution, massage and escort services have overdeveloped so some customers come and demand to watch, in other words voyeurism is being catered to. Second, in some other places, prostitution is strictly prohibited.

One type of sexual service is the association sexual service and refers to 'escort services' in the general sense. Usually this service offers no sexual caresses or sexual shows but merely offers an opportunity for association between the opposite sexes. However, even in 1997, there was no definite rule about such services in the red light districts. I discovered that in some places a 'blow job' (oral sex) was much more expensive than 'open fire once' (one-time intercourse), while in other places it was much cheaper. In some parts of Beijing, 'on-the-spot' broadcast was even more expensive than 'all-night sex.'

THE BUSINESS RATE OF PROSTITUTION

In Town A

I adopted the method of compiling fixed time and fixed place monitoring statistics to discover how many female sex workers and customers there are operating in some typical sex industry venues. I have done this because the Chinese always exaggerate the rate of the prostitution business. In ten different barbershops, during the total of thirty-four hours that I monitored, although there were 900 men who stopped and took a look at the 'goods,' there were only 200 who actually entered. Also, there were no more than ninety girls who were really taken away by the customers. That is, an average of only nine girls were really taken away by the customers at each barbershop during these thirty-four hours. Each girl was only taken away 1.6 times average and less than 0.26 time each day. What this means is that a barbershop girl has to wait four days on average to get a customer if she merely stays inside the barbershop expecting customers to call. At this point I should like to point out that the employment of such a method has hitherto been unprecedented in China.

Those who come for the barbershop girls want to have 'open fire once.' Barbershop girls who 'follow your escort' carry out a sort of piece-work, charging by the hour. In actual fact one hour consists of forty-five minutes, the remaining quarter being regarded as the girls' rest time. A barbershop boss usually collects about $6 from the customers, but $12 may be asked for good-looking girls as 'charge for visiting a parlour girl once.' The barbershop girls themselves, generally charge $37 as a tip. When business is slack, a $12 tip is acceptable to better-looking girls while the girls who are deemed less attractive charge $6 only. Local labourers earn about $0.4 an hour. Escort girls in singing and dance halls, who usually look better and offer 'all-night sex' (over two hours), have more opportunity to bargain with the customers because there is no set rule. Usually the girls ask at least $100, and the customers will pay them $62. The escort girls may demand $125 from overseas customers and earn at least $75, equal to the monthly wage of a local labourer. A massage girl charges the highest price. Regular massage takes two hours and the typical tip is $25. If a massage girl wants to be a 'follow your escort,' $62 is charged, at least for 'open fire once.' Less than $125 is not acceptable for 'all-night sex' service. However, most of the customers who go to the massage girls think it worthwhile, because a massage girl is rated more highly than an escort girl. Pertinently, massage girls are not only more beautiful but also give their customers better service as they have been more highly trained in sexual techniques.

In Town B

In this developing zone, the red-light district centres are located in the area of the roadside stores. In total it is 1,200 metres long and encompasses 116 various sexual service places, ninety-seven of which are in operation. About thirty of them are run principally as hotels and almost all other sixty-seven are specially prepared for sex work. Along the whole length of the stretch of the road there were no patrol pumps, no car repairs or car-washes, no parking lots and no acceptable restaurant. It is purely and simply dedicated to the sex industry. Such roadside stores are the chief means of operating prostitution in China because they are the domain of the local peasants. It is most convenient for them to open roadside stores and it is most difficult for the government to control. There are two major reasons that make this red light district successful: one is that being located on the border between two administrative districts, it forms a sort of twilight zone administratively. The other is that local power is so strong that it may act of its own volition. Under a prostitution prohibition policy as strict as that in China, the buyers and sellers of the sex industry have put safety and secrecy at a premium. In the roadside stores, a prostitute's client feels as safe as if he were an ordinary passerby. Roadside stores provide low-priced sexual services that happen to fill in the blanks left by the high-priced escort services in the city. Take a barbershop as an example. Of all the six girls there, each sells only seventeen times per month and once per 1.8 days average. Given all customers demand 'open fire once' (one-time intercourse), a girl may earn a $205 income each month. Given 'all-night sex' customers are half of the overall clients, the monthly income of each girl may reach $255 or something in that region. All the barbershop girls prefer customers passing through, because there is greater possibility that they will ask for all-night sex.

In Town C

This was originally a residential area which housed forty people, dispersed over nine houses. This town is located in the mountains on the borders between Hunan and Guizhou Provinces. Although it lies only 1500 metres above the sea level, the relative height above river level thirty miles away is 500 metres. In other words, the terrain is precipitous and it is very inaccessible for traffic. The first gold-mine was excavated between 1995 and the winter of 1996. In the summer of 1997, there was a total population of only 28,000 in this gold-mining area, taking into account those coming up the mountain to work during the day and going down the mountain when they went off work at night. Nevertheless, there were twenty-nine recreational facilities with a capacity to hold about 1,500 persons, about 5 per cent of the total population of this community. They are eight dance-halls, seven karaoke halls, five hairdressing parlours, five video show parlours and four snooker halls. The proportion of the female sex workers is about 0.3 per cent to 0.5 per cent, a relatively large figure for such a remote mining area. Because there are rarely even tourists visiting from outside, this area does not provide the usual facilities that a city does, and all social classes here are relatively very humble.

The market prices of the female sex workers are $6 asking price for 'open fire once' and $3.60 counter-offering price or even $2.40. For 'all-night sex': the opening price is $18 and the haggling price may be $12 or even $6. For escort service the opening price may be at $3.60 and the haggling price may be at $1.20. To assess the frequency of the sex trade and the overall volume of it, I used the same methods I applied in Town B. I noted down the number of clients visiting thirty-eight prostitutes. Therefore, I got a lower limit: in two places, nine female sex workers received thirty-eight customers over six days and five nights and each received 0.8 clients on average each day. On the basis of this, I have made the following estimate. There were 80–130 female sex workers on the mountain. If all of them behave as I have sketched above, then the sex trade occurs about 60–100 times on average each day and 1800–3000 times per month in this mining area. Given that each commercial sexual exchange was made by only one person at one time, about 6 per cent to 10 per cent out of the 28,000 strong population had ever participated in a sexual transaction.

THE STRATIFICATION OF PROSTITUTION

In Town B

There are a number of ways of soliciting customers. In the first type, one to three 'hens' heads' (male pimps) are responsible for luring customers and the prostitutes usually do not come out to solicit themselves. 'Hens' is the slang for female sex workers. Most of them only solicit in front of the gates of the premises to which they belong. The second way is to await customers. Very few pimps go out especially to lure customers inside. The prostitutes usually wait in their rooms to receive the customers and then see them off at the door. The third way is to go in search of customers. There are about thirty to forty prostitutes who do not belong to any fixed spot. They rent a room from a hotel and then go out to solicit customers themselves and take them back to their rented room afterwards.

There are a number of service types. The first is known as 'eating fast food.' Most spots offer only 'open fire once' service. Therefore, the whole set-up of the bar and the decorations is designed without embellishments for a one-time sexual intercourse standard. The bedrooms are very small, without any parlour and living-room or other facilities. The second type is called 'boiling down gruel' ('long-time sex'). This usually refers to the prostitutes' clients staying with a prostitute for 'one hour' (forty-five minutes) or 'two hours.' 'Fast food' culminates in ejaculation, however long it takes. 'Boiling down gruel' is counted by time span whether or not the prostitutes' clients ejaculate or how many times they ejaculate. This difference is significant to both prostitutes and the prostitutes' clients. Underground sex workers have a propensity to work harder and employ more sexual techniques (if they know any) to speed up the whole process and then to find another customer. Nevertheless, in 'boiling down gruel,' they are likely to loaf on the job and be ordered to get on with it. Not unnaturally, the prostitutes' clients are just the opposite. Many young customers prefer 'boiling down gruel' because they believe (or hope) they are able to achieve two ejaculations at least, or perhaps even more, during the negotiated time. This makes it much cheaper than to 'eat fast food' twice. In this red light district, the price of 'boiling down gruel' usually follows this pattern: the 'hens' heads' usually ask for $50 or so, but in most cases, the charge has not risen above $25 for 'one hour.' However, because of the business depression since 1997, $12 is accepted nowadays. The third service type is 'hire one night' (all-night sex): prostitutes' clients select prostitutes from the roadside stores first, then head for the rooms already prepared in the residential buildings. The rooms have been especially reserved by the roadside stores beforehand. In this case, the other fees do not change, but rooms may be much more expensive to rent. It is $12 at least and usually $25. So the prostitutes' clients overall expenses may reach $50 or so. It is said that the clients who choose this style are mostly men with power or a reputation, who come in from the urban area.

In Town C

The initial 'hencoops' (brothels) are only gradually beginning to appear on the mountains. In fact, they are no more than self-built little sheds in which 'hens' spread several pieces of paper and then began their business. There was not even plastic sheet. If no one visited, they just went out to 'drop around another coop' (to call on other hencoops) either to poach customers or simply had sex with customers out in the fields or even in the wilderness. There were two main characteristics of the prostitution in Town C in 1997. First, the soliciting of customers was very covert, while the love-making was very overt. Second, there were sexual services offering opportunities for voyeurism or cunnilingus.

GENERAL CONDITIONS OF FEMALE SEX WORKERS THROUGHOUT CHINA

About half the female sex workers from villages had made psychological and practical preparations before becoming prostitutes, even before leaving home. A so-called 'village young sister' ('peasant girl') is not synonymous with a virgin. According to 'hens' head' or pimp E, who often went to villages in another province to 'recruit workers,' at least half of the peasant girls had been married very young indeed. In choosing those who are not married, E looks specially for those who are not 'good' according to the traditional sexual morality. E believes that most of them have already had premarital sex, so turning them into prostitutes is not difficult. Undoubtedly, before they leave home many rural girls are determined not to sell sex so they go to restaurants to be waitresses instead of working in dance halls or massage parlours. Pertinently, such peasant girls often take quite a large amount of money with them when they leave home. For instance, in Town B, one girl brought $37, of which $6 was given by her parents and the rest of which she had saved herself. The money the other three girls brought with them was not less than $12 per girl. On the basis of the costs and the standard of living of village sisters, this $12 may enable them almost to afford food for one month. Five dollars is enough to take the bus back home, including meals taken on the road. So, such girls were under no great economic pressure to become a prostitute, unless they had other reasons – they had lost their virginity, because premarital sex or had indulged in extramarital sex. Prostitutes are made by the traditional value placed on a girl's virginity. This is true, at least in present-day China. Most female sex workers always move in a wider radius looking for better job opportunities. Few of them stay in the same town for up to half year. At present, more and more female workers laid-off from ailing state-owned enterprises in the northeast have streamed into various service occupations in the towns and cities of northern China. Growing numbers of them are entering prostitution and are becoming increasingly conspicuous. They have a tendency to move more frequently and venture further afield.

'I want to have my own home and family.' These are the words spoken from the bottom of their hearts by almost all women in present-day China. Almost none of the female sex workers should be excepted. However, they may not readily admit it as their problem is they cannot get rid of a feeling of self-debasement, self-consciousness and being fully aware of what they are doing, as they are fully aware of what social public opinion has to say about them. Even in their private chats, they prefer not to mention such desires. Conversely, I have never heard any female sex worker complaining about the hardship or bitterness of her life except when she haggles with the customers. Pertinently, I have never heard any female sex worker say that she derives happiness from such a life, except when she tries to 'keep up appearances' or talks back, but this does not often happen. One word may summarize their most general feeling – that is 'light,' meaning here tasteless and insipid. Feeling light is feeling dull, void, aimless and having no alternative. I have doubts about the claims that women sell sex for the sake of sexual pleasure. This is because there is a huge gap between their accidental sexual response while selling sex (few of them really had an orgasm) and their aim in selling sex. I suspect such stories of satisfaction are fabricated by customers. I believe my suspicion is true at least in present-day China. Indubitably subjected to the pressure of social opinion, clients are not willing to refer their soliciting behaviour as bullying or shopping. They need be able to say: 'I have given the girls what they want.' Even though they admit that it is only a market exchange, by nurturing this idea the exchange may appear in a somewhat fairer light.

In Town A

All prostitutes possess health certificates. However, since nominally they work for hairdressers, the Hygiene Immune Department can only check whether they are infected with such infectious diseases as tuberculosis and hepatitis B. The service does not inspect STDs, since hairdressing has no direct relationship to sex. Nevertheless, some prostitutes capitalize on this health certificate to deceive newcomers from beyond the border, making them think the health certificate proves its holders are free from STDs. At times they convince their clients that it is a certificate issued by the Chinese government. At least the certificate exists. Now it may not signify much but, as with many other situations in China, it may be given content later. It might be said the Chinese are very good at 'filling the old bottle with new wine.'

In Town B

There is a whole group of hometown girls active as female sex workers in Town B and they tend to stick together. This fact does not mean the sex workers do not want to keep what they do secret, or that their families or hometowns condone what they are doing. The most probable reason for their herding together may lie in the feeling that they are out of tune with the world outside this development zone. They are forced to what they do and all they can do about it is to resort to strengthening the reciprocal relations between themselves. This helps them to preserve somehow their ego intact in a marginal group. It is clear families, fellow townspeople and acquaintances appear especially significant in their lives.

In Town C
Of the eleven female sex workers whom I met and talked to in this town, the first sociologically significant characteristic they possessed was that all of them were from nearby rural areas. The farthest of which is no more than seventy-five kilometres away. The second trait was that when they did not have their own regular clients, their boss usually assigned them to do whatever work needed to be done at whatever hour. They were more like a combination of waitress and sex worker. The third trait was that all of them had a marital history. It seems the people, regardless of whether living here or living in the women's hometowns, believed that only divorced women and wives who ran away from home would want to join a female sex workers' team, and that only such women would be acceptable to it. This leads us to the issue of divorce in China. Although divorce is considered morally decadent, prostitution is thought to be even more so. People here may think that divorced women may or even should take up sex work. By thinking like this, people are actually equating the women's divorces with prostitution. This may explain why, up to now, local custom still stubbornly refuses to accept divorce and the people are capable of beating the hell out of divorced women, indeed assigning them to the very lowest, eighteenth layer of hell, as the Chinese would say. There may also be a second explanation, which is that the women themselves may encourage this. It is not that people really think divorced women may or ought to sell sex, but divorced women engaged in prostitution have invented this scenario to cover their behaviour, semi-consciously in order to have the opportunity to be able to earn a livelihood to support themselves. However, I have yet a third explanation. In their dramatic arts, the Chinese habitually display great sympathy for the tragic scenes involving orphans and widowed mothers, the homeless and vagabonds. Divorced women and the wives who run away from home are part of that theatrical tradition. Therefore, that people think these women may and even ought to sell sex is in fact to show a kind of generosity and sympathy towards them. That is to say, as long as the prostitutes have proper reasons to for taking up their profession, their prostitution is comprehensible and forgivable. I tend towards the third explanation because from daily experience I have found that the moral evaluation criterion that ordinary Chinese use to weigh up ordinary events is a 'fair and reasonable' one. Usually, fairness is put on a higher pedestal than reason. That is, as long as there is a fair explanation for it, it deserves forgiveness. People are prepared to be generous about it, and no one pays

much attention to chastity or righteousness. Those who are easily persuaded to embrace some sort of morality are usually people from the upper echelons who know about moral commandments and tend to be sanctimonious, and not the common people.

LOCAL PEOPLE'S ATTITUDES TOWARDS FEMALE SEX WORKERS AND THE ISSUE OF KEEPING A SECOND WIFE IN TOWN A

Estimations of the income of female sex workers are exaggerated. Nowadays most people are discontented with their income, and this feeling of dissatisfaction tends to plague their minds. Therefore they vent their spleen by and expend their energy on wildly overestimating what prostitutes earn. The people most likely to indulge in this sort of behaviour are those on fixed pay in the state system, and it is they who form the main stream of popular opinion in society.

A traditional disparagement of female sex workers implies that local residents, both men and women, despise these ladies heartily. Why are they so denigrating? The contempt has nothing to do with upholding the values of marital morality or with regarding their occupation as illegal, it is simply born out of prevailing negative feeling towards them, casting them as dirty, ominous, and unlucky.

More detailed investigation shows that local people are hostile to the female sex workers and do indignantly accuse them of harming the institution of marriage, a convenient peg on which to hang their own frustrations. The so-called angry denunciation of the female sex workers by the local residents, especially the local women, is mainly and really directed towards the second wives instead of towards prostitutes in general. The younger, more intelligent local women think the biggest danger the female sex workers represent is only that they make these ordinary women doubt the chastity of their men.

There is a widespread anger about those who are stigmatized as decadent officials. What local people talk about most is the 'moral generosity' of the leaders at various levels. For instance, it is said that one local leader even remarked at a meeting that it is quite normal for men to visit prostitutes and that prostitutes had to have food to eat.

Despite the furore, local people tend to demonstrate a relative degree of tolerance, in view of the actual benefits accruing. There is a symbiotic circle in the local sex industry. The local common people have been renting rooms from which to sell food and clothes and cosmetics to female sex workers and fill their pockets from customers who come here with money to spend. A saying popular is: 'One flourish brings the prosperity of a hundred trades.'

In Chinese this is a play on words as the Chinese character for 'to flourish' is pronounced in precisely the same way as the word for 'prostitution.' This has, in fact, become common knowledge in this community. So by and large people are actually tolerant of the female sex workers, and the desire to abolish prostitution is but an assumed attitude, which is why the present government policy is actually continuing to urge people 'to do but not to say.'

The price of keeping a second wife ranges from $610 per month at the highest to $61 per month. According to the local people, the average price does not exceed $244 per month. Surely, what we are talking about here is the cash men pay directly to the second wife and that does not cover all the costs. Apart from the cash in hand, men need to provide housing and daily necessities for their second wives, but these benefits are usually not bestowed in cash. Therefore, the aforesaid price is almost pure profit accruing to the second wife. Keeping a second wife falls in between taking a concubine and visiting prostitutes. It is a purely business arrangement but it is none the less tinged with a little touch of matrimony. For instance, it may be a long-term co-habitation, and it may indeed encompass tender emotions, but the major criterion is money. A man may stop this relationship any time he wants; it does not require any divorce procedure nor does it have any after-effects. A legal concubine or legal second wife is perpetually locked in competition with the first wife for the favour of the man, and sometimes the situation becomes so chaotic men are very befuddled. An unlawful second wife will not and cannot act like that because she is only as it were letting herself and is never qualified for nor does she desire to be promoted to the position of first wife. In Town A there are many second wives which leads to the question, what do the wives think about this? Indubitably what the women in the Town A hate most is keeping a second wife, instead of visiting prostitutes. This raises one very pertinent point: it seems that only the policy of forbidding the taking of concubines struck a chord in people's thoughts. Does this mean that the prostitution ban perhaps went too far?

OWNERS OF RECREATIONAL FACILITIES: MALE CONTROLLERS OF FEMALE SEX WORKERS

The basic definition of a prostitute's pimp or 'hens' head' refers to those men who organize the activities of the prostitutes. However, they differ from those owners of recreational facilities, who perform the same function on specific premises, in three ways.

Hens' heads usually go to the home village of female sex workers purely and simply with the purpose of recruiting them for the job or they coax them without deceiving them about the nature of the work. Once the girls are in their employ they usually escort them to the place where they will ply their trade in person. They generally restrict the prostitutes' freedom as individuals throughout the whole process of their being recruited, taken away and introduced into prostitution. All the income of the hens' heads is obtained from what the sex workers earn, like skimming the cream off the milk. Undoubtedly under Chinese statutory law, 'to force, seduce, retain, and introduce others to sell sex' carries an extremely severe penalty. The most severe punishment for these crimes is the death penalty. Some such pimps have indeed been executed by the firing squad. However, most female sex workers nowadays engage in the sex industry willingly or semi-willingly. They regard the hens' heads as guides or leaders. Most prostitutes accept the exploitation and control of the hens' heads as the unavoidable price they have to pay for their being launched into the business. Therefore, the underground prostitutes seldom report their hens' heads; even those who were in effect captured will not 'bite' the hens' heads. This being so, the hens' heads feel increasingly at ease and justified in doing what they do.

Furthermore, in Town B, where there is no secondary industry offering employment, the sex industry offers the sole employment opportunity. Thus, there are only two choices open to the female sex workers: to sell sex or to lose their jobs and go back to their villages. Despite their dominating role, the hens' heads are not naturally tyrannical. They observe the same 'fair and reasonable' moral rule embraced by the common people. It is in their own best interest not to harm or ruin the workers under their control. One hens' head said: 'I do this to earn money, not to grow rich at the cost of the shipwreck of others, so I do not bully the girls.' With the growth of the sex industry, especially the upswing in the intensity of competition in the same trade, the relationship between many prostitutes and their hens' heads has tended to become a sort of partnership, superficially at least.

Recruitment fees are the initial income the hens' heads earn. They are entrusted by the owners of various spots with the recruitment of the peasant girls in the villages where these girls live. The owners pay them a $25 'introduction fee.' The hens' heads rely mostly on the clues offered by the female sex workers already working for them or who have worked for them in the past. They go to their home-village to recruit workers in a process resembling a snowball effect. The routine work of the hens' heads is to recommend workers, that is to lure customers in front of the gates of the premises where the girls work. When and where it is more difficult for the female sex workers to go out to solicit customers overtly or when circumstances require that they are even required to hide themselves, the practice of recommending workers is deeply entrenched. Again, the stricter the policy of abolishing prostitution is, the more serious the control, exploitation, and risk of personal harm the female sex workers run at the hands of the hens' heads. If a hens' head cannot operate on his own, he has to 'help others.' Should he work for an owner of a store or restaurant then he depends for his income on the owner for whom he works. He has the right to a proportion of the fee the clients pay the owners of the premises. Usually this amounts to no more than $2.4 each time. Very importantly, he cannot monopolize the right to lure customers for the whole premises. In the red light district I investigated, there are only four to five hens' heads who work independently. The rest had already become the helping hands of the owners of recreational facilities. They can earn $125 for a month if they are lucky.

The way the prostitutes are controlled can be defined in terms of the severity of that control. The first degree can be classified as 'tyrannical.' Owners resort to various means to force the girls to sell sex. The second degree is 'dictatorial': the owners employ 'economic coercion' to urge the girls to sell sex. For instance, in many areas, massage girls do not have any fixed salary; their income depends solely on the tips from their customers. What is more, they have to pay the owners their board and lodging. This being so, can they live without selling sex? The third degree is 'the policy of benevolence.' Some owners only provide working premises for underground prostitutes and then collect a specified sum. They do not participate in organizing prostitution directly nor do they force the girls to prostitute themselves. This is called to 'support prostitution' and the severest punishment for it under Chinese Penal Law is also the death penalty. Nevertheless, the owners do not actively harass the girls who do not sell sex. They believe when 'some become rich,' other girls will follow naturally. Why should they force them?

The key to these above three internal administration modes is how the benefits gained are distributed between the underground prostitutes and the owners. Undoubtedly, the owners exploit the underground prostitutes, but their exploitation differs in means and in degrees. My research has shown that the lowest proportion deducted by the owners is 15 per cent and the highest is 50 per cent.

In Town A, the overall monthly income of the owner of a dance hall averages $2,320 to $4,260. The overall monthly costs he incurs average at least $2,060. His pure profit ranges between $266 and $2,200. In Town B, the one-time investment of the boss of a barbershop is roughly $1,500. The fixed overheads and daily running expenses are around $255 per month. In December of 1996, the high point of her business then, she earned about $870. The worst period was the Spring Festival of 1997, when all of her eight girls went home for the New Year holiday, and she earned less than $125 in all. On the basis of these figures her monthly income averaged between $245 and $305. That is to say, her pure profit fluctuated between

0.8 to 1 times the operating costs. This female boss treated her girls like pigs; the meal fee for each girl is only $0.27 daily, not enough to buy even a bowl of boiled noodles at the market. Therefore, part of her pure profit is the ill-gotten gains of this 'feeding pigs' management style. This is not just exploitation, it is systematic destruction of one's employees! I hope the government legislate to ensure that they receive at least the same food ordinary people have, instead of imposing so-called re-education programmes or the penalties meted out to them when the government has a burst of what is called 'wiping out the blue.'

In Town C, the same official procedures ranging from a permit for special lines and the security and administration certificate for public places to the land occupation certificate, hygiene certificate and epidemic prevention certificate are also to be found. One house even possesses no less than seven certificates. For each certificate, the owner must hand over $36 to $87 at one time. One female owner had to spend about $490 on invitations and gifts to others, even though she was backed by a cadre. All this took about 8 per cent of her total investment. Her one-time investment was $6,330 in total. Her monthly depreciation charge is as high as $106. Her monthly routine expenses are $1,105 in total. Her direct income comes from the $2.5 given by a customer who had 'open fire once.' If a girl keeps a man company all night, the boss may get $3.6 to $6.2. This, however, is not all of the boss's income. When a girl offers sexual services, she will always persuade her customer to consume something else as well. If it is an all-night escort, meaning being with the man the whole night, there is always a big meal to follow. So, the gross income of the female boss each month is about $1,125. If her business can be kept at that level, a girl can earn her boss about $880 direct income, alongside the extra income they create. This means that the bulk of the owner's income is from the girls, even though they manage a dance hall, restaurants, video halls and hairdressers. To make a rough estimate, the profit rate of the boss hiring the girls is as high as about 330 per cent. In contrast to this, the gross profit rate of the boss' restaurants is but 90 per cent or so and that of her dance hall and video hall should be around 130 per cent. This is the explanation pure and simple of why, although some owners of brothels and the like have been executed by firing-squad, there are still plenty willing to follow in their footsteps. No sooner does one bite the dust than another steps into the breach.

The emergence of the red light district in Town A owes much to the government's assiduous activities to wipe out vice. In the Zhujiang Delta, one town began to run a sex industry as early as 1985 but, because 'a tall tree catches the wind,' it was cleaned up by police sent directly from the Security Ministry. After 1990, the sex industry began to flourish in another town and this was an open secret. The upshot was it was decided that this threatened the collective interest of the whole delta area. So after 1992, the Provincial Security Department sent in police officers and basically swept away the sex industry there. At this point, the sex industry in Town A was just in its teething phase. It commenced just in time to fill a gap in that area and therefore started off on just the right foot. Why did it not collapse amid the competition from other businesses in the same line? The first reason is that the situation in the Zhujiang Delta area has provided conditions conducive to accommodating any expansion in the sex industry since 1993. The main reason is that the local people of the delta area began to turn to keeping a second wife rather than visiting the girls. Simultaneously, the sex industry of many other inland places began to develop, so the delta was no longer the only 'paradise.' The second reason is that there was no role available for anyone wanting to take a punt in the geographically disadvantageous conditions. The third reason is that since 1993, the central government has been making systematically concentrated efforts to abolish the vice industry. So it is impossible for the local governments at various levels to tolerate any 'new boomers,' because such official bodies have to be conscious of the essential interest of the whole. The fourth reason is that after more than ten years, many people in the delta have become aware that many other places that did not take the trouble to develop the sex industry have attracted no less investment. This forced them do a bit of cost accounting. Was it really beneficial for them to devote so many extra resources and to run bigger and bigger risks just to make use of the sex industry to attract and introduce business and investment? This situation is the product of the 'mounting on the steps,' the steady progress of the market economy. Economic growth is spreading gradually and has imperceptibly weakened the prime motive force of the local governments in many other places in the competition to establish red light districts. The fifth reason is that because the sex industry relies more on capital from the power system than other sectors, from the point of view of the individual operators, the profit rate of the sex industry is falling rapidly. To top it all, by the end of 1996, production of pirated CD and VCD introduced a new hot point, holding out the promise of colossal profits. As a result, many businesspersons and investors turned to other businesses, promising tempting profits at a much lower risk.

INTERNAL REASONS FOR THE DEVELOPMENT
OF THE SEX INDUSTRY

In Town A

There are four limits that will always stymie the sex industry here. Essentially, it cannot operate in crowded or centralized places. Therefore, the establishing of a set of matching services such as food, massage, sexual services and drugs is impossible. It is proving impossible to set up unitary management in places where there are a number of operations. The emergence of obviously profitable groups is an insuperable barrier because in Chinese politics any such trend in this matter provokes an essential issue that threatens the very existence of the actual political system. The local interest groups in the sex industry have been carefully avoiding these three mine-fields. First of all, escort girls at various local recreational premises are present in sufficient numbers. They are under the guidance of two to three or four to five 'mummies' (procuresses) respectively. Barbershop girls form another independent category and they operate from barbershops or hairdressers. This mutual exclusiveness means that escort girls and the barbershop girls do not work together, so it cannot be said they match set services in centralized places. Secondly, various female sex workers are basically managed by a 'mummy' and are seldom directly under the control of bosses or managers. There are only a few instances when the pimps interfere directing in the process. In other words, the boss who owns the property rights to the recreational premises has little to do with 'mummy' who manages female sex workers. At the same time, the control of the 'mummies' over female sex workers has been greatly weakened and the relative freedom of female sex workers has been greatly increased. Relative separation has been making an ever stronger appearance. This is the first tentative display of self-confidence, independence and self-decision shown by female sex workers. The outcome of these centrifugal forces is that no centralized, planned economic administration system and operating mechanism can take root in the noisy, teeming sex industry of this town.

Thirdly, in the initial period, those individuals who established the sex industry had made full use of the power system and capital they possessed. This probably caused the line to develop continuously as a combination of both official and business interests, which eventually formed a more politically significant interest group. However later, the original development route seemed to have been shelved. It would be fair to say it was abandoned. People seemed to take the reins into their own hands, and began to earn money with money. This obviated the clear cut growth of any interest group in the local sex industry, which could then profile itself as a visible organization with political clout.

45

In Town B

The most salient development here has been the appearance on the scene of outside competition. In the autumn of 1996, a new red light district began to emerge in the nearby city. Because it is not as convenient for passing traffic as the development zone, it has taken the form of a holiday village and villa district that offers mainly long-time sex and all-night sex. The prices here are much lower than that in the development zone. For $25 it is possible to buy all-night sex. As a result, economically conscious clients have streamed into the newly developed red light district. This has forced the prices in Town B down to the point that it has been possible to buy an 'hour' of 'long-time sex' for $12. Internal development then stagnated. Three to four years after the beginnings of the sex industry, there were still only two karaoke halls. No sauna, massage or any form of escort service was to be found there. Its reputation was made by its highly simplified interpersonal sexual association like straightforward 'open fire once.' This red light district has provided for a need which was there but unsatisfied. The clients have a need and the prostitutes satisfy it. There is reciprocal support and the two blend together. Furthermore, neither side has enough independent power to break this solid mould.

Basically there has been no sweeping away of prostitution. If any such attempt were to be made, the direct sexual services here will simply be transmogrified into various expanded sexual services. If there were any faulty attempt at abolition, the sex industry might well be helped to train its team, expand its ideas, make technical innovations and go for a more comprehensive occupation. In fact, no such clean up campaigns have been undertaken. So the sex industry lacks any challenge and stimulation from outside. Paradoxically this has held back to its development. The biggest harm done to the local sex industry is that when threats of abolition are in abeyance, its reputation is safe. Any potential customers within a hundred square mile radius know it is safe here so nothing restrains them from making use of the facilities. As they do not have to tout for custom, all the people engaged in this line here lack a kind of customer and service sense. Any sense of enterprise which might have kept them on their toes has been stifled. This means it is an uphill battle to introduce improvements and changes.

In Town C

Here the local sex industry is largely patronized by the local residents. All the people engaged in the sex industry are also locals, instead of workers brought in from far away. There is a symbiotic relationship between the sex industry and the whole community of this place; they develop and promote each other. The sex industry here is of a type peculiar to such a newly booming, swiftly and violently developing and rather special gold-mining area. It is still in its developmental stages. I have not found any trace of the sex, gambling, drug industries forming any block, nor is there any interest group with a large slice of the sex industry. The sex industry here is a relatively closed shop and is unlikely to expand any further. Although its reputation has spread far and wide, it seems it is unlikely to be a model that the nearby areas will strive to imitate. The sex industry here was born under special circumstances and its birth was expedited by the natural demand of the local community, a fair proportion of whom work in the gold-mines. It was not deliberately launched by the local government. It has never engaged in any special connivance with or sought protection from the local government. It has also never formed any solid alliance with the administrative and managerial class of the whole community either. The relationship between the local sex industry and the local government has only manifested itself in the 'slipping into the water' or falling into evil ways of very few officials. Pertinently, it has not and will not present any obvious and colossal realistic financial interests to the local government or to the managerial class.

THE INTEREST GROUPS IN THE SEX INDUSTRY

The interest groups in the sex industry are comprised of those owners of recreational facilities who organize prostitution either openly or secretly. The pornographic spots in many cities and counties in North China have been monopolized by 'prostitution VIPs' who have rushed in from bigger cities. The majority of the prostitution VIPs run a joint operation with investment from outside and the connivance of the local powers-that-be. Each owner will exaggerate the potential clout of his joint owner or ally, building him up to be a threat to big establishments, especially cogent if he happens to be connected to one of the various dictatorial organs. For example, fifteen of the nineteen recreational spots in the six counties and two villages of north China I have investigated claimed they allied with big establishments in other parts of the country, which ultimately involve almost all the component parts of the dictatorial system such as public security, safety, armed police, army and the judiciary and so on. Therefore, in some places, the owners dared to claim that no one from the public security bureau is not allowed to enter such places without the signature of the highest local leader. For instance, there are 223 restaurants in one county, sixty-seven of which have an official background. Nevertheless, the police has failed to discover any prostitution cases among the 300 waitresses working at these restaurants. By contrast, the police tried 275 cases and imprisoned 550 persons and collected fines to the tune of $157,300 from the other, non-official restaurants over a one-and-a-half year period. With the development of the underground sex industry, members of various related interest groups may form themselves into some sort of power block. A covert political struggle may even emerge. In any consideration of this development, it has to be remembered that there have always been basic secret societies and various trade unions throughout the thousands of years of Chinese history.

THE COST OF BANNING PROSTITUTION

Research carried out in 1993, in the periphery of a certain city in central China showed to arrest a prostitute with substantial proof required 7.5 hours of a security worker's time. Therefore, according to the survey I did in 1994 in a large southern city with a population of 6 million, 450 full-time policemen would have had to work in an all-out effort for 900,000 hours to arrest all the underground prostitutes and their customers. Any such attempts require that the government actually would have to employ a very large social services staff alongside the regular police. This is the economic cost of banning prostitution. Recently, people's confidence in such repressive policies has been greatly undermined. In the survey of the three cities I carried out in 1994, I asked: 'What would you do were you unintentionally to run into a man and a woman who are obviously not married but are having sex and whom you do not know?' The result was that only 3.75 per cent answered 'I would stop them, warn them, or reprimand them.' while 5.8 per cent replied 'I would report them to the relevant departments.' Those who gave the above answers were only 9.5 per cent of all respondents and they are mostly older people above fifty-five years old. The remaining 90 per cent replied 'I would pretend I had not seen anything' or 'I would hurry away.' These answers imply that the magic weapon the government used to wield to maintain security, the public monitor, no longer works. The people's inert attitude towards illegal sexual affairs is a sign that their confidence that prostitution can be effectively banned, if indeed that is what they really wanted, has weakened. In the above survey, only 9.7 per cent of the respondents believed that 'all the underground prostitutes could be discovered (not speaking of whether they are arrested).' Also, only 3.75 per cent believe that 'almost all the prostitutes' clients might be discovered.' In contrast, 42.85 per cent believed that 'the underground prostitutes are seldom to be discovered' or even 'none is to be discovered'; 63.1 per cent believe that their clients are seldom or never to be discovered. These answers suggest that another magic weapon the government used to employ to maintain security, namely 'to kill one in order to warn all,' has basically lost its magic.

The message which seems to be coming through loud and clear is that the more unwilling people are to poke their noses into other people's business, the more difficult it is for prostitution to be discovered. As the number of prostitutes and their potential clients swell, the less the general public is likely to interfere, as legal sanctions are weakened. Concomitantly the more slogans such as 'eradicate' or 'liquidate' are yelled, the slacker the law-bearers become because they feel the situation is out of control. The social cost of banning prostitution may well be an undermining of people's respect for the law. It all boils down to a cost-benefit analysis. Even if the state can pay out the money, what will be the social cost? There is also a strong element of practicality involved. Is it worth expanding huge sums to try to eradicate something as deeply rooted as prostitution?

THE REALITY OF 'SWEEPING AWAY PROSTITUTION': GOVERNMENT POLICY

There is a kind of quasi-police in China. Its staff is not composed of officially hired government employees and its members cannot arrest citizens. Nevertheless, in most places, it is their task to apprehend female sex workers.

In Town A
As neither on-the-spot escort nor massage is forbidden, the police are not obliged to arrest the girls involved. However the quasi-policemen do know which girls are on the game and go to their homes to arrest them deliberately. Another method the quasi-police use to arrest the female sex workers is to intercept those who look like prostitutes in the streets between 4 a.m. and 7 a.m. on the pretext of checking their identification cards and temporary residence permits. These hours happen to be when those all-night sex girls go off work and are heading home. It is impossible for them not to walk through the streets or not to take their ID cards with them while selling sex. Usually, after being fined $365 (equivalent to three months' wages for a professor in Beijing), female sex workers are released. As the girls do not have such sums on them, they are allowed to call someone or give a message to someone asking them to bring the money. Most of the quasi-police members in Town A were peasants from nearby villages. Their usual income is no more than around $240 monthly (upper-middle level income locally). This quasi-police team has dug itself a nice little niche. They have a

protected status. No one will investigate the fines they collect from female sex workers. They are respected in the local community, of which they represent the collective interest, but most of the people they deal with are outsiders. They form a well-organized team recognized by the community and this provides social solidarity. The community is now pretty immune to official corruption, so they are not open to either threats or seduction by the prostitutes or the brothel-keepers. In its own general interest the local community is willing to sacrifice the interests of individuals members. It also likes to keep up a pretence so the red light district can continue to flourish, but prostitution is putatively banned, with what resembles a private army or vice squad whose intention is eradication to prove it.

The local officials have played the social role of a buffer, mediator, and arbitrator between the government and the interest groups of the lower sex industry so well they have become rich on the proceeds. Many of them have become Hong Kong residents and come back only to engage in the sex industry. As a result, they have had to cede political power and resources and have to compete with those owners who stick to the old style sex industry. Their innovations have already been foiled. It is an interesting illustration of the fact that those who promote the development of the Chinese sex industry are neither the government at the higher level nor the businesspeople at the lowest level, but the so-called 'parental officials' in the middle. If the sex industry in a place has matured, only these parent officials have the power to determine its fate.

In Town B

The public security officers from the city and from the county were in heavy competition in the arrest of gamblers. After that, matters reached a stalemate. There was no police to carry out any duties. Then, in the summer of 1998, provincial leaders ordered armed police in and this later effectively eradicated the sex industry.

In Town C

One policeman was in the pay of one of the dance- and singing-halls. He was simultaneously the personal bodyguard of the owner and also of the customers and the female sex workers. He threatened hooligans but also warded off the competitive invasions and harassment from the owners of other premises. He ensured his premises escaped any clean-up campaign and also spread propaganda praising its safety and reliability in the hope of luring more customers. His pay depended on two things: he was the ticket collector and second, he slept there as a guard. Is it the sort of town where 'officials prostitutes themselves when they take down their trousers and clean up prostitution when they have their trousers on ?'

ATROPHY OF THE OFFICIAL IDEOLOGY ON PROSTITUTION

Since the beginning of the 1980s, government policy, issued regularly every three years has been beating a gradual retreat on prostitution. At the very beginning, it objected to bizarre dress, thick make-up and sunglasses, but three years later these had become popular. The next target was disco and rock-and-roll and the same pattern repeated itself. The prohibition on heterosexual massage was formally launched at the end of 1988 but by 1992 it had become popular in the South. Objections to escort service were preached by a central newspaper in 1994. By 1997, many places had begun to levy taxes on escort services.

I once interviewed an official from Town A, a college graduate, born and raised in that place. His analysis concluded that among the five major reasons for the formation of the local red light district a major one was that foreign investment had brought in many foreigners and people from Hong Kong and Taiwan. Besides this it was easy for the local men to earn money, the local girls were young and beautiful, and the men were willing to spend money on them. The high income to be made from prostitution attracted more and more girls from other places to engage in the sex industry. The fact they were strangers, far away from their home towns, helped alleviate any inhibitions they may have had. The local government connived at and supported this development in various ways. He thought that this set of circumstances, which could be applied to most of China since the 1980s, explained the lack of success of the campaign for the eradication of prostitution. The government is in a dilemma. It is confronted with a widespread essential tolerance towards prostitution in Chinese society. Official dogma does not dare to associate prostitution with foreign investment because the latter is the engine for the open policy, the gateway to new found prosperity. Where the shoe pinches is the fact that any admission of the existence of prostitution is an acknowledgement that the long-term education of the Party has accomplished nothing. Official discourse is bound to object to the idea that girls are driven to take up sex work because they are just the tip of the iceberg of unemployment. Many more people are driven by poverty to do whatever they can to fill their stomachs. Any glimmer of acknowledgement that prostitution is lurking in the background is no more than an admission that some corrupt members of the government succumb to this vice. But this argument does not even sound plausible to some ears.

ANOTHER KIND OF PROSTITUTION IN CHINA: EXCHANGING SEX SERVICES FOR POLITICAL POWER AND VICE VERSA

Visiting prostitutes and paying with public money is very common. Lower-ranking officials entertain their superiors with escort and/or sexual services. Corrupt officials take bribes, and buy escort services, indulge in prostitution, and take a second wife. One newspaper reported that an official had spent 500,000 Chinese dollars (about $61,000) on a female sex worker. Capitalizing on their official powers, they offer various perks to the women (almost never cash) in exchange for their sexual services. The real value in such a sexual exchange is usually much higher and more useful than the money income earned directly from sex work. This sort of buying and selling of sex is confined to the upper classes. This is why prostitution is not proscribed by law. A central tenet of Marxism was that all laws serve the interests of the ruling class. Why should a prostitution prohibition law be any exception?

There are plenty of discussions about whether prostitution should be banned, and how this might be achieved, but the subject of what kinds of people become prostitutes is left unspoken. The upper echelons of society foster illusions that only the women of the lower classes who serve the poorer men are prostitutes. The VIP club girls, sexual private secretaries, extra-marital girl lovers, and second wives are not sex workers. They are transmuted to the realm of participants in romantic affairs and the frisson of sexual scandals.

This testifies to an unequivocal double standard. Generally, ordinary people require only equality before the law and expect punishment, even severe penalties for the upper class men who really look for wild prostitutes. So far, such hopes have been baseless as VIP activities involving the purchase of sexual favours are not counted as prostitution. The upshot is that no crime has been committed, so no punishment can be enforced. Therefore, almost no man with power who indulges in extra-marital sexual activities even though frequently and frivolously, has ever been dealt with in the same way as a lowly client of a prostitute. The heaviest reprimand is disciplinary action within the Party or an administrative disciplinary measure for having committed a 'style problem,' or perpetrated a 'living issue' or 'man and woman relation issue.' Only those male cadres who are foolish enough to go out into the real world to look for real secret prostitutes may run the risk of being treated as a prostitute client. Certainly, there will always be some brave persons who will stand up to denounce and punish those VIP sex buyers. But, as long as the law banning prostitution stands and remains unchanged, these brave persons may be suspected of 'committing crime,' and those VIPs may turn their tables on them.

It may well be those brave enough to adopt a stance are not doing so out of compassion for the underdog, but to try to undermine the VIPs. Therefore, we should quote the attitude held by the Chinese government in 1963 with the 'Treaty of Partly Prohibiting Nuclear Experiment': 'Prostitution prohibition? Good! But – all or none!'

CHAPTER 3

JAPANESE SEX WORKERS: BETWEEN CHOICE AND COERCION

WIM LUNSING

As I have described in an earlier paper, one may look at love and sex as commodities that can be exchanged for others, such as money, food, security or goods, regardless of whether it takes place in a marriage, a love affair or in the context of prostitution (Lunsing 2000). This view goes hand in hand with a very practical outlook on life, in which power and money are the central ruling principles. Recent developments in Japan suggest that the economic aspects of sex have become more explicit than they may have been for some time, which may be closely related to a change in discourse. While prostitution has not featured prominently in the media for a long time, nowadays it has come to the forefront. This media attention does not go so far as to prove that there is an actual increase of sex being traded for money. My fieldwork findings, however, suggest that, indeed, there is.

In any investigation of sex work, the question of whether people engage in it of their own choice or because of coercion is asked more than in the case of most other occupations. A major reason for this is that sex work is widely regarded as demeaning and humiliating. In this sense Japan is no different from most countries. As Jo Doezema suggested, this question may be divisive, as it glorifies the victims of forced prostitution and damns those who engage in prostitution by choice. As a result, international organizations like the UN have focused entirely on forced prostitution, while neglecting any problems of those who chose the occupation whom they may encounter (Doezema 1996). This is not an open and shut case as I believe that choice of occupation is often limited and that therefore some measure of coercion is usually present, as is some measure of choice. After all, the vast majority of people are forced to make choices about what to do with their lives. If given the option, many would choose to be millionaires but few are. For most the choice simply is not there. Therefore, I believe that the question of whether people do what they do by choice or coercion provides an excellent angle from which to highlight differences among the various types of sex workers.

In this paper, I first provide a historical background to which my investigation of the actual situation of various sex workers in relation to their freedom to choose their occupation can be related. On the basis of interviews and written sources, I discuss the present situation of sex workers in Japan, concentrating first on legal regulations, in particular where minors are concerned, and then investigating various types of sex work. It appears that in many cases people make a positive choice of their occupation as a sex worker, in which finance, time, and the pleasure of being able to engage often in sexual activity are the major pulls. At the same time, many people feel trapped into sex work. In particular in the case of foreign sex workers, there is also a proportion of them who live in virtual slavery, made to work in order to pay of debts to the *yakuza* who helped them travel to Japan.

SEX WORK IN HISTORY

William LaFleur discerns two types of sexual activity in Tokugawa Japan (1603–1868), one for procreation and one for pleasure. Sex for procreation took place inside the household and as such was beyond the scrutiny of the Japanese government. Obviously, this concerned only heterosexual activity. Sex for pleasure took place mostly outside the household. Typically, sex for pleasure was seen as a 'natural need' of men. People (in practice mostly men who were not poor, although there are also cases of women enlisting the services of male prostitutes) could obtain sexual gratification by paying for it. This traffic was open to the scrutiny of the shogunate that made repeated efforts to limit it to particular quarters of the city and to make it less publicly visible, in particular in cases where it might lead to social unrest. At the same time, this recreational sexual activity may have been permitted because it functioned as a safety valve to help people cope with the rigidity characterizing the overall social structure (LaFleur 1991).

Sex for pleasure or *iro* (colour; Fushimi 2000:77–92, Saeki 1996) was available in two ways, sex with women (*joshoku/nyoshoku*) and sex with men (*danshoku/nanshoku, shoku* being the Sino-Japanese reading of *iro*), terms that show that sex was seen as something to be enjoyed by men only. Gary Leupp carried out comprehensive work on sex with men in the period, coming to the far-reaching conclusion that during the Edo period bisexuality was 'the norm' in urban Japan (Leupp 1995). Members of the Japanese gay activist group Occur, however, criticize such a position for presenting a much too optimistic view of the position of homosexuality in Japanese culture. While I have had my own disagreements with Occur (Lunsing 1997, 1998, 1999, 2001a, 2001b), in this case I agree with it, as the quarters of sex central to Leupp's discussion are obviously limited to some parts of urban Japan only and usually characterized by prostitution, as Gregory Pflugfelder (1999) makes clear. If the numbers of male and female prostitutes and the numbers of brothels where male and female services were provided were to be counted, I have no doubt that one would find that the quantity of straight sex far outweighed that of gay sex. Apart from this, outside such quarters heterosexuality ruled.

More importantly, Leupp had little eye for those who were penetrated and had, according to discourse, to be convinced either by romantic love, by financial means, or power in equality to allow their partners to have their way. Anal penetration was seen as painful and therefore it was not conceivable that people could engage in it for their own physical pleasure (Leupp 1995:41–3, 55–6, 268–9). Although Leupp noted the fact that most of the sex he discussed actually concerned prostitution, he barely paid attention to negative aspects such as young men possibly being forced to sell themselves, like girls were sold into prostitution by poor parents (Harada 1997:129–130). It seems that Leupp, indeed, has been idealizing the historical situation in Japan.

The Tokugawa period ended in 1868 with the American naval officer Commodore Perry figuratively shooting open the walls Japan had erected against the intrusion of the outside world. The US forced Japan to enter into diplomatic relations with foreign countries other than those with which it had been dealing during the period of national isolation, i.e. the Netherlands, China, Korea, and the Kingdom of the Ryukyu Archipelago. Initially, the treaties with the foreign countries were not on a parity. Japan was forced to give foreign countries access to its markets but gained little in return. In this period, Japan developed extremely fast under a strong leadership of oligarchs, stimulated to reach Western industrial standards and to be taken seriously as an equal in partner negotiations (Reischauer and Craig 1989).

In order to reach this goal, the government felt a need to counter various practices that the Victorian Western eyes viewed as indecent. In his concluding chapter, Leupp (1995) also writes about the importance of discourses in which homosexual activity was seen as criminal and of people calling for its criminalization. Mistakenly, Leupp writes that this never happened. Japan did experience a period in which homosexual activity, in particular anal intercourse, was criminalized in 1873. This resulted partly from the influence of Western discourses concerning decent behaviour but the law itself was modelled after the sodomy law of Qing dynasty China (Pflugfelder 1999:159–62). The law was little applied and scrapped in 1882 under the influence of the French lawmaker Gustave de Boissonade who was hired to supervise the compilation of a new code of laws, the Keihō (Pflugfelder 1999:170–2, Furukawa 1994), underlining again that Western influence had its limits in reshaping reality. It appears that the Japanese authorities chose those what suited them best from the various Western discourses available.

During this period, writings on homosexual activity changed qualitatively from matter-of-fact like description, romantic treatises, and humorous stories to depictions of rape and abuse, for instance among students in dormitories (Furukawa 1992). During the same period medical discoures began to develop, largely along lines similar to those in Europe of the period (Pflugfelder 1999). To what extent this reflected an actual change in activity taking place is, however, not entirely clear.

Similarly, prostitution came to be dealt with in terms of a social problem, though it was left relatively untouched by the authorities. Here too, the discourse changed but actual practice seemed to have remained largely intact. While the gates around the pleasure districts such as Yoshiwara in Tokyo were opened up and the scrutiny of the authorities lessened, the districts remained intact. As Sabine Frühstück (1997) wrote, discourse on sexuality was greatly influenced by translations of Western, she claims mostly German, work. Publications on sexology had a relatively large readership, to such an extent that she speaks of the popularization of sexological knowledge.

Reliable material on changes in actual sexual behaviour is rare. The important book by Robert Smith and Ella Lury Wiswell on the women of Suemura, a poor village on Kyushu, the southernmost of the four main islands of Japan, in the 1930s has a chapter on sexual practice. Sex was engaged in both within and outside of marriage and in those cases where the women were not married to the men with whom they had sex, with they could expect to become the subject of lively gossip. Bastards abounded as did visits to the *geisha* in the local town by the men. These visits were not characterized by the high-class entertainment *geisha* are often supposed to offer.[1] The *geisha* in this case hardly differed from regular prostitutes (Smith and Wiswell 1982). It appears that the popularization of sexological knowledge had its limitations. The only reference I found which explicitly referred to change was that a daughter of a couple living in Suemura sent a package of condoms with the admonition that her parents use them, as they already had so many children (Smith and Wiswell 1982:89, also quoted in Frühstück 1997:167). Indeed, birth control spread throughout Japan (Frühstück 1997:158–70)

More information about change during the years from the Tokugawa period is contained in a book by the Japanese anthropologist Morikuri Shigekazu (1995), concentrating on *karayuki-san*. He conducted fieldwork during the 1980s and 1990s on Amakusa, an island off southern Kyushu, again a remote and relatively poor region. Though *karayuki-san* are typically cast as Japanese women who went first to China, to which *kara* refers,[2] and later also to other parts of Asia to work as prostitutes, Morikuri ineluctably demonstrates that the first of them, originating from Amakusa, went to trade other goods. However, later *karayuki-san* did go abroad to work as prostitutes and were often forced to do so by parents selling them to brokers, like girls had been and were still sold to the pleasure districts.

The main thesis of Morikuri's book deals with a change in sexual practice away from the practice of *yobai*. *Yobai* was the practice of young men sneaking off at night into the house of a woman he fancied in order to have sex with her, with much local variety in how it was actually carried out. It can be regarded as a form of dating, in which marriage could be postponed until pregnancy when the fertility of the couple had been proven. This system gradually lost ground as the ideal of the bride being a virgin gained ground, an ideal that could have stemmed from high class Japanese values as well as from Western influence. According to Morikuri, straightforward prostitution replaced the sexual outlet for the men who, as in the Tokugawa period, were still expected to have a 'natural' need for sex and a *karayuki-san* could engage in sex work in Japan after she had returned home.

During the Second World War, the Japanese government did not appear to have changed its attitudes towards sexual activity much. For men, sexual intercourse was still regarded as a natural need and a system was set up to provide for this need: the system of *jūgun ianfu*, comfort women in the army. This system was set up in the first place to keep the troops in good health. The comfort women's health was monitored. Another goal of this system was to prevent the military from raping/engaging in sex with civilian women with all the problems that could entail. Most comfort women were not Japanese. Foreign women, in particular Korean former comfort women, have been vocal in demanding compensation for what they see as sexual slavery from the Japanese government (Ueno 1998:99–144).

After the war, Japan was destitute. In the period right after the war, prostitution abounded, in particular around the American bases. This embraced both straight and gay prostitution.[3] In Japan, like in many European countries, the post-war years were characterized by a major effort to redevelop. During the 1950s and early 1960s the rate of marriage increased to an extent never seen before or after (Lunsing 2001b). Sex outside marriage was frowned upon in the case of men as well as women. The housewives' movement was particularly vocal in demanding a prohibition on prostitution.

In 1956, a law prohibiting prostitution was adopted. Pleas by a prostitutes' union, which had formed from networks of female miners who lost their occupation after the war and moved into sex work (Shiga-Fujime 1993), could not prevent this. Officially, the law led to the closure of all the brothels, the *yūkaku*, that had survived since the Tokugawa period and the *akasen chitai*, the red light districts, in which they were located. Prostitution was seen officially as a social evil. Although the law stipulates that sex workers must be resocialized and that they not their clients are committing a crime, in practice sex workers are most at risk of being arrested and detained, albeit for short periods only. Eventual pimps and other managers can expect prison sentences, while patrons are generally not prosecuted.

With the *yūkaku* officially closed, and most of them did actually close, prostitution diversified in manifold ways. Infamous for upsetting the Turkish government is the *toruko*, borrowed from Turkish baths. Diplomatically, they have been renamed *sōpurando* (soapland), but the activities engaged in remain essentially the same, bathing and vaginal intercourse. Other establishments range from the *pinku saron* (pink salon), where fellatio while seated in a dark corner is the most common activity, to call-girls working from private apartments. At the same time, some of the less conspicuous *yūkaku* did remain operational. The prohibition on prostitution remains largely superficial. As long as no problems arise and no official complaints are made, the police are unlikely to intervene (Lunsing 2000).

MINORS, SEX WORK, AND THE LAW

One of the cases in which problems are more likely to occur than in others is that of minors engaging in sex work. Japanese law does not recognize an age of consent as such. Article 176 of the Penal Code (Keihō), however, does provide for something similar by implication. Rather than making a positive statement about the age at which people are free to engage in sexual activity, it states that it is illegal to force sexual activity upon people of any age or to engage in sexual activity with persons below the age of thirteen. Sexual activity is represented by the term *waisetsu no kōi*, which translates literally as 'indecent behaviour' (Koh 1988) but here is generally understood to refer more specifically to sexual activity. The penalty for transgression is forced labour for at least six months and at most seven years. In Article 177 only females under the age of thirteen are mentioned as people with whom it is forbidden to have sexual intercourse. Here the text uses the term *kanin shitaru* (Nakadono 1993:142), which translates as 'to misconduct oneself' or 'to commit fornication' (Koh 1988), which, although it is not further defined legally, is also generally understood to refer to sexual activity (Nakadono 1993:142). The fact that only women are mentioned here reflects the incomprehensibility of men or boys becoming the object of sexual attention to the lawmakers of the period just after the Second World War.[4]

Apart from this, the Child Welfare Law (Jidō Fukushi Hō) forbids the use of people under eighteen in for either pornography or nude photography, but does not say anything about the possession and distribution of pornography or nude photography in which children appear (Tsunoda 1992:223–33). Furthermore, it forbids making people under the age of eighteen engaging in sexual activity, represented by the term *kanin kōi* (acts of fornication). This is directed at preventing children from being made to work in prostitution and the like. It does not, however, prohibit people below the age of eighteen from engaging in sex if someone older has not forced them to do so (Nakadono 1993:143).

As prostitution itself was outlawed in 1956, one may wonder why special rulings were deemed necessary to forbid child prostitution. The position of law in Japan is dissimilar to that in some Western countries. Rather than offering strict guidelines to be adhered to, it appears that Japanese laws are used as guidelines to fall back on in the event of trouble occurring. Since trouble is more likely to occur in the case of younger sex workers, whose parents are more likely to interfere than those of older ones, apart from including a prohibition of the use of young people in pornography, the Child Welfare Law may be seen as stressing the fact that the prostitution of young people is under closer scrutiny than that of people over the age of eighteen. Otherwise, prostitution is generally tolerated as long as it does not become too visible to people who might take offence (Lunsing 2000).

Prefectures and municipalities throughout Japan do not seem to have considered these laws enough protection for young people and therefore passed a number of local regulations, called *jōrei*, to offer additional protection, in particular directed towards sexual activity with people under the age of eighteen. These rulings are part of what is generally known as Seishōnen Hogo Ikusei Jōrei (Regulations for the Protection and Education of Young People), or in short Seishōnen Jōrei (Youth Regulations; Nakadono 1993:143), of which those concerning sexual activity are known as Inkō Jōrei (Obscene Acts Regulations; Nakadono 1993:143). An interpretation of the terminology of these regulations, which vary from place to place, could be that they forbid the seduction, the overwhelming by force or by words, or the deception of children and such, i.e. the abuse of people under the age of eighteen for one's own pleasure rather than engaging in mutually consensual sexual activity with them (Nakadono 1993:144–5). In other words they are not much different from the Child Protection Law. These *jōrei* have gradually been adopted nationwide, with the exception of Nagano Prefecture, although its capital, the city of Nagano, has a municipal *jōrei* (Tsunoda 1992:229). As just mentioned, the actual contents of the *jōrei* vary to a great extent from place to place with penalties as tiny as a fine of a maximum of 30,000 Yen to imprisonment for up to two years (Nakadono 1993:145).

Parents may find out about their children engaging in sex work and go to the police, which can ultimately lead to places where prostitution is engaged in and organizations that manage prostitution being closed down. The managers are arrested and are given prison sentences, although this does not appear to happen very frequently. To prevent this, such organizations may ask their sex workers to show proof that they are at least eighteen years old, an age after which the influence of parents in these matters is thought to be less strong. One reason for this, apart from the Child Welfare Law and the *jōrei*, may be that people from the age of eighteen are more likely not to live at home with their parents. In the case of male prostitution, the proof of age that is usually asked is a *gakusei shōmeishō*, a student card, the possession of which may imply that the owner is living in a city other than that of his parents and thus has more privacy in his use of his own time. Another option is a driver's licence (*unten menkyoshō*), which can only be obtained by people eighteen years old and upwards.

Pertinently, a *gakusei shōmeishō* is easy to forge and instances in which gay prostitution houses run into trouble because the parents of one of their workers has put the police on their trail occur every now and then. When found out, the usual procedure is that the whole place is closed down (Lunsing 2000). Similarly, a girls' prostitution ring, which functioned under the guise of a type of escort service, called *konpanion* (companion), and was supposed to be a service consisting of pouring drinks and offering conversation, often carried out by young students or high school girls, was shut in Osaka. This was because it was discovered that most of the girls were minors and had been engaged for sexual activities rather than pouring drinks (Sano 1995:65–6). While it is even illegal to engage minors in the *fūzoku sangyō* (the entertainment industry), which includes work as a *konpanion*, it appears that when sexual services are involved, the police is more likely to act of its own accord instead of waiting for complaints from parents and the like.[5]

In recent years, one of the most prominent ploys has been *enjo kōsai*, which literally translates into 'support relations.' The 'relations' here does not necessarily refer to sexual relations but to social relations. Typically, it consists of a girl or young woman associating with an older man in exchange for money. The woman is supposed to accompany the man to have dinner or to some other form of social activity. This is somehow similar to the idea of the *konpanion*, which consisted mostly of female university students serving groups of men in after meetings. In both cases, however, the men had the option of trying to engage the women in sexual activities. In the case of *enjo kōsai* in particular, sexual activities have increasingly been expected to be part of the deal, by both the women and the men in question. While the *konpanion* usually worked through agencies, in the case of *enjo kōsai* the girls may either work through an agency or set up for themselves, in which case telephone clubs, through which people can find each other anonymously, play an important role (Miyadai 1997:40–6).

There are also advertisements placed in gay magazines by young men searching patrons for *enjo kōsai*. In this case, it appears that a form of financial patronage is expected for social services including sex. It distinguishes itself from straightforward prostitution by the desire for a continuation of the arrangement over longer periods, similar to the relationship between a mistress and her patron. An important characteristic of *enjo kōsai* in both the straight and the gay context is that it often involves young people, including teenagers as young as fourteen years old. Indeed, the younger they are, the higher the prices they can demand. It is apparent that this fact, at least partially, accounts for the media hype, in which it is often stressed that the young women concerned are often daughters of 'good' families.

My friend Momocca Momocco,[6] a sex worker who spoke as such at the Yokohama World Aids Conference in 1994, said that she initially felt that minors should not be allowed to do this sort of work, but after some major reconsideration, she thought that this was a rather patronizing, or perhaps matronizing, attitude. Having consciously chosen sex work as an occupation because it meant that she could often have sex, which she desires, plus earning a good income in a short time so that she had more time for other activities, she realized that her young colleagues had equally cogent reasons for choosing to work in prostitution and that their age did not really matter much in this context. As long as they chose it freely, she failed to see much of a difference between them and herself.

Sex work exists in an infinite variety in present-day Japan, from very casual contexts to rigidly arranged ones, whereby the latter are often managed by the Japanese mafia, the *yakuza*. In more casual contexts, however, it may hardly be organized at all. A young lesbian friend, for instance, wore a *sērāfuku*, a sailor suit, which in Japan is a common uniform for school girls, in front of men who paid her to do so. Her clients were recruited by them soliciting her on the streets, without her having to approach them in any way. The most sexual part of her performance was to lift up the skirts of her *sērāfuku* so that the men could have a peek at her panty hose and for an extra sum she would sell them the pantyhose she had worn. While my friend thought it to be sad that she had acquired no skills, meaning this to be one of the few ways open to her to earn a living, she was adamant that her patrons were real gentlemen and that she did not run the risk of them even so much as touching her.

The sale of used panty hoses, supposedly at least, by school girls has become a rage in Japan, with shops specializing in buying them from the girls[7] and selling them to male customers (Lunsing 2000:53). A scholar who specializes in this form of fetishism acknowledged that he himself was also attracted to panty hoses and even stole them from clotheslines every now and then. Cogently, when homosexuality was discussed at a meeting of a study group of sex and sexuality, he wondered why it was not placed in the framework of mental illness, while he thought that panty hose fetishism was merely an exciting and innocent hobby. This confirms the limited dispersion of political correctness in Japan, while at the same time it betrays a lax attitude towards what is seen as sexual play.

Another young informant asked two of her older female friends, both of them graduates from art universities who engaged in sado-masochistic lesbian performances, which they regarded as a form of artistic expression, for the telephone number of a nude photographer. She was under the age of eighteen and the friends made a show of being hesitant about giving her the number, wondering whether she knew what she was getting herself into and such. She was adamant that after having modelled for pictures in clothes, she now thought it to be interesting to see how she would cope with nude modelling. Eventually her friends gave her the number, having run out of arguments about why she should not do it, other than her age, which they felt they could not really use without being maternalistic.

This easy-going attitude towards sex and sex work is not necessarily new to Japan, although it may have been pushed aside during the years of rebuilding and high economic growth after the Second World War, only to resurface recently. Japanese Buddhism was quite positive about sexual activity for its own sake rather than for reproduction and there even was a sect, the Tachikawa sect, which saw the pursuit of sexual satisfaction as a method to reach Enlightenment (LaFleur 1991). In Japan today, sex is often not regarded as being of much consequence. Apart from sex as a means for reproduction, which has become very limited, given the low number of children that are born nowadays (Jolivet 1997), sex is widely seen as recreative, as a form of play, in Japanese *asobi*, in which people may choose to engage if they wish to, without being greatly concerned about moral aspects relating to it (Lunsing 2000, 2001a, 2001b). And if sex is not bad for adults, then why should it be so for younger people?

While recognizing that young people nowadays are sexually much more developed than some time ago, the psychologist Sano Akira feels uneasy with the readiness and ease with which some teenagers engage in sex work. Although he does not want to say that they must not have sex except for love, he wants them to be more serious about it than what he perceives as an attitude towards sex that makes it not much different from doing 'radio gymnastic exercises.' Unfortunately, he fails to elaborate upon the question of why it should be more than that. It seems to have something to do with the way he regards his own daughters. He betrays how upset he felt upon finding that a case of teenage prostitution, involving a junior high school student who was asked to have sex by a journalist, was problematized not because of the prostitution itself but because the customer failed to pay up the promised amount of money (Sano 1995:53–4). This may be similar to the reaction of the father of a friend of mine upon discovering that she was a sex worker. While he was not opposed to prostitution as such, he dreaded the idea of his daughter being treated in the manner he had treated prostitutes. Indeed, this appears to be patronizing.

ADULT SEX WORKERS AND EFFORTS AT ORGANIZATION

During my last fieldwork periods in the winters of 1996 and 1998–9, I was confronted with the fact that increasing numbers of my informants, who I had known since my long-term fieldwork period lasting from 1991 to 1993, had taken up some type of sex work or other. Sex work has become widely publicized in the aftermath of what the media have coined 'gay boom' (see Lunsing 1997). Part of this is definitely attributable to the fact that the media are forever in search of new themes to fill their pages. Nevertheless, there is an undeniable link between discourses on homosexuality and those on sex work. One of the more powerful constructions of homosexuality in Japan argues that it is characterized by prostitution. On being informed that I was investigating homosexuality, a straight male informant even warned me to take great care as many of the workers were actually not gay themselves and did not really want to prostitute themselves but rather to rob their clients.

Men and boys engaging in sex work, are relatively free to choose the hours they want to work and to quit when they choose to do so. This is stressed in some articles in the gay magazine *Bádi*. The establishments in which they work are always advertising for staff and they try to keep the staff they have by providing for them relatively well, including in many cases offering them a place to stay. Their most usual reason for engaging in sex work is money, which they may want for a specific goal. One such example is Yuki from Gunma, who wanted to go abroad to study (Henshūbu 1999a). Curiosity about the actual work can also draw them (Henshūbu 1999b). Ages can vary from the late teens to men in their forties and the types in demand vary greatly. Lately, for instance, a market for chubby male sex workers has gained ground (Henshūbu 1999c). *Bádi* staff members even investigate all the places that place advertisements to check whether they are 'decent' businesses that do not exploit their employees unduly. This may help to account for the fact that all the men found that they had little to complain about, except perhaps the occupational necessity of having to deal with men they dislike (Henshūbu 1999a, b, c). Thus, it is not surprising that the interviewers were impressed by the fact that the hosts of the establishments who co-operated in the articles were doing their jobs with pride (1999c).

However, as Momocca Momocco said, there are, indeed, many settings in which people are pressed to engage in sexual activities with clients and also in those cases where they decided to engage in prostitution. It often happens that they are pressured into engaging in sexual activities they abhor, such as the practice of *gansha*, ejaculation in the face, which has become a popular part of the menu brothels offer.[8] Another informant said that a friend of hers, who protested about having to engage in particular sexual activities she did not like, such as anal intercourse, was made to work in another brothel, which specialized in providing '*hentai* sex.' *Hentai* may be translated positively as queer (Lunsing 2001b), but in this context was used fairly negatively as inclusive of activities such as anal sex, sado-masochism, and sex involving excrement, all of which the woman concerned abhorred. She felt she could not refuse this because she thought that she was dependent on sex work for her income and that her opportunity to work depended on her co-operation with the *yakuza*, who organized her work. They threatened to make it impossible for her to work, unless she agreed to have anal sex.

A friend working at a brothel advertising as specializing in sado-masochism said that most of her customers did not have much of a clue as to what sado-masochism is. The actual specialization of her brothel consisted of anal sex rather than sado-masochist activities. Most of her clients wanted to be dominant, but she usually managed to talk them out of this by asking questions as to what sort of activity they liked. As a result, most of the time she succeeds in playing the role of the master/mistress and in effect teaches her clients about sado-masochism, which she herself had learned about in Copenhagen. Her interest in developing the experience she gained in Copenhagen led her to take up this particular type of sex work, but this was also inextricably combined with financial pulls.

It appears that the question of whether people possess the freedom to engage in prostitution in the way they wish to depends very much on their own assertiveness as well as on the particular surroundings in which they work. The less organized may generally seem to offer more freedom as to what is expected to be done. The problem is that, given the fact that prostitution in Japan remains illegal, it may be easier to engage in sex work in a setting 'protected' by the *yakuza* who are experienced in keeping the police at bay, possibly making use of bribery or blackmail. There are clearly hostess bars and other settings in which people are lured into becoming sex workers, as an example of a woman working in a *pinku saron* (pink salon), where sexual activity is usually confined to fellatio and masturbation, showed. She came in answer to an advertisement seeking hostesses and had no idea that it concerned sex work. Once she arrived, however, she decided to give it a try anyway, having travelled all the way from the countryside and being eager to remain in Tokyo. The upshot was she found herself fellating men with 'tears in her eyes' (Kakinuma 1991, Lunsing 2000).

Momocca Momocco decided to engage in sex work because she saw it as challenge and for practical reasons, like time, money, and the opportunity to have plenty of sex. She was already in her thirties when she began working in a pink salon. Gradually the power structure began to grate on her. The men that were there to protect the women against misbehaving clients and to tout for costumers were on the top of the hierarchy. On the female side, the woman who was the girlfriend of the top of the man was the top of the hierarchy among the women. She felt that she and her colleagues were being played out against each other. Eventually she found employment in a *yūkaku*, a traditional-style brothel. The work here was more demanding, as vaginal intercourse was the core of the business, but she felt that the atmosphere was much better. There was a great deal of solidarity among the women, a fact which she related to men playing much less of a role in the establishment, the management of which pivoted around an older woman.

The question of whether people engage in prostitution of their own free will or not does not seem to have much relation to their age. If there is any relation at all, it is most likely that people under eighteen years of age feel less compelled to engage in activities in which they do not wish to partake than those above, who feel they may have less of a choice, especially if they have a relationship with a pimp or if they are in debt. Furthermore, as I discussed before (Lunsing 2000), it appears that men who engage in prostitution have more power over themselves than women. Cogently, many transsexuals and transvestites engaging in prostitution feel that they have less power to refuse any activity because they believe that they can do no other work. Their perception is often that they have no choice.[9] Nevertheless, in their case, too, there are gradations. Transgendered sex workers are popularly known as *nyū hāfu* (new half). The archetype of the new half is similar to that of the Latin American *travesti* (Lunsing 2001b), in that they have acquired breasts while retaining their penis. In common parlance, post-operative male to female transsexuals are usually included.[10] A new half may work in establishments where the putting on of shows is the main attraction and sex work is not part of the contract. Nevertheless, many of them do engage in various types of sex work, including prostitution and pornography. Besides the idea that they cannot work in regular occupations, one reason for engaging in sex work is, that this way they can earn large sums in relatively a short period, which they can then use for sex change surgery (Matsuo 1997, Nekome 1998), usually carried out abroad.

Worst of all is clearly the position of a group of foreign sex workers, who are forced into virtual sexual slavery in order to pay off debts they incurred with the *yakuza* who shipped them to Japan. An informant said that as a rule their passports are taken from them after their arrival and they are not allowed to leave the brothels in which they work. In order to avoid them establishing relationships with patrons, they are often moved from one place to another throughout the country. In a case in which some of them escaped and fled to the police, they were rounded up and returned to the brothel. They enter the country either on a tourist or an entertainment visa and they often remain in Japan illegally after their visas expire.

People engaging in sex work often derive pride from being good at satisfying their customers. This pride can be related to the service industry at large, where such features have, for instance, been described for the case of hostesses whose main task is to pour drinks and make pleasant conversation with customers. Although the latter may not be pleasant at all, it not being unusual for them to harass the hostesses sexually with remarks about their breasts as well as with touching them in intimate places.[11] This makes the whole concept of *sekuhara bā* (sexual harassment bar), a novel type of bar introduced after sexual harassment became a hot topic in the Japanese media, not as novel as it may seem. In the case of *sekuhara bā* it is made explicit that one of the features on offer is the possibility to harass the hostesses sexually, mainly finding expression in touching and pinching them, but in reality such features were part and parcel of many, if not most, hostess bars all along. Even the common practice of expecting female employees to make and pour tea for their male colleagues in most work settings, has been called the beginning of sexual harassment, for it clearly indicates that women are not treated as people but as women and more explicit forms of sexual harassment can be seen but as a consequence of this view (Keiko 1991). Placed in such a context, one may, indeed, wonder why sex work is so often singled out as problematic.

When I attended meetings of the sex worker network *SWEETLY*, short for 'Sex workers! Encourage, Empower, Trust and Love Yourselves!' (Momocca 1998), there were non-sex workers present, including MTF transsexuals and lesbian women. Their major concern was the freedom of sex workers to determine whether their pictures are used in advertisements and such, their freedom to determine in what types of sexual activity they wish to engage, and protection in the case of violent patrons. Sex workers often feel unsafe to the extent that they avoid travelling by train at night and, even when making use of taxis do not let themselves be taken to their actual addresses but are usually dropped off a little distance from there so that they can walk home without the taxi driver learning where they live.

Furthermore, such a network provides proper knowledge concerning STDs, in particular HIV. It was discovered that the majority of sex workers maintain no sensible policy concerning safer sex. Speaking about her colleagues, Momocca Momocco said that they still nurtured the illusionary idea that, since they refused 'dirty' customers, they had nothing to fear. On the other hand, Momocca herself invited a man who called to ask whether he could come, even though he was HIV-positive. She said that she takes pride in not refusing any client. Akira the Hustler, who had a column in the gay magazine *G-men*, decided to engage in sex work for reasons similar to Momocca. He began as a call-boy through an organization in Kyoto but later he decided to move town and set up business for himself in Tokyo, advertising in gay magazines. He always insists on using a condom with anal penetration but, even in his case, it has happened that a man with a small penis ejaculated inside him even before he noticed that he was being penetrated. On another occasion, when a client stealthily took off the condom before ejaculating inside him, Akira told him that a friend of his died a year ago of AIDS, which was actually true, though this friend was not his lover. The face of the client froze and Akira hoped that he may have prevented him from doing the same with other sex workers (Akira 1998a). A telephone councilor who informs people about HIV said that there had been a recent increase of gay sex workers who called because they were worried about unprotected anal intercourse. It seems that consciousness may be on the rise.

The successful monthly sex education club nights in clubs, such as *Club Love+* (*Kurabu rabu purasu*), in Kyoto and Tokyo, have paid attention both to sex work and to homosexuality. The audience attracted was highly mixed. Discourses relating to sexual activity in both the context of gay activists and of sex workers were strongly characterized by the idea of sex for pleasure. Sexual activity was primarily engaged in for the pursuit of lust. Sexual techniques were, hence, an important topic of discussion. Procreation was an issue hardly discussed at all and, when I began asking questions about what love has to do with it, this seemed to be a largely unexplored topic. Akira just replied that he loved his clients, though he also maintains that he does not sell his love (Akira 1998b). The people present depicted sexual activity solely as good and pleasurable, if only the right knowledge was applied. In the case of sex workers, there is of course a great deal to be said about problems encountered with pimps and with johns. Pertinently, these problems were typically seen as a deplorable result of society having turned its back on sex workers rather than being inherent occupational hazards.

Recently, the free-lance reporter specialized in sex work, Matsuzawa Kureichi, has been instrumental in bringing the opinions of sex workers to the fore by publishing several books in which sex workers write about their occupations in an effort to engage a debate on sex work. In the first one, they question the writings of a number of scholars and journalists who generally condemn sex work (Matuszawa 200a) and the second is more descriptive with regard to actual work situations (2000b). The number of people concerned here is limited. They form an elite. Nevertheless, they have many links to the rest of society and are possibly quite influential in shaping talk about sexual activity, since not many other people venture into dealing with such topics when taking themselves seriously. Thus, they are clearly linked to the progressive writing on a whole plethora of sexuality activities. This discourse is very highly developed. People like Miyadai Shinji (1994), defending the choice of women engaging in *enjo kōsai*, can also be seen as part of this discourse.

CONCLUSION

It appears that male sex workers tend to have an edge over their female counterparts in embracing these freedoms, which can probably be attributed to the fact that their brothels and escort clubs are constantly in need of personnel. MTF trans-gendered sex workers tend to feel trapped in their occupation more than their female counterparts. While lately in Japan much media attention has been devoted to minor/teenage sex workers, it appears that their position is actually better than that of their older colleagues, because of a combination of by-laws and the fact that they tend to engage in it more for their pleasure than out of financial necessity.

It is apparent that there are many matters amiss in sex work in Japan and that many people are made to do things in which they would rather not participate. However, this is the case in most occupations, including for instance, that of the housewife. I do not believe that coercion and lack of choice is any more of a problem here than it is in many other occupations. If people do not like what they are asked or told to do, they can take the liberty to refuse, even if that could mean an end to their occupation. There are, after all, other occupations. It appears that personal characteristics are of major importance in this context, as is the case in most occupations.

Rather than condemning sex work and criminalizing it, sex workers would be helped by legalization and public support to help them arrange their affairs free of the influence of the *yakuza*. This could help their self-organization grow and gain influence, which would be beneficial not only to their own work situation but would also limit the spread of STDs, something from which the entire population eventually benefits.

A major change I wish to note is that the youngest generation of Japanese women appear to have taken their fate in their own hands. Undoubtedly, in the Tokugawa period and later young women were sold into brothels to lead a life of virtual slavery, nowadays young women choose to engage in sex for money of their own accord. Even the prohibition on prostitution can be circumvented by not working in the traditional context under the protection of the *yakuza* but by arranging one's own appointments. In addition, it appears that age has become less restricted, with men as well as women working in the sex industry well above the age of forty. Notwithstanding beliefs to the contrary, the increase in sex work can hardly be attributed to foreign influence. It seems instead to have its roots in a Japanese tradition of sexual permissiveness, in which sex was not seen as danger but as something to enjoy.

Acknowledgements

I am indebted to the support of Ueno Chizuko and my many informants among whom in particular I wish to thank my dear friends BuBu, Momocca Momocco, and Akira the Hustler. Frans Verwayen has been most helpful in guiding me through some of the legal issues. The Japan Society for the Promotion of Science provided a research fellowship to support fieldwork concerning sexual activity.

NOTES

1   See Dalby (1998) on the more high-brow type of *geisha*.
2   *Kara* is written with the character *tang* of the Tang dynasty.
3   Notwithstanding my finding of an abundance of male prostitutes selling their services to the American military, Watanabe Tsuneo wrote that only years later did homosexuality re-emerge in a different shape from that assumed during the Tokugawa period, in which case he characterized it as love of young men by older men (Watanabe and Iwata 1987). In agreement with this, Benedict found that among Japanese in American camps during the war, people there found homosexuality in that form understandable, but thought that homosexual attraction between men of the same age was quite incomprehensible (Benedict 1977). However, it seems to me that this change is not as pronounced when actual activity is concerned as it may be in discourse.

4 The lawyer Tsunoda Yukiko said at a meeting in Tokyo in December 1993 that the fact that marriage law stated that marriage was a contract between a man and a woman merely reflected the ignorance of the lawmakers when it came to homosexuality and that this did not necessarily signify that the law prohibits same sex marriages (Lunsing 2001b).

5 The managers of an organization that let high school girls work as *konpanion* in resort hotels in Arima Onsen, a famous hot spring resort north of Kobe, were arrested for violating the Jidō Fukushi Hō (Children's Welfare Law), which prohibits letting minors (namely those under eighteen) work in the entertainment industry. The resort hotels claimed that they were unaware of the age of their staff and could therefore not be penalized. Asahi Shinbun (1990), reprinted in *Faito Bakku*, 2, Summer 1990.

6 Any Japanese would understand instantly that this name is not her real name, for its meaning is Peach-River Little-Peach, and peach is a word with strong connotations of sex work.

7 While I realize that it is generally believed to be politically incorrect to use the term girls instead of young women, I decided to use it here anyway, because it is the term that is used in Japan in the field. People speak of *onna no ko* (girl), *otoko no ko* (boy) or *ko* (child or girl or boy). While political correctness is not unknown in Japan, knowledge of it is much more limited than in Western contexts and people often have little understanding as to why it should matter which wording one uses.

8 Since vaginal or anal intercourse or fellatio cannot be shown close-up or even from some distance in pornography, other ways of representing actually sexual activity have had to be sought and found in, for instance, the practice of *gansha*. What is shown is a man's sperm squirting over the face of a woman or, in gay pornography, of a man or a boy. It may not actually be sperm but something that looks similar. Here it is obvious that pornography exerts its influence on sexual behaviour with *gansha* often being on offer in the menus of brothels and, as Momocca Momocco said, being expected by customers to be part of the service even if it is not on the menu. She said that in particular younger customers often seemed to think that *gansha* was the proper way to finish having sex.

9 This is similar to the perception of work options transsexuals and transvestites in England appear to have (Perkins 1996).

10 Jennifer Robertson (1998) grossly misrepresented new half by failing to draw clear lines between them and transvestites and gay men. In addition her notion that the term *nyū hāfu* somehow suggests a foreignness because of a relation to the term *hāfu*, which means someone from mixed

Japanese and foreign parentage, is false. New half are by no means seen as foreign to Japanese culture. The *hāfu* of *nyū hāfu* refers to a halfway status between male and female. See also Matsuo Hisako (1997) and Lunsing (1998, 2001b) on the term.

11 See on bar hostess work for instance Allison (1994), Louis (1992) or Mock (1996).

REFERENCES

Akira (1998a) Akira no daiseikō nikki 7 (Akira's great diary of successful sexual intercourse, 7), in *G-men,* 29, August, pp. 74–5.

– (1998b) Akira no daiseikō nikki 1 (Akira's great diary of successful sexual intercourse), in *G-men,* 23, February, pp. 96–7.

Allison, Anne (1994) *Nightwork: Sexuality, pleasure, and corporate masculinity in a Tokyo hostess club.* Chicago and London: Chicago University Press.

Benedict, Ruth (1977 [1946]) *The chrysanthemum and the sword: patterns of Japanese culture.* London: Routledge and Kegan Paul.

Dalby, Liza Crihfield (1998) *Geisha.* Berkeley: University of California Press.

Doezema, Jo (1998) 'Forced to choose: beyond the voluntary v. forced prostitution dichotomy,' in: Kamala Kempadoo and Jo Doezema (eds) *Global sex workers: rights, resistance, and redefinition.* London and New York: Routledge, pp. 34–50.

Frühstück, Sabine (1997) *Die Politik der Sexualwissenschaft: zur Produktion und Popularisierung sexologischen Wissens in Japan 1908–1941,* Beiträge zur Japanologie, 34, Vienna: Institut für Japanologie, University of Vienna.

Furukawa, Makoto (1992) 'Kindai Nihon ni okeru dōseiai no shakaishi' (A social history of homosexuality in modern Japan), in: *Za Gei* (The Gay), May, pp. 24–60.

– (1994) 'The changing nature of sexuality: the three codes framing homosexuality in modern Japan,' *U.S .– Japan Women's Journal,* English Supplement 7, pp. 98–127.

Fushimi, Noriaki (2000) *Sei no rinrigaku* (Ethics of sex, sexuality and gender). Tokyo: Asahi Shinbunsha

Harada, Rumiko (1997) *Shōjotachi to manabu sekushuaru raitsu* (Learning sexual rights with girls). Tsuge Shobō Shinsha.

Henshūbu (ed.) (1999a) 'Shutchō hosuto intabyū' (Interviews with 'visiting hosts' [call boys]), in: *Bádi* (Buddy), January, pp. 424–5.

– (ed.) (1999b) 'Shutchō hosuto koborebanashi' (Gleanings of 'visiting hosts' [call boys]), in: *Bádi* (Buddy), January, pp. 426–8.

– (ed.) (1999c) 'For the guys chubby-chaser boys loved: Fat Max 28,' in: *Bádi* (Buddy), February, pp. 248–9.

Jolivet, Muriel (1997) *Japan: the childless society? The crisis of motherhood*. London: Routledge.

Kakinuma, Chisato (1991) 'Pinku saron: Shasei sangyō no "saiteihen"' (Pink salon: 'The lowest' of the ejaculation industry), in: *Sekkusu to iu oshigoto* (Sex work), Bessatsu Takarajima, 124, JICC Shuppan, Tokyo, January (second print), pp. 66–71.

Keiko (1991) 'Onna no Fesutibaru ni sanka shite' (Participating in the Women's Festival), in: *Faito Bakku* (Fight Back), 5, spring, pp. 8-11.

Koh, Masuda (ed.) (1988) *Kenkyusha's new Japanese–English dictionary*. Tokyo: Kenkyūsha (revised fourth edition of 1974).

LaFleur, William R. (1991) *Liquid life: abortion and Buddhism in Japan*. Princeton: Princeton University Press.

Leupp, Gary P. (1995) *Male colors: the construction of homosexuality in Tokugawa Japan*. Berkeley: University of California Press.

Louis, Lisa (1992) *Butterflies of the night: Mama-sans, geishas, strippers and the Japanese men they serve*. New York and Tokyo: Tengu Books.

Lunsing, Wim (1997) '"Gay boom" in Japan: changing views of homosexuality?' in: *Thamyris: mythmaking from past to present* 4(2), pp. 267–93.

– (1998) 'Lesbian and gay movements: between hard and soft,' in: Claudia Derichs and Anja Osiander (eds) *Soziale Bewegungen in Japan, Mitteilungen der Gesellschaft für Natur- und Völkerkunde Ostasiens e.V.*, 128, Hamburg: OAG, pp. 279-301.

– (1999) 'Japan: finding its way?' in: Barry D. Adam, Jan Willem Duyvendak and André Krouwel (eds) *The global emergence of gay and lesbian politics: national imprints of a worldwide movement*. Philadelphia: Temple University Press, pp. 293–325.

– (2000) 'Prostitution, mating, dating and marriage: love, sex and materialism in Japan,' in: Michael Ashkenazi and John Clammer (eds) *Material culture and consumption in Japan*. London and New York: Kegan Paul International, pp. 163–190.

– (2001a) 'Between margin and center: researching "non-standard" Japanese,' *Copenhagen Journal of Asian Studies* 15, pp. 81-113.

– (2001b) *Beyond common sense: sexuality and gender in contemporary Japan*. London and New York: Kegan Paul International.

Matsuo, Hisako (1997) *Toransujendarizumu: seibetsu no higan* (Transgenderism: the other side of sex difference). Yokohama: Seori Shobō.

Matsuzawa Kureichi ed. (2000a) *Baishun kōtei sengen: uru uranai wa watashi ga kimeru* (Declarations in support of prostitution: I decide whether I sell or not), Tokyo: Potto Shuppan.

– (2000b) *Watashi ga kimeta* (I decided), Tokyo: Potto Shuppan.

Miyadai, Shinji (1994) *Seifuku shōjotachi no sentaku* (Choices of girls in school uniforms). Tokyo: Kōdansha.

– (1997) *Seikimatsu no sakuhō: owarinaki nichijō o ikiru chie* (How to write the end of a century: the wisdom to live and endless everyday). Tokyo: Media Fakutorii.

Mock, John (1996) 'Mother or mama: the political economy of bar hostesses in Sapporo,' in: Anne E. Imamura (ed.) *Re-imagining Japanese women*. Berkeley: University of California Press, pp. 177-91.

Momocca, Momocco (1998) 'Japanese sex workers: encourage, empower, trust and love yourselves!' in: Kampala Kempadoo and Jo Doezema (eds) *Global sex workers: rights, resistance, and redefinition*. London and New York: Routledge, pp. 178–81.

Morikuri, Shigekazu (1995) *Yobai to kindai baishun* (Yobai and modern prostitution). Tokyo: Akashi Shobō.

Nakadono, Masao (1993) *Sei no hōritsu: Kekkon, furin, rikon* (Laws on sex: Marriage, immoral conduct, divorce). Tokyo: Asahi Shinbunsha

Nekome, Yū (1998) *Nyūhāfu to iu ikikata* (The lifestyle of the new half/*travesti*). Tokyo: Goma Shobō.

Perkins, Roberta (1996) 'The "drag queen scene": Transsexuals in King's Cross,' in: Richards Ekins and Dave King (eds) *Blending genders: Social aspects of cross-dressing and sex-changing*. London and New York: Routledge, pp. 53–62.

Pflugfelder, Gregory (1999) *Cartographies of desire: male–male sexuality in Japanese discourse 1600–1950*. Berkeley: University of California Press.

Reischauer, Edwin O. and Albert M. Craig (1989) *Japan: Tradition and transformation*. St. Leonards: Allen & Unwin.

Robertson, Jennifer (1998) *Takarazuka: sexual politics and popular culture in modern Japan*. Berkeley: University of California Press.

Sano, Akira (1995) *Dokyumento sekuhara* (Document sexual harassment). Nishinomiya: Rokusaisha.

Saeki, Junko (1996) '"Renai" no zenkindai, kindai, datsu kindai' ('Love' before the modern time, in the modern time and after the modern time), in: Inoue Toshi, Ueno Chizuko *et al.* (eds), *Sekushuariti no seijigaku* (The politicology of Sexuality). Tokyo: Iwanami Shoten, pp. 167–84.

Shiga-Fujime, Yuki (1993) 'The prostitutes' union and the impact of the 1956 anti-prostitution law in Japan,' in: *U.S. – Japan Women's Journal*, English supplement 5.

Smith, Robert J. and Ella Lury Wiswell, (1982) *The women of Suyemura*. Chicago and London: Chicago University Press.

Tsunoda, Yukiko (1992) *Sei no hōritsugaku* (The jurisprudence on sex). Tokyo: Yūhikaku Sensho.

Ueno, Chizuko (1998) *Nashyonarizumu to jendā (Engendering nationalism)* (Nationalism and gender). Tokyo: Seidosha.

Watanabe, Tsuneo and Junichi Iwata (1987) *La voie des éphèbes: histoire et histoires des homosexualités au Japon*. Paris: Éditions Trismégiste.

CHAPTER 4

TIFUL DAUGHTERS AND TEMPORARY WIVES: ECONOMIC DEPENDENCY ON COMMERCIAL SEX IN VIETNAM

IAN WALTERS

Much of the literature on prostitution in Asia contains horror stories: how girls are duped, trafficked, made to work as sex slaves, and exploited in various other ways. This is a literature of outrage. But it is also inextricably linked to development and policy changes to ensure Asian governments and bureaucracies conform to current Western or Northern standards of morality, public policy, and political behaviour. For example, many forces are constantly applying pressure on Asian governments to become signatories to United Nations and other international conventions and instruments. Some of this horror is indeed true and justified. But as some authors have recently begun to write: do not believe all the hype (Murray 1998).

The global commercial sex scene constitutes a booming market, involving a multi-billion dollar industry (Kempadoo 1998:16). As an example from the region, the Thai sex industry is said to be worth about 5 billion US dollars a year (Kempadoo 1998:16). However, the economic aspects of sex industries are rarely discussed. Because of the dominant influence of discourses on morality in characterizing the sex industries of the world as evil and abounding in horror stories, the economic contributions made, particularly to poorer countries in regions like Southeast Asia, are rarely considered. In this paper I put aside moral concerns to concentrate on another aspect of the issues concerned with the sale of sexual services: to examine the scale of economic dependence on prostitution in one of these Asian countries, Vietnam.

In an insightful paper on tourism and the sex industry in Vietnam, Cooper and Hanson (1998) make two important points. The first is that the sex industry is an important component in the economy of many countries, and it could be so in Vietnam should the government seek to value the work of prostitutes, decriminalize their services, and recognize their contribution to the economy. The second point is that research, outreach and support work done with prostitutes should be responsible to people involved in the sex industry rather than to government or its bureaucracies. I wish to take up both these points here. Initially, to take an empirical step beyond the claims of Cooper and Hanson (1998) that the sex industry contributes significantly to the economy of Vietnam, by asking: does it? My aim will be to investigate if this is indeed so. I ask: What is the scale of economic dependence on prostitution in Vietnam?

Secondly, I aim to set this investigation against a backdrop of what such an issue means to those involved in the sex industries of Vietnam, in order to be responsible to people actually involved in the industry, to interpret empirical findings from their perspective rather than that of government and its bureaucracies. Here I ask: What are the implications of this for Vietnamese involved in sex industries (economically/socially/culturally/ politically)?

My essay attempts to reflect the language and moods of the encounters with people involved in the sex industries, in their places of trade. In this sense, in places the essay will take on a familiar non-academic tone, which is exactly what I am striving for. My data for this paper come from Hanoi, Ho Chi Minh City and a beach resort in northern Vietnam, near the capital, which I prefer to keep anonymous, so that people who provided information are not compromised.

To show the scale of economic dependence on prostitution is difficult. How can reliable surveys be conducted on a set of illegal industries in a totalitarian country like Vietnam? It is very difficult for researchers to obtain accurate survey data in such a complex field. Because of such difficulties it becomes meaningless to talk about numerical estimates with any reliability. Rather, my aim involves giving some insights which will suggest the scale of industries and the amount of money involved. This means showing the scale of prostitution itself. My work is ethnographic, involving participant observation. Ethnography has been used successfully as a research tool to understand the motivations and behaviours of people in the sex industries of Asia (e.g. Cohen 1982, 1986, 1987, 1988; Murray 1991; Fordham 1995; Lyttleton 1995, 2000; Askew 1999). I made my observations on several short field trips to the country. I made contact with sex workers at their work stations. Many were wary of providing information, and worried about the police. Some were curt, seeing me as taking up their valuable time. But some were happy to talk, and on occasions I was able to arrange to meet them out of working hours to chat. To compensate for their time, I generally gave sex workers who talked to me money. Other people in the industry provided different interactive situations. I was able to talk to clients, hotel staff and so forth, in the relaxed atmosphere of lobbies, clubs, and other locations.

Prostitution is illegal in Vietnam yet, following its supposed resurgence in the 1980s (Le Thi Quy 1993), it thrives and grows. The Vietnamese government is justifiably proud of its record in being effective at keeping its country from becoming – in their eye – another Thailand or Manila. It has done this through an attempted prohibition involving a heavy concentration on policing and punitive measures, backed by moral social campaigns and policies declaring sex industries to be a social evil (Le Thi Quy 1993, 1997; Mai Thuc 1997; Walters 2004, in press). Despite the emphasis on morality, there have to be economic considerations as well. The paper is set in terms of economic dependence, but I seek an anthropological interpretation of what these issues mean to the Vietnamese. To do this, I draw upon two major scholarly ideas from the literature on Asian prostitution: dutiful daughters and temporary wives.

DUTIFUL DAUGHTERS/TEMPORARY WIVES

Muecke (1992) has shown that growth in the Thai economy has been accompanied by an increase in commercial sex services. Yet this has enabled female prostitutes to conserve the basic institutions of society. Prostitution has flourished at least in part because it allows these women, through their financial remittances home, to fulfil traditional cultural functions of daughters, conserving the family and village level Buddhism, as well as institutions of government. Her study demonstrated the ideologies of family and religion 'have not been changed by the growth of the sex trade in Thailand' (Muecke 1992:898). In fact these ideologies ensure the perpetuation of prostitution because of the 'conversion of wages into consumer goods for families' (Muecke 1992:898).

Andaya (1998) showed how cultural attitudes towards sexual relations which prevailed in Southeast Asia throughout the early modern period (1500–1800) were vastly different from those of more recent times. Here I summarize Andaya's important insights, quoting from her paper at some length. As I need to set out her ideas and data in detail, I will draw extensively from this important work. In the early modern period there was no shame attached to casual or premarital sex for money, any use of women's sexuality to gain economic advantage being taken as sensible, respectable, and admired behaviour, rather than the opposite. Being in a relationship with a foreign trader, for example, who could bring wealth, was seen as something of value, even if the relationship was only short term. There was no slight on women who moved on from one temporary relationship to another as foreign merchants or sailors came and went. There was no 'stigma attached to common law wives' and 'condemnation of women who exchanged sex for material gain was not a traditional feature of Southeast Asian societies' (Andaya 1998:1). The 'attitudinal shift' producing more recent stigma and condemnation is as yet an 'unresearched aspect of the history of sexuality in this part of the world' (Andaya 1998:1). She relates it to the 'spread of world religions, rise of patriarchal states, increased foreign presence, coin currencies, and emergence of towns' (Andaya 1998:11).

When Europeans arrived they were struck by the hospitality they received from locals who assumed they would need assistance, and were keen to incorporate them into kin networks. This was most effectively achieved by 'providing a local woman as a companion, and if desired, a sexual partner' (Andaya 1998:1). Sexual relationships were used to welcome traders into the community (Andaya 1998:2). 'Southeast Asian men always preferred to trade in places where they already had relatives who could furnish companionship and assistance, and assumed others would feel the same' (Andaya 1998:2).

Andaya (1998:2) relates how when Miguel de Legazpi arrived in the Philippines in 1565 female traders converged on the camp to exchange wine and sexual services with his soldiers. One of the local customs, he said, was to provide outsiders with women. A hundred years later Dampier noted this offering of women as the custom in the East Indies, Pegu (southern Myanmar), Siam, Cochinchina, and Cambodia. In Tonkin 'most of our Men had Women aboard all the time,' it being 'Policy to do it,' the captains of ships having 'the great men's Daughters offered them' (Andaya 1998:2). And importantly, the custom of temporary marriage could not have persisted for such a long time and so extensively in pre-modern Southeast Asian societies without the compliance, co-operation, and active involvement of the women concerned (Andaya 1998:2).

Where foreigners were a rarity, 'considerable prestige accrued to those possessing a lover or husband from overseas' (Andaya 1998:2). 'Perceived wealth was certainly a factor in the popularity of foreigners' (Andaya 1998:3). 'By receiving valuable or unusual gifts from foreign traders, women and their families acquired prestige items that could be displayed or exchanged, significantly enhancing their status within the community' (Andaya 1998:3). 'Basic to most Southeast Asian cultures was the belief that access to a woman's body was part of a reciprocal process in which the exchange of gifts was critical' (Andaya 1998:3). In Burma, in an undated example she mentions, 'gifts from a man to an unmarried woman were regarded as the prelude to sexual intercourse and legally belonged to her if the act occurred' (Andaya 1998:3). In the fourteenth-century law code of northern Siam, 'it was quite acceptable for a husband or parents' to have a woman 'go and live with another man in order to get money and goods from him, with a limit on the period' (Andaya 1998:3).

Alexander Hamilton, a trader, noted that Vietnamese nobles had previously 'thought it no Shame or Disgrace to marry their daughters to

English and Dutch Seamen, for the Tune they were to stay in Tonquin [sic]' (Andaya 1998:4). The 'departure of a foreign husband could thus mean social advancement rather than the stigma of being an abandoned wife' (Andaya 1998:4). She had 'increased her economic resources and was assumed to possess new knowledge as a result of her association with a European' (Andaya 1998:4). Far from being condemned as loose or amoral, Hamilton said a 'woman who had been passed from one European to another' was in her own society 'rather the better looked on, that she has been married to several European husbands' [sic] (Andaya 1998:4).

By the sixteenth century there was a 'marked rise' in the number of single males, especially Europeans, in the port cities of Southeast Asia (Andaya 1998:5). Short-term financial transactions by women became common. This was 'an acceptable way for the very poor to make a living as long as all parties agreed' (Andaya 1998:6). A 'flourishing trade in sex was already developing' (Andaya 1998:6). Li Tana and Anthony Reid report how in 1694 a Chinese monk remarked of Hoi An: 'The women were very good at trade, so the traders [from Fujian, southeastern China] who came here all tended to marry a local woman to help them with their trading' (Andaya 1998:6). In 'a compelling example of cultural misreading,' this willingness of Southeast Asian females to sell themselves for economic gain, led the Europeans to see the women as promiscuous and wanton (Andaya 1998:7).

But the 'increased visibility of prostitution in historical records is not just a product of European preoccupations' (Andaya 1998:9). A 'feature of this period is the growing indebtedness of ordinary Southeast Asians as economies became increasingly monetized' (Andaya 1998:9). Prostitution 'presented one solution to economic hardship since then as now it was customary to channel to the family resources earned in this manner' (Andaya 1998:9). In eighteenth-century Vietnam Barrow records how 'mothers often helped negotiate sexual liaisons for their daughters' (Andaya 1998:9). Young women, said Barrow, 'dispose of personal favours to procure articles of the first necessity for themselves and their families' (Andaya 1998:9). Neither the husband, he continues, 'nor the father seems to have any scruples in abandoning the wife or the daughter to the gallant' (Andaya 1998:9).

There are also present-day temporary wives. A very dark-skinned girl comes to the hotel at which I am staying in Ho Chi Minh City (Saigon). She is with a big Singaporean guest, who is here with three of his associates. She is from a provincial city. He met her there when he and his colleagues went down there on business the previous week. A long-time friend of one of the businessmen is a go-between, and introduced this big shot to the girl. I am told she is a prostitute, and said to be a sexy dancer at some club in her home town, where she is reputed to dance with no clothes on. She is very young, nineteen, and speaks not a word of English. The Singaporean man speaks little or no Vietnamese. When I saw them in the lobby one night she looked bored and sullen while he, his Singaporean friend, and one of the hotel receptionists talked in English. Another hotel staff member joked with me that the relationship involved communication in body language. The receptionist was translating some things into Vietnamese for the girl, but mostly she was ignored. At one stage she went to the reception counter and made a phone call, then silently resumed her place. When they leave for Singapore she will apparently take a bus back to her home town. In the interim he has taken her around, eating with her at restaurants, going shopping, to clubs and so on. And of course she sleeps with him at the hotel. She has been his temporary wife for the duration of his stay, and has been paid handsomely for it.

One foreigner I met in a club told me he finds it difficult to distinguish prostitutes from girls who are just trying to go with foreigners, girls who are looking for a foreigner to marry. He says, for example, he slept with one girl for a week and never paid her anything. She never asked for money. While other girls with whom he has sex negotiate prices straight away, some look on themselves as girlfriends, becoming temporary wives for these men.

CONTEMPORARY FORMS OF PROSTITUTION

Some impression of scale can be gained from the variety and diversity of forms and outlets of prostitution. In Vietnam the industry is 'booming' (Franklin 1993:1) and 'on the rise' (Population Council, Vietnam s.d.:7). In recent years it has 'developed at a galloping pace and reached alarming proportions' (Le Thi Quy 1993:1). It is practiced 'in almost all hotels, inns, restaurants, dancing halls, beauty and massage parlours, beer houses, cafeterias, public parks, street pavement, bus station, railway station, and any other places such as dyke embankment or sea beach' [sic] (Le Thi Quy 1993:4). To this can be added hairdressing salons, manicure and beauty parlours, nightclubs, bars, and karaoke establishments. Some outdoor homeless people also work as prostitutes (Nguyen Van Chinh 1997).

Ngo Vinh Long (1993:338) reported on girls in what he calls the high-class category, operating 'out of villas, private apartments, and hotel rooms.' Often they 'work out of their own houses and apartments through contacts and through meetings at the various four-star and five-star restaurants and hotels in the city,' or they work in 'the so-called villa cafes' which are 'located in the private villas located in the more exclusive city residential areas' (Ngo Vinh Long 1993:339). Some of these girls attach themselves to foreigners as temporary wives, in the fashion of women in early modern period.

ESTIMATES OF NUMBERS OF SEX WORKERS

Hiebert (1992) reported police estimates of 50,000 prostitutes in Ho Chi Minh City, up from 40,000 when the communists took over in 1975. The 'public security service' estimated nearly 40,000 prostitutes and 1,000 brothels in the country in early 1990, rising to more than 200,000 and 2,000 by 1992 (Le Thi Quy 1993:1). A footnote reference to this security document says that after 1954 there were 11,800 prostitutes in North Vietnam, with forty-five brothels. After 1975 there were 200,000 prostitutes in the South. An unofficial estimate for the country may be 500,000 prostitutes (Khuat Thu Hong 1998:45–6). The

> current total number of prostitutes in the whole country is, as estimated, equal to the figure recorded in pre-1975 South Vietnam. As released by public statistics, there are about 176,000 prostitutes across the country. Yet, many people hold that this figure is far from reality. As for sex buyers, the number is uncounted (Hoang Ba Thinh 1999:5).

By 1990, according to interviews Ngo Vinh Long (1993:336) conducted 'with officials knowledgeable about prostitution,' the estimates were 160,000 to 200,000 in the country, of whom 100,000 were in Ho Chi Minh City. According to reports given to Do Thi Ninh Xuan (1997:289) 'there are now 76,000 prostitutes in the country,' but she thinks it may be higher, given that it is estimated by some to be 200,000. According to a Southeast Asia e-mail list news item from 1999, the Director of the Department of Social Evils Prevention in Vietnam is quoted as saying they have 'some 185,000 prostitutes' on their files.

As can be seen estimated numbers vary widely and are probably pretty worthless. The estimates never seem to be linked to a rigorous survey method and are presumably all flawed. But they do give some idea of the scale of the sector, and allow an acknowledgment that the numbers involved are indeed high.

INCOMES AND NUMBERS OF CUSTOMERS

Massage girls in Hanoi earned 800,000 to a million Vietnam dong (VND) per month (then about US$80–100), 'much higher than manual labourers' wages' (Nguyen Van Chinh 1997:53). One man I got to know, Mr Vang, says the girls who come to the mini-hotel where he works, charge the customer US$50. Hien, one sex worker with whom I am acquainted, told me she charges US$50 per trick and usually makes about VND15 million per month, which is about US$1,000.

A motorbike taxi driver (*xe om*) took me to a bar he knew where I met some girls, and began talking with one for whom I had to buy drinks. This driver later told me bar girls like those to whom he introduced me go for VND500,000 (US$35). A Westerner I met in a dancing club tells me he takes girls all the time. He usually pays US$50 for girls from this place, but he points out some women drinking at the bar and says they are far too expensive: US$100. At other dancing clubs, according to my *xe om*, the girls also go for VND700,000 (US$50). One male go-between (*moi gioi*) said the current price range for girls in his 'stable' was VND200,000 (US$14) on up to US$100.

On one of Ho Chi Minh City's main thoroughfares, where I went on the back of an *xe om* motorbike taxi, I encounter the girls on motorbikes about whom Mr Xuan, an Overseas Vietnamese, had told me. Exactly as he said, they cruise with you in the traffic and move up alongside you to talk. No sooner did I ask one the price, in Vietnamese, than I had a pack of six all surrounding us. I had quotes of VND300,000 (US$21) from the first girl's driver, and the second girl tells me, also in Vietnamese, twenty dollars (*hai chup do*).

As I walked back to the hotel from a dancing club, at about two in the morning, a woman alone on her motorcycle draws alongside at walking pace, talking to me. This girl puttered beside me for five hundred metres, persisting with her sales pitch, as though she refused to take no for an answer. In English she offered me a massage for twenty dollars: 'the whole thing, you can have everything, twenty dollar. We go to a hotel, a mini-hotel.' Mini-hotels are private hotels often run by families.

In some areas of the city girls still stand in the darkness on footpaths, awaiting custom. Potential clients approach, mostly on motorbikes, but also on bicycles or in motor vehicles. They negotiate prices and if a deal is made, will take the girl to a mini-hotel or resthouse for sex. We cruised, checking out the scene, approaching one girl who was standing alone. She offered VND200,000 (US$14) for a fast one (*lam nhanh*) or VND300,000 (US$21) for the night (*dem*): 'Where? At a resthouse (*nha nghi*) near here. It will cost VND50,000 (US$3.5) to rent a room for a fast one, VND100,000 (US$7) for the night. Or we can go to a restaurant hotel (*nha hang khach san*) and rent a room for the night for VND200,000 (US$14).'

Another girl came over to join in. She was twenty-three, and she went for VND100,000 (US$7). She also took customers to a resthouse.

Others work through minders or pimps, middle-aged women who front as vendors or fruit-sellers. I met two of these in a quiet street late at night. Both minder women wore the street-sellers' gear of floral pyjamas. Two street girls were there with the minders, who were vigorous in their negotiations. One actually butted in to change the prices the girl quoted, doubling the VND100,000 she had said, obviously catering to the fact I was a foreigner.

Still others stand on footpaths adjacent to parks, where they take breaks on benches, eating and smoking, talking to their friends. One I talked with, Dung, said she is sixteen, though she is solidly built and looks more like twenty-two or twenty-three. She said she had an evening target of VND300,000. If she could earn that, she would go home. I asked her about this. She said she took customers at VND70,000 or 80,000 (US$5 or a bit more) per customer. That means you have to have three or four customers a night, I say. No, she replies, two or three. How? I inquire: three customers at eighty thousand each is VND240,000. She then said she targeted three hundred thousand a night. But no, she then contradicted herself, two or three hundred thousand, and two hundred thousand would usually do. And that usually meant two or three customers a night. But two was only VND140,000 or at best VND160,000 I say. The matter remained unresolved, but one young man, who frequented the park, raised the subject of Dung with me, as he saw me spending a lot of time talking to her. He insisted he saw Dung regularly take eight to ten clients per night.

At a beach resort in the north of Vietnam, a cafe drink stall (*giai khat*) madam accosted me as I walked past, with the offer of a young girl, seventeen, for VND100,000. I could take her to a *nha nghi* nearby, in the back streets. Some nights later, on another evening walk around, as I approached shops from the beach side I was accosted by a girl who grabbed me and would not let go. She wanted me to go into the back of her café, and wanted to have sex with me for VND200,000. I would have to pay an extra VND100,000 to rent a room nearby, and then some more for drinks at the café. She was eighteen years old.

A group of Singaporean businessmen were staying in my hotel. They were there for a week. One arrived with a girl from the country town where they had been doing business. A hotel receptionist told me the girl is with one of the businessmen. He has paid her US$500 as a fee for the week, to be his companion and sleep with him. Plus he gave her about VND1.1 million (US$80) when they all left; the men for their country and the girl back to the countryside. This was all for five nights and five days. During that time he also bought her meals, maybe some small gifts, and took her on outings as well.

RAMIFICATIONS THROUGH THE ECONOMY

First site of dependence (and ultimate site also): family
Beyond the girls themselves, who are benefiting from the income of their own sex work, there is a massive superstructure of dependency, beginning and ending with the family. The families of workers constitute the first and principal site for financial benefit from the gains of the industry. The girls remit money to their families, and are seen as dutiful daughters for doing so. For example, one worker named Vui told me she remits VND2 million (US$125) every month to her family who live in one of the poorer socio-economic areas of another large city. Another girl, Hien, told me she remits US$500 a month to her mother who lives in the countryside near yet another large city. Such earnings were used therefore to 'support themselves and their families' (Nguyen Van Chinh 1997:53). This is similar to the situation in Thailand described by Muecke (1992, see also Cook 1998), where girls gain the status dutiful daughters for contributing to their families' material life circumstances, building them better houses, buying consumer goods, educating siblings and the like. In Thailand they also contribute to temples and monasteries, and earn Buddhist merit, improving their life chances in this and the next life. Muecke (1992) suggests that in this way sex workers are actually helping to conserve important traditional institutions of Thai culture and society. The Vietnamese girls are also fulfilling the roles of dutiful daughters, supporting mothers, fathers, siblings and extended families. As good daughters who increase the material prospects of their families, they will increase their own chances of making a better marriage, eventually becoming wives and mothers in respected and respectable social situations.

Go-betweens/minders/pimps
A hotel-worker named Vang talked to me about going to a dancing club, saying I should go at least once, just to experience it. I said we should go together. This was what he had been waiting for. Yes, he said, he sometimes took foreigners to clubs to introduce them. He also has a list of phone numbers for girls and can help clients such as hotel guests who want a girl. On several occasions he subsequently demonstrated this to me, ringing girls from reception to check their availability for arrangements clients desired. He took a cut of the fee when this happened, the one time I witnessed it, the amount being VND50,000 (US$3.5).

I was standing outside the hotel drinking a can of beer when to my surprise an *xe om* pulled up and asked if I wanted to go meet some girls. Girl boom boom. He had that kind of street English the hustlers here have: 'Where? Not far from here.' He repeated this over and over again: 'Not far from here. Hotel have girls. Very young. Beautiful. You can choose. Thirty dollar. Thirty dollar girl boom boom. Ten dollar for room. I take you, one dollar. Yeah, we go, yeah.'

I was stunned when he pulled out a laminated card with some hotel or something on it, which I could not read in the street gloom without my glasses. He turned it over to reveal a photo of five young women standing in a line facing the camera, the outer four in ordinary dresses, the centre one in her underwear. He showed me other cards for cafés which have girls. I could choose. He took me there. One dollar.

Then there are the street girls the Overseas Vietnamese reject. They continue to come around to the hotel to be rejected. Always hopeful. One is a girl who kept circling the hotel the other night after being among three the Overseas Vietnamese had turned down. Her driver, who is the same guy as that other night too, was very pushy. All the drivers were young boys younger than twenty-five. None looked like sleazy *xe om* at first, but more like an average Vietnamese student, shirt worn outside trousers, wearing scuffs (*dep*) on their feet. They all earn cuts from any work they can get for their girls, and any transporting of them they do to and from hotels and like places. Xuan said that earlier in the evening he had gone up past where I saw the fourteen-year-old on an *xe om*, and had immediately been accosted by six or so girls, themselves all on an *xe om*. Up there they were thick on the ground. A local vendor bore this out for me, saying normally there were hundreds of them up there.

One street girl, standing waiting, offered my driver a go-between cut of VND50,000 for bringing me, if I took up her offer. That represented a quarter of what she was asking as a fee on that occasion, a pretty big cut. Two other street girls I encountered were with minders, both middle-aged females, who were boisterous in their negotiations. One actually butted in to change one girl's quoted price, doubling it to VND200,000 (US$14). The young girl was presumably inexperienced at dealing with a foreigner, and was asking too low a price. The sixteen-year-old from the park, Dung, and her young man minder, Mr Thuoc, lived together. Dung paid him nothing because of that partnership. As children they had been young lovers in their village, she told me. He said that pimps like him normally get five to ten percent of the girls' take. We stopped where the cucumber seller was and I talked to a woman in pyjama bottoms and tee shirt who had looked really young as we passed by, but on stopping, I could see she was well into her thirties. She did not go, but was a go-between, she told me. She claimed she had beautiful girls cheap.

All these go-betweens represent a significant component of the sex industries of Vietnam. They assist the sex workers, and for their services take their share. They provide transport, contacts, arrangements, and sometimes protection. Sometimes they are husbands or brothers, or mothers or aunts, but usually not. In such cases they represent the first ripple of economic dependence extending beyond the immediate family of the prostitute.

The next ripple of dependents is composed of hotels, police, bureaucrats, taxis, phone companies...

Colimoro (1998:197) says sex workers 'generate a lot of indirect employment' for 'we are a world of people.' Sex workers, she said, need support in their struggle from those supported by them, such as people in hair and beauty salons, massage parlours, bars, brothels, and cafeterias, plus such figures as taxi drivers, parking attendants, as well as those implicated by bribes, such as inspectors or firefighters (Colimoro 1998:198).

Let us say five girls on average work in a mini-hotel per night. Take the mini-hotel I lodged in on one trip. There were seven people living and working at the hotel, and all have dependants. Even members of the main nuclear family who were the bosses would remit to their parents, especially to those of the proprietor himself. These staff members either have a spouse and child or parents, or a parent and sibling, dependent on them. Let us then say two dependants per person, that is fourteen dependants. Then there is the old man who comes to collect the garbage and sift through it for things he can use and items worth selling. There are the drivers who bring and take the clients to and from the place. Let us say four out of five girls also have drivers, either taxi cab drivers or motorbike taxi drivers. That is up to eight drivers. There is the health certificate man, the fire safety man, the phone company man, and the electricity man. Let us say four of them all up. Then there are the police who monitor the place and even raid occasionally. So for the hypothetical five girls who worked here on that hypothetical night, there were forty people dependent at least in part on their trade. That is a ratio of 40 to 5, or 8 to one.

Over and above this there is other indirect dependence to be added: those who make money from the electricity the girls use, for which hotel pays, airconditioning, lights; there is the phone company for both internal and mobiles, there is the petrol company for all these vehicles, there is the beer and other drinks companies for the beverages the clients consume in the rooms; there is the garment companies who make and fit those thoroughly modern clothes the girls wear; their makeup and perfume suppliers, hairdressers, nail painters, jewellers, the motor-bike suppliers, or – dare I say it, for at least one girl we have talked to has intentions in this area – car suppliers. I have mentioned petrol, and this leads to other additional products, like tyres for cars or bikes for example, material for clothes, right back to the primary producers or the import/export company workers, shipping and transport companies and so forth. And the customs officials, the tax collectors, and the government itself through any such taxes.

Hotels

Yes, the place at which I am staying in takes hookers. As I had thought it should, but was surprised when it seemed at first it did not. My friend was telling me all those girls I was seeing arriving were girlfriends of guests. But there had to be more to it, especially as some of them only remained a short time. Sure enough they were all hookers, every one of them. One Overseas Vietnamese man has a regular girl, but as he has been here playing around six weeks it can only be that long. And it will end when he goes back to the USA in three days time. Then she will be off to the clubs again to find another good paying client. In effect she is a hooker, but may be on the lookout for a husband as she is over thirty. At least she is a kept woman, one of those to whom Andaya (1998) refers as temporary wives.

Mr Vang informs me that one room alone, the most expensive in the hotel, which therefore is the one least occupied, often draws a million Vietnam dong a night from hookers (US$70). They have to pay VND200,000 for the room each time, so that is five occupations. And when they arrive in pairs or numbers, more than one room is occupied at a time. Even if the hotel only averages a million a night, that is a good income.

Do they ever get raided? I asked. Never, was the answer. They paid and were not raided. How much? I ask. Plenty. How often? I ask. Whenever the police require it. Not a monthly thing, but when the police feel it needs the money it simply phones up or sends word around.

Last night again the place was full of East Asians. I was at reception talking to staff. The girls were telling their clients the rooms are US$30 and the suckers are paying (the actual hotel charge is VND200,000, some US$14). Three men handed over the US dollars as they went upstairs. When they came down, they were sat down in the foyer while the girls outrageously passed money back and forth at reception, to the staff there, getting the amounts right. One had the good sense to keep her hands beside and below the counter as she deals out the notes. Another, next to me, turned her back on the clients. But it was still so obvious, they were so bold and blatant, taking their VND210,000 or so refund back from reception (US$30 minus VND200,000 comes back on the sly). Mr Vang described it to me as the hotel keeping US$15 and the girls taking US$15, but with VND going back and forth it was more probably the girls getting VND210,000 and the hotel the rest, as US$15 is currently some VND210,000. The Japanese clients did not even appear suspicious. They chatted desultorily, one drank some water from a La Vie mineral water bottle. A cab was called and they departed.

The girls supply by far the bigger share of hotel income. They outnumber other room renters by a ratio of at least 60:40, I would estimate. On average here, Vang says, they take eight to ten girl-related rentals per night. Sometimes they have bad nights, but have an average of eight. They usually seem to have about the same number booked by full night clients like myself. One night while I had been there, they were fully booked, but that was unusual. In addition, of the full nighters, at least three were Overseas Vietnamese there for sex. They were here for other things as well, business or family visits, but they go out to play every night, and every night return to the hotel with the girls they were paying for sex. Other Overseas Vietnamese friends of theirs, who were staying with family, joined them here at the hotel on various nights, also with girls. So my estimate is based on renting for sex versus other renting, and it comes down to a ratio like 10 rooms to 6, or 8 to 6.

Clubs and bars

Vang went as far as saying the only women who go to dancing clubs are girls. Girls was the common English term many of my Vietnamese contacts, including Mr Vang, used to refer to prostitutes. It may be a shortened version of other expressions such a taxi girl, or money girl. For them to say someone is a girl, is akin to saying someone is a hooker. This may be an overstatement, but it is a very interesting claim. If it is anywhere near the mark, it also gives an indication of how thick on the ground the sex workers are, because there are so many clubs.

A Vietnamese friend led us to a karaoke bar of his choosing. It hired out rooms for singing and girls come as a component of this. We were quoted VND50,000 an hour for the room, and VND50,000 for each girl. An hour with girls and a few drinks, I estimated should all cost about a few hundred thousand Vietnamese *dong*. They sang for two hours or so, and I had to really fork out. Of course, no one throws you out or calls time after an hour, and as there was no clock, time just passed and there you are having to pay for a second hour. But the really expensive aspect is the drink. These girls poured their way through fifty-two bottles of yoghurt drink. I could not believe it. But the empties were lined up for counting on the floor, and they formed a veritable slab of glass. What could they have done with the stuff? Altogether I had to pay out more than VND700,000 (>US$50).

My *xe om* suggested I went to a place on the main drag and drink a cup of coffee, and the girls would come to me. I did not know what he had in mind, and was in half a mind to decline. But I acquiesced. Knowing I was short of cash, I thought a coffee could not bank the balance too much. I could not quite imagine what would happen. We ended up in a bar he pointed out to me on the initial ride around. Girls waved from the door. We dismounted and entered. It was dark inside. I ordered a lemon juice, scared of the cost. I was shown no menu or price list. He sat beside me, and at the invitation I had to make, he ordered a beer. Then I was set upon by one of the hostesses. Which was why we were there, of course. He discreetly got up and ambled to the bar. There he explained his role as go-between to ensure his cut of what I paid. The place had a small bar and four or so of those stand-alone tables and high stools, one of which I sat at. Upstairs was a pool table and even greater discretion, I guessed. One other foreigner was in the place, it seemed. Or perhaps the clack of the pool balls indicated more upstairs. Later several would in fact emerge from upstairs and leave. The lone man then went away too. But his place was soon taken by another. There were about six or seven girls, and two older women behind the bar, one smoking. A couple of guys were also present. When I finally called for the bill my girl was dismayed. She asked if I would like two girls, that is, for another to join us. I said no. Frightened of the unknown but mounting cost I called a halt. The bill amounted to VND180,000 (US$13) for my lemon, the beer, and three of her drinks.

If a bar like that has on average one customer every minute of its ten hours of opening (quite possible given that I overlapped with three others at one stage, one other at other times, and was on my own there for a few minutes), that is a gross taking of around US$300 per night or US$9,000 per month, for an annual profit of US$108,000. A two-customer average doubles the annual gross to US$216,000.

Assume that the city has a hundred such places: some of which are far more packed than the little joint I was in that night. Assume they each have only a one customer average throughout. This still represents a gross annual profit of US$10,800,000. A two-customer average pushes it up to nearly US$22,000,000 and so on. Assume that there are city and town, and country outlets which can be seen to amount to the equivalent of five times this amount. It means the clubs and bars of Vietnam – even if they had only a two-customer average – are taking over one hundred million US dollars a year from sales attracted by and linked to the provision of sexual services. The profit made from the actual sexual services themselves then has to be added to this.

The customer average is actually far higher, it has to be, given the density of the crowd at some of these places. And there are bound to be more than 100 venues in the largest cities. But I am concentrating only on the high profile foreigner venues for my hypothetical example. Across the city there would be thousands of such places for Vietnamese customers. And then there are the other cities as well. The country is making money hand over fist on the back of prostitution: for no girls, no custom; or very little.

There is another aspect of the bar culture: the girls are obviously trained and given instructions to order plenty of drinks (they do not have to drink them, just order them), keep the customer there till closing time, then go with him for sex. The girl I met was in no hurry to leave my side, and kept insisting I relax and stay there, even after I had finished drinking and was commenting that the bar was closing. She knew the boss would appear, to arrange for her to go for sex with me, yet she said nothing.

Cafés

Two girls lounged in a café. As we approached I heard instructions being given to them to sit down on the lounge near the door, apart, adopting an obviously come-hither pose. Here come foreigners! Yet when the offer came, it was for neither of them. This woman told me the café is just a meeting place. We went in, drank coffee or whatever and the girls talked to us, and then went with us after a price has been negotiated.

On the beach after dusk we were invited to sit down in rented deck chairs and meet beautiful young girls. Only VND50,000. I said we would look see (*xem thu*). The proprietor agreed and sent out for girls. Eventually some arrived, but we left. All along the beach we were made the same offers. All the touts were old women, grandmother vintage, the ones who man the strand stalls during the daytime. The deck chairs are arranged behind their stalls, down near the water line. On another occasion we rented the chairs and sat for hours it seemed, but not one girl ever materialized. When we left, I had to pay VND85,000 for rental, and for the beers and coffee we drank.

Rooms for rent

We encountered a fat older woman in pyjamas on a bicycle who called out to us. We went straight over to talk to her. It turned out she was not on the game. She had a house with rooms to rent. She thought my Vietnamese friend was a sex worker who had picked me up already and was in the process of taking me somewhere for sex. Matters were explained to her. Ever hopeful she gave my friend her name, her husband's name, and their address, just in case. She said her rooms are cheap, only VND20,000 to 30,000 (US$1.6 to US$2.1) for the night. She was cruising the streets late at night offering people she encountered, presumably prostitutes with clients, rooms to rent for sex. These women who rent rooms may also be cigarette-sellers, or may sell condoms and aphrodisiacs, all part of this sex economy.

Police and local authorities

Street workers are directly involved with the police. One I talked to suggested we go to a resthouse nearby for sex. She told me the name. She said the place was good because it was safe. It was safe because the owner is a policeman.

One girl told me they paid the police VND300,000 (US$21) to be allowed to work without fear of arrest or harassment. I could not ascertain how often. But she says recently there was a raid, and she and another girl, who stands nearby, got off free because they had paid the police already. One girl who had not paid was arrested and taken away.

Dung from the park pays the police VND300,000 a month. Mrs Thuong from the local karaoke bar confided to me she pays the police, but did not say how much. She said her payments for the bar total the amount of VND20 million a month (US$1,250), including rent.

A young Ward (phuong: administrative level below district) civil police worker in uniform came to the hotel reception, and called one of the hotel staff over to their office just across and a little way down the road. It turned out he and his colleagues wanted drinks. For he returned, took a can of Tiger beer and a soft drink from the foyer fridge, and carried these back for them. I asked if he had to pay money. Not this time, he said. If you gave drinks like this when they asked, there was less trouble. Without the drinks, there can be even bigger trouble. Obviously they sat over there in their office and watched the girls come and go. I was told they know everything that is going on. Hotels are required to register room occupancies with the police daily. The hotel owners pay some police individually. But they also have to be in league with everybody who counts so they will not get reported or closed down. For example, in addition to the police, they pay money to the heads of the District (Quan) and Ward, to the medico who carries out health inspections of the hotel staff, to the people who check or service phones, faxes, and so forth, to the tax collector himself over and above the state taxes he comes to collect, to the tourism company which covers all hotel business in the city, to the fire people when they come to check fire safety. And so it goes on. All this keeps them in operation and keeps gangsters out of their hair. Without friends in high places on the take, they may be open to gangster harassment.

Mr Vang says the money they pay the police each month amounts to VND500,000 (US$>30) per policeman stationed at the Ward office (five men in all). That is, two and a half million VND per month, a little over US$150. This is less than I expected, but when this is placed in the context of the hotels they are taking it from, it is a very large amount of money. Vang estimates there are 140 or so hotels in their ward. So that is some VND70 million per man per month, or more than US$3,500. And that means over US$42,000 per policeman per year, amounting to the salary of a very wealthy person in Vietnam.

Midnight, the night before last, after we went to bed, between one and two in the morning, there was a police raid. The doorbell rang. Vang opened the roller door to three policemen. They asked: 'Are you concealing anything?' In other words were there any prostitutes, unregistered with the station, working in rooms. Somehow one of the night staff managed to get upstairs while this was going on and smuggled some couples who came in late up on to the roof. There was a flurry of clattering and banging above us. Lights went on. The police demanded to be taken upstairs to the sixth floor, where the proprietors lived. Ensconced there, instead of the regular proprietors, a married couple who are away on holiday, was the actual owner, mother of the regular resident, an elderly and formidable matriarch. She merely confronted the invaders with VND1 million, cash in hand. They went straight downstairs and left, pausing to issue a certificate of inspection before they departed, showing the place to have been inspected and found clean. Next day Vang showed me this document, red stamp and all. Vang said had the old lady come down to reception straightaway with the million, they would not have even bothered to go upstairs.

At the beach resort I had a conversation with the owners of our guesthouse about the possibility of customers bringing girls back to their rooms. Not possible, they said, for the police do not approve. A few nights later at the karaoke bar with our Vietnamese friends, the girl who was entertaining me asked where we were staying. I told her, and then said: 'Do you know you cannot come back to my room, as the owners said the police do not approve.' She just laughed and replied: 'We simply pay the security people of your hotel and all is OK, no problem. They in turn pay the police. The police understand, because all the policemen know it is a poor place and we all have to get what money we can.'

I talked with a senior plain-clothes detective, a member of a squad responsible for karaoke, casino, prostitution, and drugs. He had a very insightful perspective on things. Yes, he admitted, he is on the take. Owners of premises, prostitutes and others came to him once a month and gave him money, depending on what they could afford. If they did not, he would have little money, because his salary was very meagre. And what they did give him had to be split with his superiors, as he passed on a percentage to higher-ranking officers. If the police closed down all such places, these people too would have no money, and there would be even worse unemployment and economic problems in the city and the country. If karaoke bars, for example, did not have girls there to entertain, they would not get any customers. They had to have girls. Yes, he agreed, the police could shut all these places down, but to what end? The upshot would be massive economic dislocation, and all these people including himself and his own family, would be far worse off economically, perhaps even out of a job.

DISCUSSION

The forms of prostitution in Vietnam are many and varied, with sex being for sale in a vast array of social and industrial situations in towns and in the countryside. There are large numbers of people selling sexual services in the country, with estimates suggesting maybe up to half a million providers at any one time. Sums of money being paid for sex services are also highly variable, but at the top end of the market prostitutes are making high incomes even by industrialized world standards. Those operating in many other sectors are also making plenty of money, much of which is being distributed through a network of kin and business relationships. The amount being taken throughout Vietnam has to be astronomical. No Vietnamese government could be blamed for giving such an industry the nod. At present the government seems to be taking pragmatic steps towards the toleration of the sex sector, while at the same time pursuing a legislative, media, cultural (moral) and policing agenda of discourses and policies which are supposedly intended to combat it.

Prostitution is illegal in Vietnam. It can only continue to exist and indeed flourish with support from the various levels of government, bureaucracies, and the police. Many in power do not want prostitution expunged, despite the vast amount of government, research, and police rhetoric to that effect. This is essentially because they see the economic value in the sex industries. Where this contradiction occurs it is generally interpreted as arising from corruption. But is it corruption in Vietnam? What may seem on the surface to be corruption can, with more insight, be interpreted as little more than a form of income substitution, replacing what Westerners or Northerners would define as taxation or welfare.

Vietnam has no effective state-sponsored welfare system. It is a totalitarian one party state, an administration with little by way of effective taxation mechanisms. People must generally find their own means to provide for their own welfare and this mostly comes down to support from the family. The major implication from this paper is that necessary financial support ramifies from sex workers to family and on to other levels of society, all the way up to the level of state economy itself.

There is an important consequence arising from this: the government and its international financial backers could do well to set aside their discourses and moral stance on prostitution, acknowledge the industry, and recognize the money flow as an important contribution to the economy and to the struggle of individual citizens to survive and live as best they can. Viewed from the perspectives of those involved, prostitutes to police, the economic dependency is crucial and the flow of money equates to salaries, taxes, levies, and welfare.

This study provides quantitative as well as qualitative support for the claims made by Cooper and Hanson (1998) that the sex industry contributes significantly to the economy of Vietnam. Prostitution makes a huge contribution to the Vietnamese economy. Those involved in the sex industries see themselves as making sensible and filial contributions to family, to employer, and the country. Sex workers are perceived by families and their own communities as dutiful daughters and temporary wives, providing not only comfort, support and sexual services to men who reward them with money or material culture, but also crucial financial support for families. Money and materials are moved on in a ripple effect beyond families to surrounding layers of society which are also dependent upon them to a significant degree.

Acknowledgements

The Department of Social Evils Prevention, Ministry of Labour, Invalids and Social Affairs granted me permission to research sex industries in Vietnam. Thanks to all of you involved in the industries, those mentioned by here by the names I have created, and those unmentioned, who gave their time and their insights.

REFERENCES

Andaya, Barbara Watson (1998) 'From temporary wife to prostitute: sexuality and economic change in early modern Southeast Asia,' *Journal of Women's History* 9(4), pp. 11–35.

Askew, Marc (1999) 'Strangers and lovers: Thai women sex workers and Western men in the "pleasure space" of Bangkok,' in: J. Forshee, with C. Fink and S. Cate (eds) *Converging Interests: Traders, Travelers, and Tourists in Southeast Asia*. Berkeley: University of California, Centre for Southeast Asian Studies, Monograph 36, pp. 109–48.

Cohen, Erik (1982) 'Thai girls and farang men: the edge of ambiguity,' *Annals of Tourism Research* 9, pp. 403–28.

– (1986) 'Lovelorn farangs: the correspondence between foreign men and Thai girls,' *Anthropological Quarterly* 59(3), pp. 115–27.

– (1987) 'Sexuality and venality in Bangkok: the dynamics of cross-cultural mapping of prostitution,' *Deviant Behaviour* 8, pp. 223–34.

– (1988) 'Tourism and AIDS in Thailand,' *Annals of Tourism Research* 15, pp. 467–86.

Colimoro, Claudia, interviewed by Amalia Lucia Cabezas (1998) 'A world of people: sex workers in Mexico,' in: Kempadoo, Kamala and Jo Doezema (eds) *Global Sex Workers: Rights, Resistance, and Redefinition*. New York: Routledge, pp. 197–9.

Cook, Nerida (1998) '"Dutiful daughters", estranged sisters: women in Thailand,' in: Krishna Sen and Maila Stivens (eds) *Gender and Power in Affluent Asia*. London and New York: Routledge, pp. 250–90.

Cooper, Malcolm and Jody Hanson (1998) 'Where there are no tourists … yet: a visit to the slum brothels in Ho Chi Minh City, Vietnam,' in: Martin Oppermann (ed.) *Sex Tourism and Prostitution: Aspects of Leisure, Recreation, and Work*. New York: Cognizant Communication Corporation, pp. 144–52.

Do Thi Ninh Xuan (1997) 'To prevent and combat social evils a contribution [sic] to women's progress,' in: Le Thi and Do Thi Binh (eds) *Ten Years of Progress: Vietnamese Women From 1985 to 1995*. Hanoi: Phunu Publishing House, pp. 287–96.

Fordham, Graham (1995) 'Whisky, women and song: alcohol and AIDS in Northern Thailand,' *The Australian Journal of Anthropology* 6(3), pp. 154–77.

Franklin, Barbara (1993) *The Risk of AIDS in Vietnam: An Audience Analysis of Risk Factors for HIV/AIDS Amongst Men and Commercial Sex Workers in Hanoi and Ho Chi Minh City*. CARE International in Vietnam, Monograph Series 1.

Hiebert, Murray (1992) 'More vice, investment,' *Far Eastern Economic Review* (15 October), p. 51.

Hoang, Ba Thinh (1999) *Sexual Exploitation of Children*. Hanoi: The Gioi Publishers.

Kempadoo, Kamala (1998) 'Introduction: globalizing sex workers' rights,' in: Kamala Kempadoo and Jo Doezema (eds) *Global Sex Workers: Rights, Resistance, and Redefinition*. New York: Routledge, pp. 1–28.

Khuat, Thu Hong (1998) 'Study on sexuality in Vietnam: the known and the unknown issues,' *South & East Asia Regional Working Papers* 11. Hanoi: Population Council.

Le, Thi Quy (1993) 'Some ideas about prostitution in Vietnam,' paper presented at the Conference on 'Joining Forces to Further Shared Visions,' Washington DC, 20–24 October 1993.

Le, Thi Quy (1997) 'Social policies to prevent and contain prostitution in Vietnam,' in: Thi Le and Binh Do Thi (eds) *Ten Years of Progress:*

Vietnamese Women From 1985 to 1995. Hanoi: Phunu Publishing House, pp. 297–310.

Lim, Lin Lean (1998) 'The economic and social bases of prostitution in Southeast Asia,' in: L.L. Lim (ed.) *The Sex Sector: The Economic and Social Bases of Prostitution in Southeast Asia*. Geneva: International Labour Office, pp. 1–28.

Lyttleton, Chris (1995) 'Storm warnings: responding to messages of danger in Isan,' *The Australian Journal of Anthropology* 6(3), pp. 178–96.

Lyttleton, Chris (2000) *Endangered Relations: Negotiating Sex and AIDS in Thailand*. Amsterdam: Harwood.

Mai, Thuc (1997) 'On the model of women's participation in the fight against prostitution,' in: Thi Le and Binh Do Thi (eds) *Ten Years of Progress: Vietnamese Women From 1985 to 1995*. Hanoi: Phunu Publishing House, pp. 311–8.

Muecke, Marjorie A. (1992) 'Mother sold food, daughter sells her body: the cultural continuity of prostitution,' *Social Science and Medicine* 35(7), pp. 891–901.

Murray, Alison J. (1991) *No Money, No Honey: A Study of Street Traders and Prostitutes in Jakarta*. Singapore: Oxford University Press.

Murray, Alison (1998) 'Debt-bondage and trafficking: don't believe the hype,' in: Kempadoo, Kamala and Jo Doezema (eds) *Global Sex Workers: Rights, Resistance, and Redefinition*. New York: Routledge, pp. 51–64.

Ngo, Vinh Long (1993) 'Vietnam,' in: Nanette J. Davis (ed.) *Prostitution: An International Handbook on Trends, Problems, and Policies*. Westport, Connecticut: Greenwood Press, pp. 327–50.

Nguyen, Van Chinh (1997) 'In search of work: socio-economic change and seasonal migration in northern Vietnam,' in: 'Social Change in Rural Vietnam: Children's Work and Seasonal Migration,' *Political and Social Change Working Paper Series* 13, pp. 39–65. Canberra: Department of Political and Social Change, Research School of Pacific & Asian Studies, ANU.

Population Council, Vietnam (nd.) *Access to Reproductive Health Services of Sex Workers in Ho Chi Minh City*. Research Report 7.

SEASIA LIST (1999) Child prostitution. SEASIA-L@LIST.MSU.EDU, 11 June.

Walters, I. (2004) 'Prostitution: trends and policy implications for Vietnam,' in: L. Husson Olivier-Vial and J. Baffie (eds) *Prostitution in Southeast Asia*. Marseilles: IRSEA/CNRS, in press.

CHAPTER 5

WHAT IS KNOWN ABOUT GENDER, THE CONSTRUCTS OF SEXUALITY AND DICTATES OF BEHAVIOUR IN VIETNAM AS A CONFUCIAN AND SOCIALIST SOCIETY AND THEIR IMPACT ON THE RISK OF HIV/AIDS EPIDEMIC[1]

PAULA-FRANCES KELLY

Vietnam at the dawn of the twenty-first century is continuing to experience the effects of the dramatic economic changes which commenced in 1986. The social changes taking place in its society are of the type that support the economic changes. Therefore this is a case study of a country in transition during an era of increasing globalization which is ominously accompanied by the HIV/AIDS pandemic.

The context can be briefly described as one in which Vietnam, a society developed from feudal roots, is undergoing rapid economic change resulting in changes in personal values, still inexorably linked to the rhetoric of traditional values as they pertain to gender, sexuality, and the family. Vietnam is a country which has been plunged into conflicts for centuries. It has been colonized, annexed, and controlled. Each invading group has influenced the prevailing cultures of the time, but, in the areas of sexuality and gender, there is an abundance of evidence to show that it has been the Chinese who have stamped their culture most deeply on the Vietnam psyche. As rulers for ten centuries (110BC–AD 902) and for two other short terms, 1407–27 and 1788–9, they instilled the precepts of Confucian philosophy which fitted well into the framework of the feudal society. It is a philosophy and structure which has much to say about the 'natural' roles of men and women, women being of less importance than men. The label 'Confucian' refers to Imperial Confucianism, defined as an ideology with the ritual support of the emperors, i.e. the justification of the patriarch's right and the delegated authority imbuing those who exercised power on his behalf. Nowadays in modern but in many respects, still feudal Vietnam, this patriarchal privilege tends to be bestowed on all men in general.

Gender and sexuality are social constructs. Acceptance of the status quo is the result of a process of educating formally and informally from birth: parents, society and institutions are the base educators. They pass down and maintain rules based on sex segmentation and the constructs of what it is to be male and female bounded by specific 'appropriate' behaviours.

Gender as a social construct is a new concept in Vietnam. In fact, there is no word in the Vietnamese language which can encompass the concept. It has been introduced to academic, welfare, and development circles by Western professionals. The word *gioi* (a classifier in the linguistic sense) is used by those who have learned about the concept of gender, but is not common currency among the general population. Unfortunately this misunderstanding has meant that the research results of studies by non-Vietnamese have not generally taken this into account. In work on sex, sexuality, and gender, the writer has found that only well educated people with health or development backgrounds are likely to have the Western understanding of the concept. Even now, when discussing gender it usually refers to the roles of men and women, especially the unequal situation of women in relation to men.

The category of study called 'sexuality' is still rather new outside Vietnam, although a substantial amount of work had been done on it in Europe, the United States, and Australia. It seems that its importance has emerged more unequivocally since HIV/AIDS has loomed large as a serious health and social problem:

> The urgent need for a state response to HIV/AIDS has placed sexuality much more firmly and explicitly on the public agenda then on any previous occasion (Ballard 1992).

A definition of sexuality appropriate to Vietnam[2] could be along the following lines:

> Sexuality is a social construction of a biological drive; it is multi-dimensional and dynamic. An individual's experience of sexuality, therefore, is mediated by 'biology,' gender roles and power relations, as well as by factors such as age and social and economic conditions. Perhaps the most profound societal influence on an individual's sexuality comes from prescribed gender roles – the social norms and values that shape the relative power, responsibilities, and behavior of women and men (Zeidenstein and Moore 1996).

Because of concern about gender equality expressed by the government, international NGOs (INGOs), multi-lateral, bi-lateral agencies, and Viet-namese agencies and institutions, most research has been carried out into the roles of women, the construct of women's sexuality, changes in women's entrance into decision making bodies, and gender in the family, the society and history with an emphasis on the crucial roles played by women. What these analyses have missed is:

... a men's studies' perspective that seeks to understand how men in Vietnam understand and experience themselves as part of 'having to be a man' in Vietnamese society (Harris 1998).

Hanh of the Women's Union in Hanoi calls for the current policy agenda to:

... Increase men's responsibility for and access to reproductive health care, impact of HIV/AIDS on women, and domestic violence (Hanh 2001).

Delving into the area of current gender inequalities, this paper presents what is known about the constructs of sexuality and how these constructs have allowed a situation in which HIV/AIDS amongst sexually active young people and adults will continue to develop. The paper emphasizes the role of men and masculinity within the cultural framework of a society strongly influenced by Confucianism. Regardless of awareness campaigns, which admittedly do not take into account the very reasons for the dominant values, or of behaviours and inequalities of gender, the constructs of sexuality for men and women are ignored and little is even known about masculinity.

This paper emphasizes masculinity because, whilst the construct of sexuality for women has been very well researched over the years as noted in this text, virtually nothing is known about the construct of sexuality for men – what is known are no more than the results of the construct i.e. men's attitudes and behaviours and patriarchal institutions as Connell (2000) puts it:

Masculinities do not first exist and then come into contact with femininities; they are produced together, in the process that makes a gender other.

Cogently Caplan's warning needs to be heeded because in Vietnam masculinity is not actually researched, as a topic although aspects of the 'world of men' have been documented. In society masculinity is treated as 'fixed' i.e. natural. This is certainly still so in Vietnam. Caplan (1987) sees the problem as one of lack of theory:

The problem is that masculinity is so often treated as an ontological category which is fixed because of the power which men share in relation to women. The alternative view, which would see masculinity as a social role defined by the expectations of other, tends to assume it is easier for men to change than it has proved to be. This is partly because of the institutional and social power men share, but it is also related to the forms of inherited masculine identity which have so rarely been theorized.

RETURNING TO 'TRADITIONAL' GENDER ROLES

Having posited the problem of the neglect of a conceptualized masculinity, it is time to return to 'traditional' gender roles as these developed under Confucianism. Barry (2001) argues that globalization has reinforced traditional behaviour and values. She supports this with a distinction between two contradictory forces: 'universalism' and 'particularism.' She sees the latter a force against globalization, as a:

> ... Resurgence of traditional beliefs combined with renewed emphasis on traditional cultural practices ... as ... peoples' efforts to maintain their own cultural particularity in the face of globalization that homogenizes and depersonalises, renewed emphasis is on cultural traditions, beliefs and practices.

While this phenomenon she states, can be found everywhere, it is particularly noticeable to a writer in Vietnam where, regardless of socialist policies, laws, and the community rhetoric of equality and egalitarianism, women and men are aspiring to traditional gender roles which can be presented as a reversion to 'patriarchal feudalism,' a turning back of Vietnam to the era of Confucian dominance.

There is evidence to argue that in Vietnam, globalization is but one force driving society towards particularism. The other major force could be the collective fear of the reality of HIV/AIDS: the laying of blame on women and the lack of any official or societal responsibility placed on men for the spread of the virus. Returning to the traditional cultural roots is thus a smokescreen for the rejection of the equality brought to men and women in the north of Vietnam in the era of the post-French occupation and in the south in the post American Vietnam war period (1975). Now at one level the rhetoric is of equality, but the common attitudes, and consequently behaviour, are otherwise.

This situation continues to have dire consequences for the population at risk of HIV/AIDS, as this paper reveals.

The direct link to these attitudes, values, and behaviours is the construct of sexuality in society for both boys and girls which enables the status quo to reject those sorts of social changes which could address the current economic injustices of aggressive globalization. It could put men into a situation in which they must take responsibility for HIV/AIDS and it could promote equal social decision making, including those in personal relationships, such as in the family (as prescribed by law).

RECENT RESEARCH INTO HIV/AIDS, GENDER, AND SEXUALITY

A paper presented by two CARE Vietnam staff at the Regional AIDS Conference in Manila in 1997 outlined the perceived limitations of the HIV/AIDS programme. There were stated as: '... Mainly a lack of natural and human resources at all levels and across sectors.'

Like other papers based on research into the epidemic, at no time was there any mention of the huge limitation of information on which preventive programmes could be based. They would include information on why men and women behave in ways which augment HIV spread. What are the messages which girls and boys have received as they grow into adulthood about their sexuality i.e. social definitions of masculinity and those of femininity?

Since 1997, there has been such a wealth of research pursued in Vietnam by institutions, academic centres, and International NGOs into childhood messages for girls in the social areas of gender, health and family – but nothing of substance about boys. The writer research into the construct of sexuality for women who was the HIV/AIDS co-ordinator for CARE Vietnam to 1997, proposed and was funded in 1996 through AusAID within CARE. This was completed and other research publications have followed (papers presented by P. Kelly at conferences in 1997, 1999 and 2001).

The major body of research into relationships comes in the form of history cast in the scenario of a comparison between then and now. The 'then' leans heavily on Confucian values and systems. All research published is vetted for its philosophical stance by the Ministry of Culture. Little wonder that most research, which is passed as official discourse, compares the present very favourably with the grim past of colonialism and feudalism. This has become the official discourse. However, some academics, while agreeing that it is much better now, still note some problems. In her book *The Rule of the Family in the Formation of Vietnamese Personality*, Dong Thi Hoa (Le Thi),[3] ex-professor of philosophy, ex-director of Centre for Family and Women's Studies and ex-editor-in-chief of *Science on Women and Family Today*, has a statement in the forward that her work is to be:

... A contribution to the carrying out of the Human Strategy laid down by the Vietnam Communist Party Seventh Congress and the objective of promoting the rule of the family, which is set forth in the National Plan of Action for the Advancement of Vietnamese Women Toward 2000 (Le Thi, 1999).

A publication by Khuat Thu Hong (1998) gives the history of the changes in attitude and behaviour throughout different historical periods and reviews the literature. She emphasizes the strength of the Confucian traditions. Her work is a social cultural history of recorded anecdotal descriptions of changes in aspects of sexuality. It shows that culture is not static. Although it does not give evidence of why masculinity or gender is as it is, it certainly makes the point, perhaps not overtly, that Vietnamese culture has not been static but has been influenced to different degrees by Chinese, French, American, and Russian values. She too sees deficits in current research.

For over a decade, Le Thi Quy has written extensively and convincingly on the position of women as sex workers, victims of domestic violence, and trafficked persons. Her work shows bravery in its forthrightness and the ability to present research facts that are not culturally or politically palatable is for a large part attributable to her forging 'new ground' fearlessly. Her work leaves no one in doubt that there is very little, if any, gender equality in current society, its families, and its institutions. Pertinently, her research covertly points to the increasing vulnerability of women to infection with HIV/AIDS as a direct consequence of the social conditioning of men and women. Again the method of conditioning – the construction of the eventual inequalities – are not part of her research on women. She is, as is the writer of this paper, now turning her mind to this void in research.

Reports stemming from 'Save the Children Fund' (SCF, UK) in Vietnam on HIV/AIDS issues in the period 1995–8 have information on the behaviour of men who cannot necessarily be identified as 'gay' or 'bisexual' but simply as 'other.' SCF conducted projects with such men, followed up by research into their knowledge, attitudes, and behaviour relating to the HIV/AIDS risk. Although these reports remain unpublished, they point very clearly to the pressures exerted in families pushing boys to follow the norms of the masculinity constructed by the culture. Also they point to the strongly homophobic attitudes in the culture, which are manifested in discourse about sexuality, homosexuality, and behaviour. Behaviour related to this includes the ridiculing and the ostracizing of those who do not conform to male norms in public.

In research circles what would indubitably assist and will need to be officially encouraged is a focus on ethnographic research into the systemic causes behind the gender situation which leads to increasing numbers of predominantly young people, but also older people, entertaining attitudes and behaviour which are risky in the era of HIV/AIDS. The symptoms of inequality, at structural, social, and familial relationship levels, can be a point of departure for their research. Addressing symptoms afresh themselves will be a never-ending fruitless task which can only militate against efforts to prevent HIV/AIDS spread. Addressing the causes has the potential to stop symptoms in future amongst newly sexually active young men and women.

In the footsteps of Harris (1998), this paper call for: '...Significant, indepth, inter disciplinary research on gender in Vietnam that includes men.'
One place to start is the construct of masculinity and femininity and the institutional, educational, and social forces that both develop these constructs in society and maintain the status quo under the banner of 'traditional culture,' namely that based on Confucianism. Phan Xuan Nam, an academic, leaves no doubt about the role of culture in the formation of personality, but refers only to that of men, not that of people in general:

> Culture is primarily to build a Vietnamese man who is featured by the following characteristics: eager for good ideals, morals and personalities; having a good soul, good sentiments and life-style; being intelligent and capable of creative work; being capable of making his own happiness of his family harmonize with that of the whole community (Nam 1998).

It is easier to research and write about gender as it exists and women (structures and the like) than to investigate what messages a traditional culture actually imbeds in the psyche of its men. Messages which lead to gender relationships and which appear to hinder new-found knowledge on gender issues being internalized by men falls on deaf ears, according to Harris (1998).

It seems that men and women are constricted within tight circles of behaviour and constraints by a framework of 'traditional culture,' which has been developed from Confucian roots, and then promoted and maintained by Vietnamese men over the centuries, a form of patriarchy in fact. Even now under a socialist rule, which has been embraced by the vast majority of Vietnamese people and is a source of national pride, men maintain behaviour and hold attitudes which they declare are 'natural.' Subjection to social conditioning means women accept, but do not necessarily agree with, the role and behaviour expected of them as women. Jamieson (1995) explains such a situation in terms of patriarchy.

> Patriarchy is male-identified insofar that it creates the ideas that core cultural ideals about what is good, desirable and preferable are embedded in the masculine and not the feminine.

Harris (1998) notes the level of gender scholarship in Vietnam. He states that:

> There is a significant and glaring duality in the scholarship on gender produced by Vietnamese scholars of gender. On the one hand, these scholars have continued to support the immutable centrality and importance of the female in 'family happiness,' while on the other hand, they have also argued that women have the duty to play a significant role in the larger public social, economic and political sectors. This complex perspective has created a theoretical and practical tension: It has resulted in the uncritical acceptance and support of Vietnamese women's 'double burden,' and concentrated on women's rights and women's welfare, without pointedly examining the dynamics of gender relations of family and work life that would require attitudinal and behavioural changes by men.

Focus groups with women from a stratified sample of city dwellers (CARE International 1996) have been shown to be in strong agreement with what Harris realized two years later. Initially, there was not one positive answer initially to the question 'Do your enjoy being a woman?' The resounding 'no' was eventually tempered in the discussions by the fact that only women can be mothers and this was the best part of femaleness – the rest was extremely difficult physically, socially, and emotionally. They are hampered by huge, unshared physical and social burdens and the responsibility for all emotional and moral aspects of the family placed on them by a male-oriented culture as part of the 'natural order.' This is verified by all research on Vietnamese women.

WHAT IS KNOWN ABOUT MASCULINITY

In a study on Vietnamese mobile men, Beesey (1998) stated four findings about masculinity. In a nutshell being a man, according to the data collected, means that: he has sexual urges that need to be satisfied regularly and quickly; he cannot control sexual urges, and thus being away from home justifies needing sexual outlets; and he partakes in the four sorts of behaviour that define masculinity: smoking, drinking, gambling, and patronizing sex workers. In the face of 'temptation,' his defence or resistance is weak. Taking refuge, he asserts that peer pressure means that others deride men who are not skilled in the 'four pleasures' as being effeminate, sick, or abnormal.

There is no tolerance for a variety of masculinities. The four pleasures bind men and one, in conjunction with the others, according to Beesey, appears to act as a way to define male relations as well as to imbue a notion of a male culture.

Previous research by Franklin (1993) and other CARE research (until 1998) is validated by Beesey's study. Among the data she has generated (1997–8), the writer also has statements from group interviews, many of which confirm the above, such as:

> He is not a man, he is like a woman and he is scared of his wife so cannot gamble or go to prostitutes if he wants to with his friends. He does not share either smoking or drinking with friends (men) so we do not want to be with him (statement collected by the writer in 1998).
>
> Men who are not men are like women – weak and have no logical thinking power or the ability to organize and do heavy work. (statement collected by the writer in 1997).

Homosexuality is mocked in Vietnam, but not outlawed.

Sex workers agree that men need sexual release quite often and that:

> As the women aren't supposed to have sex before marriage and that men are supposed to be unable to control their sexual drive, there must be somebody to please them. So the men who aren't married, who didn't have girlfriends or who can't have sex with girlfriends will end up buying sex (CARAM 1999)

Beesey (1998) concludes:

> The notion of a male culture where men have a certain visibility and superiority in public life is evident in Vietnam. This is played out in many societies by men having certain privileges, such as intimate and sexual access to more than one female partner. This is often a remnant of past traditions, mainly of the aristocracy. It seems to manifest more among the middle classes and those of a higher socio-economic status.

This of course is the opposite to what Socialism wishes to achieve.

Harris (1998) explains that the men's behaviour as outlined by Beesey is the result of the patriarchal system:

106

Vietnamese patriarchy is one in which men maintain power and privilege, and claim these as rights because they provide production, protection, and 'responsibility.' Ironically, in the public sphere, male activity can range from leading other men to the most de-based subordination by other men. But as heads of families, the role of the Vietnamese man has been that of a king.

The writer concurs with this summary by Beesey and statements (such as the above) of Harris. From her ten years of observation and formal and informal interviews she sees it as part and parcel of current Vietnamese men's norms. It must ineluctably be based on very shallow information about Vietnamese masculinity as no solid studies, which demonstrate the void in data, have been carried out.

MESSAGES ON MASCULINE AND FEMININE DESIRED BEHAVIOUR

Tracing the development of cultural attitudes and the rewarded behaviour of boys and girls from early childhood through school and social institutions to adulthood, it should be possible to explain the actual social construct of sexuality for both men and women. The great hiatus is that there is a void in the data about the messages boy-children and young male adults actually absorb. This is not so for women.

Women know from where the messages which construct their sexuality actually derive. They are well acquainted with their Confucian roots. They are taught to be 'feminine' from a very young age and many can relate examples of these lessons. These messages come first from the family, and older women are custodians of traditional values and practices. Later they are reinforced by their communities, schools, and employment or higher education. The lessons cover the three obediences and the four virtues (below), not so much as a litany but in a system of rewards, punishments, and socialization, so that she imbibes gender role tasks and skills in relationship maintenance – all regardless of her desires and her will.

The three obediences (*tam tong*) refer to women's submission to men in the context of social-cultural relations, which plainly undervalue women's status. She must be obedient: to her father when unmarried and still living at home (*tai gia tong phu*), to her husband when married (*xuat gia tong phu*), to her eldest son if widowed (*phu tu tong tu*) (Kelly and Jarvies 1997, Hai 1996 and others).

The four virtues (*tu duc*), which, although they have been officially redefined by socialist ideology, still define what a woman is, what is femininity and what is her virtuous soul. Families still quote them to their children. They are:

- Employment (*cong*): Good at managing domestic activities such as housework and agricultural work.
- Appearance (*dung*): Women should strive to appear fresh and appealing, and dress correctly. She should be beautiful.
- Speech (*ngon*): Polite in speech. Not talkative or loud-always quiet.
- Morality (*hanh*): Allowing her movements to be dictated by parents, her husband, and even parents-in-law. Never noticing another man (Kelly 1997, Hai 1996).

Covertly or overtly researchers report that these rules still apply to women, more so in rural areas, but they are also alive and well in the cities (for a recent example, see Gammeltoft 1999). While some researchers see that changes have happened, the on-going research of the writer has consistently shown that the rules are still fairly solidly entrenched in reality. Indubitably it must be admitted that urban rhetoric has certainly changed among those who are interviewed by foreign researchers.

While divorce is now more common, the seven grounds which fifteenth-century Confucianism (*that xuat*) featured as rationale for men to divorce or take another wife are still quoted when discussing whether or not a wife is moral, worthy and so forth. For many centuries, a wife could be sent from the family and lose the status of a wife for the following reasons: barrenness, bad conduct, neglect of parents-in-law, being coarse and loud, theft, jealousy and ill-will, and for suffering from incurable diseases (Lilejestrom 1991, Hai 1996).

Today she can still be rejected for reason 1 and severely reprimanded for reasons 2, 3, and 4, although the new family law recently enacted should have freed her from this situation. It may still assist in changes in family and community attitudes in the long term

From childhood, women in Vietnam, like those from other Confucian influenced cultures, 'owe' their parents a moral debt that cannot be repaid, and before and after marriage they live in guilt when family members stray, and family face is lost. They accept that it is their 'fault' and so it is perpetuated (Kelly and Le 1999, Jamieson 1995, Tam 2001). Men do not shoulder any responsibility for such things. Somehow they are not taught that this is a shared responsibility or their responsibility, they alone are 'head of family'.

SOME MESSAGES WHICH MAY INFLUENCE THE CHILD'S CONSTRUCT OF MASCULINITY

Preference for boys

From conception the story of boys' and girls' sexuality and social development is different.

Boys are preferred to girls, although individual couples openly say they personally do not have a preference, their families have, so that ancestor worship – taught to boys from childhood but not to girls – will not flag. The reasons why this is a men-only duty is explained, as 'the nature of manhood.' As the saying goes 'being female is a stigma in itself' and this is certainly true in Vietnam.

> 'A hundred girls are not worth one boy.' This saying had both economic as well as moral significance: the male child ensures succession, he 'brings' to his parents, in addition to the heritage, a daughter-in-law, an extra work-hand for the family. Feeding a daughter on the contrary, is an unprofitable investment (Mai and Le 1978, quoted in Kelly and Jarvies 1997).

It is clear that as they grow up boys and girls must absorb the comments made by relatives and friends about the luck of having boys and the slight mocking, by other men and sometimes women too, albeit in 'fun,' of the father producing an all girl family.

There is often talk within families about other men who 'have to take another wife' because the first one 'cannot produce a son' (see reason 1 above). When confronted with the misplacement of 'blame' for this, men and women will explain that fluids in some 'unsuitable' women actually kill male sperm, ensuring a girl-only family. Even medical personnel have cited this as fact.

Le appeals for modification of current family preference for and treatment of boys:

> The son is always in a privileged position, enjoying more advantages than the daughter. In modern society, when gender equality and human rights are ensured by the State and society, out-dated education should be modified, first and foremost in the family environment (Le Thi 1999).

Father's Role

The treatment of boys and girls as children is very different, although in interviews this is more likely to be denied.

Most fathers express that they treat sons and daughters equally. Most families pay little attention on the methods of rearing children, therefore there is no consciousness in teaching sons differently from daughters. But, if specific questions were asked, such as 'Do you teach your daughter how to worship their ancestors?'. Most fathers answered 'no'. Some fathers said they would not mind teaching if their daughters insisted on learning (Ngan 1995).

The message of how to be an adult male must come at least in part from the boys' own role models – first fathers, then uncles. Fathers in Vietnam are to be feared. The UNICEF sponsored research by Ngan (1995) summarizes thus:

Children fear their fathers more than their mothers. Children are less afraid of their mother than their father simply because the latter is bigger and stronger. Plus, as fathers are the primary disciplinarians, they prefer that their children fear them so that obedience would naturally follow. Another reason is that mothers are closer emotionally and physically to children.

One man in the Ngan research explained why children fear fathers. His opinion is a common one in Vietnam:

Because I see so little of my children, they are more afraid of me than they are their mother. I like for them to fear me, so they can respect me. I think sometimes it is good to keep a respectful distance ... I think that mothers tend to always give in to children; it's a part of their nature, showing their gentle side. And they always forgive children, even very bad ones. Fathers, on the other hand, should be tough and strong figures. They should be the main disciplinarian in the family. Mothers tend to spoil the children. But, fathers who do this are not good.

The writer has witnessed what in her culture amounts to emotional cruelty to children (and wives) paraded under the banner of 'maintaining respect': children ridiculed, belittled, ignored, blamed for father's sorrow/anger/situation in general, and sometimes beaten.

Le Thi (1999) calls for a change in these traditional patterns of family behaviour:

In the old-type family, patriarchy was a great power in unconditionally subjecting children to their parents. This 'parental dictatorship' cannot exist in the present society imbued with democracy and equality. On the contrary, there should be discussion, exchange of views and mutual respect in considering family affairs.

Media and folk tales

Over the years films on television and indeed many traditional folk tales depict this 'respected,' 'austere' father who underneath is very kind – but this kindness is meted-out at his leisure and most unevenly. Do these cultural constructs reinforce or strengthen the messages which boys receive? Research on this topic is unavailable.

Pertinently, messages in Vietnamese media and publications are very much of a military, bellicose style in words and visuals (uniforms). Although these messages might have been expected during the American–Vietnam war, now they could be developing potentially more aggressive men than is in line with the policies of socialist Vietnam. American authors on male sexuality point to the images of military men as important in developing aggressive and 'brave,' 'powerful' aspects of masculinity. However, the 'soldier' role is less overt in the cities now so perhaps those boys currently moving towards teenage hood may not be as influenced. Rural 'boys,' it appears will continue to be influenced.

Lack of communication skills

This non-communication by and austere presence of the father most likely tells boys that to be men, in the presence of the family unit, they must behave as did their fathers before them. To some extent, this could explain why men are reported in so many studies (Beesey 1998, Kelly and Jarvies 1997, Harris 1998, Franklin 1993) as being very poor communicators. They do not need to learn intimate and relationship-building communication techniques, because they learn very quickly that this is unnecessary for men: masculinity constructs require minimum communication.

These studies report that men and women do not communicate adequately with each other and this hampers their ability to discuss issues of a personal nature, including safer sex practices. Some researchers state that the failure to discuss sex is the result of it being a taboo subject. Sex is in fact a very commonly discussed topic between same sex groups in Vietnam. Women joke about sex with other women as men do with other men. Some women's jokes actually shock some non-Vietnamese. The rub is that the verbal communication male to female is very poor and the non-verbal communication of either aggression (male) or submission (female) is better practiced and more heavily loaded on the male side. Some examples of this are: 'I get what I want by simply pretending to give in to him,' 'I do not hit my wife because she never talks too much,' and, 'in the end men must appear to be right if you want a happy home' (writer's files).

On the basis of both general development theory and of the women's own stories it can be confidently claimed this 'fatherly behaviour' influences the women's role and behaviour when, as girls grow into women, they learn to be 'indirect' in communication with men to keep them happy and avoid any possible confrontation/conflict. The girl sees the mother responding according to her own childhood role models – she is long-suffering, gentle and placates her husband. She is not talkative or nagging for were she to be so, there is a strong chance it would result in domestic violence towards her and even the children (CARE International in Vietnam 2000, Quy 1994a). Women state that this message is very strong.

Conversely, the message no doubt received by the young boys of the family is that women are 'owned,' 'controlled' and receive meted-out pleasures in the form of non-aggressive male behaviour – provided they do not 'overstep the line.' They are subject to the whims of their fathers, husbands, and elder sons as in the three obediences (above). However, the results of this behaviour on the later male ideal of the boys has not yet been researched.

Plainly, because of the hierarchical order of society, men have difficulty in actually communicating with other men when they move out of teenage-hood. Alcohol assists communication and it is very, very superficial communication and most unsophisticated. Despite its shortcomings, at least it lowers the barrier constructed by age and class, albeit only for a short time.

Men do not discuss all about themselves with other men like women do with women. They would be seen as weak and a bit stupid. We keep all of us inside us. That takes strength. We show anger, hate and joy through other than speech. This is how really strong men communicate (Writer's collected texts 1998).

Children's games
Children's games are played along gender lines and the encouragement of 'girls to be girls' and 'boys to be boy' must assist in the construction of their sexual identity.

Even now girls are not encouraged to play energetic games. 'They get sick.' Being female they have 'thin blood.' 'They get over-excited.' By the time they reach school-age they have already taken on much of what is required for womanhood (writer's interviews with families and women.)

No encouragement of difference

It is clear that there is no tolerance in Vietnamese society for any form of masculinity other than the culturally dictated variety. Conformity, thus harmony within society (Confucian values), is narrowly constrained and does not allow for different masculinities. Families, it could be argued, would do sons a disservice if they accepted patterns of masculinities developing among their sons which deviated from the norm. These sons will be ridiculed as men or by-passed as rational beings by future employers. (Cases of both of these treatments exist, one being presented as the reason for seeking refugee status in a foreign country in 1998).

The situation does not stop 'difference' and those who feel that they cannot follow the role, attempt, sometimes successfully, to lead another secret life away from the family with other like men (Franklin 1993 and writer's collected interviews 1996–2001).

Although marriage is part of being a good son, indeed as it is in many cultures, some men who do embrace different masculinities[4] and do not marry, but most do and they must, of course, produce sons. The clandestine lives of these men, unmarried or married, outside the family, are not spoken about by the community, but are well known and only brought up publicly when men drink together. Conformity in all things is any family expectation of its members.

A CARAM document (1999) describes the Vietnamese society's overwhelming need for conformity thus:

> In Vietnamese society, the pressure to conform is very high. People are expected to follow a social order that is defined quite precisely in Confucianism. One is expected to fulfill his/her duty towards family and to obey those in positions of authority. Marginality, independence and critical thinking are not valued. People often easily follow advice, with very little question, from their family, the elderly, neighbours, friends and figures of authority. People do not want to distinguish themselves from the masses ... They will consider it as a proof of respect for the social order, a proof of their respect for fulfillment of filial duty, friendship.

In research, it has been related by women that conformity starts at a very young age and this has been verified by some men (as anecdotes) and written about by anthropologists (Gammeltoft 1999, Rydstron 1998, Soucey 2000) and other men. They all acknowledge that sexuality is imprinted on the minds of girls and boys by using masculinity and femininity as extremes of powers or negatives depending on one's sex. Boys are reprimanded for being 'sissy', namely behaving like girls, and girls are reprimanded for activities acceptable only for boys – climbing trees, running, shouting, hanging-out with friends, being untidy. In fact, many mothers refuse to let sons do any housework at all, lest they become too 'sissy' or, worse still, '*be de*' which is a term for transvestites, but used in common language for gay men or those deemed effeminate. It is a derogatory term linked to the general homophobia of the culture. Harris (1998) states very strongly that:

> Masculinity and femininity become authoritarian constructions of a form of 'gender-tyranny' in which men and women become trapped. As subjects to patriarchy's arbitrary power that is supported by the fear of going against its tacitly enveloped ideology, women and men have become locked into roles; roles that have very narrow bandwidth. Through the policy and practice of male supremacy ... The socialization to the belief system of patriarchy, which is rooted in an ideology of male domination, sustains a system of gender norms that act as a mechanism for the social control of women and men.

Household responsibilities
A quick glance at the household responsibilities of boys and girls around the same age (see below) leaves no doubt that boys and girls are allocated their gender roles long before they are old enough even to define their own sexual identity. These gender roles run parallel to the messages of masculinity and femininity and must be influential in the current masculine and feminine behaviour of Vietnamese.

Table 5.1 Rural Household Activities of Children (aged 10–13 years)

Girls	Boys
6.00 – Wake up – Give mother a hand to cook breakfast	
6.30 – Eat breakfast	6.30 – Wake up – Eat breakfast
7.00 – Go to school	7.00 – Go to school
11.30 – Go home – Eat lunch – Wash up	11.30 – Go home – Eat lunch
12.30 – Have a rest	12.30 – Have a rest
13.30 – Clean up the house, root out weeds, pick up vegetables, do shopping	
	14.00 – Learn

16.00 – Learn	
	16.30 – Have rest or entertainment & bath
17.00 – Give mother a hand to cook dinner, give bath to younger sister or brother	
18.00 – Eat dinner & wash up, prepare animal fodder, have a bath	18.00 – Eat dinner – Have a rest
	19.00 – Learn
19.30 – Learn	
21.00 – Enjoy some entertainment	21.00 – Enjoy some entertainment
22.00 – Go to bed	22.00 – Go to bed

Source: Que, 1999

It must be stated that the situation depicted above continues when the children are adults with women working 15–18 hours per day and men 8–12 hours (in rural areas) as outlined in every document on women in development in which gender is raised. One quote here will suffice:

> If the woman does everything, what is the gender equality in the family? From survey figures computed of three target families of peasant, worker and intellectual, the results are almost homogeneous with only differences in degrees: customarily, husband and wife co-operate in production; in the country in the North, however, it is the wife who is responsible for the heaviest load of work and most of the phases of agricultural production; as for domestic chores, she is the sole doer (Le Thi 1996).

Stoltenberg's essays strongly suggest that the continuation of trying to live up to the socially constructed masculinity leaves women doomed to being second class citizens. As yet this has not been articulated in Vietnam, but 'hints' have come forth through academia.

> So long as we continue to try to act in ways that keep us still 'men,' we are doomed to paralysis, guilt, self-hatred, inertia. So long as we try to act as men, in order to continue to be men, in order to do our bit in the social construction of the entity that is the sex class men, we doom women to injustice: the injustice that inheres in the very idea that there are two sexes' (Stoltenberg, 1989).

115

He calls for men in general to change this absolute to allow sexual identities to be many:

> Male sexual identity is not a 'role'. Male sexual identity is not a set of anatomical traits. Male sexual identity – the belief that one is male, the belief that there is a male sex, the belief that one belongs to it – is a politically constructed idea (Stoltenberg, 1989).

Instant gratification for boys

Boys, it could be said, learn that instant gratification is their birthright. This appears to be reinforced at least in games in the comments of family and friends and in the allocation of family tasks (as above). It is necessary to discover if these childhood messages have influenced adult men in their feelings about their right to rule the family, their sexual desires and gratification for and with more than their permanent partner, and their refusal to use 'condoms' because of diminished pleasure. The strong need for approval from other men and, for some men, the fear that their wives and children have of them could also have had their origins in messages passed on through family discourse, games, and dictated roles.

Coping

There is evidence in research data from international NGO sources (CARE, SCF (UK), World Vision, CARAM) dealing with HIV/AIDS which, although not identified as such, points very strongly to a marked difference between the coping mechanisms of women and men, particularly when away from home.

When men are away from home for work or play, they require excitement and turn to drinking and sex (with sex workers). They do this when absent for longer periods too. They seek alcohol and sex when they are suffering from alienation and loneliness. Cogently in these situations they actually seek out close relationships with women in preference to casual sex (Trang 1999).

They do this because they feel unable to be emotionally or physically alone. From the data, they also appear to need the power over their own lives that they have in their families and local communities. They need to redeem their personal identities, lost when out of their own environments. The CARAM project repeatedly identified in different environments these features of men's adaptive behaviour in its research from 1997 to 2001. Research available does not throw any light on what it is about their 'manhood' constructs in childhood that leaves them in such desperate need. This situation is crucial to the effective dissemination of HIV/AIDS

116

programming at the moment and research is needed to discover how best to tackle this situation.

On the other hand Vietnamese women who travel for fun, seek gratification other than 'sexual fun.' Women's tourism is a new phenomenon in Vietnam. They usually also travel in groups as do the men, but display very different behaviour both within the group and outside it (the writer's texts from interviews 2000 and CARAM research 1997).

Women away from home for longer than holiday periods are usually there to make money for their families, in factories or the entertainment industries, and many end up in, or seek out sex work (De Bruin and Starink 2001). At times, families are involved in aiding traffickers to entice these women (Kelly and Le 1999, Schunter 2001, Tam 2001).

Pertinently, in none of the recorded cases, do women seek anything other than remuneration for families when they travel for long periods away from home. This may be internally (other provinces) or externally (Korea, Japan, Taiwan, Middle East, Libya, and others). They usually go in the capacity of overseas labourers, with the exception of these going to a marriage arranged prior to leaving home.

The women are much more emotionally resourceful and need no assurances of their sexuality when out of their usual environment. Some relationships develop, but women do not actively seek this (Trang 1999). Mobile men therefore are the prime users of the sex industry and continue not to practise safer sex.

Masculinity tied to reproductive ability

In Vietnam, masculinity appears to be strongly tied to the reproductive systems of men. If they 'do not work' i.e. cannot have intercourse or cannot father a child, somehow they believe they will become unintelligent, stupid, and unable to work using their strength. Evidence of their views can be found in explanations for why women, not men should be sterilized, as a birth control method.

> I think male sterilization may affect the intelligence of men and it also affects coordination.
> Some say sterilization makes men stupid so we dare not do it.
> A sterilized man is considered to be like a capon. They will know nothing and become stupid, their intelligence will decrease. So they don't dare to [have it done] (Population Council 1997).

Beauty cult

Women are generally viewed as beautiful toys (observation and interviews with women and men). Although this is quite common in many societies, it is particularly striking in a socialist state which, unlike its socialist counterparts in China and Cuba, has never discouraged displays of the sexuality of women and men in the public, institutional, and educational domains. People in Vietnam relate sexually. At meetings women and men make it very clear by their behaviour that they are asserting their sexuality and this is seen as acceptable. 'We think that is normal until we go overseas' (ex-student).

The writer has grown used to this too and was quite surprised to discover that this sexual interplay in behaviour was not present in the same social and work circles in China. The Chinese explained that this is a 'very Vietnamese characteristic.'

There is general denial in discourse on gender that women are outgoing and not actually shy about their sexuality (CARE sexual data 1996 and 1997). Certainly they 'play the right game.' As they grow up the virtues taught are congruent with society's attitudes, which are actually very overtly sexual. The writer described this at a conference in 1997 when she questioned how men (foreign) can say that the 'air is electric with sexuality,' when society proclaims that women are there to be beautiful, but passive playthings before marriage and honourable mothers after.

Part of the thesis she presented is reprinted here because it raises the question of what messages boys, youths, and men receive via public displays and support of the sexuality of girls and women – even within educational institutions.

> Girls in Vietnamese families display their sexuality and are encouraged to do so at an early age. Girls are taught by society to attract the attention of men in their behaviours and their decoration from an early age. Two-year-olds, as cute little dolls with make-up, are taught to stand provocatively for photographs. Six-year-olds, clad in adult style 'sexy' beach attire and full face make-up are photographed by proud mothers and the photographs are admired by both men and women amongst comments of the sexuality of the girl. School girls have as their official uniform, a form fitting white pajama style outfit (*ao dai*), which is seen as very graceful and feminine, shows off her shape, makes movement very restricted (e.g. riding a bike) and is often see-through, displaying the undergarments carefully selected by the young student to be 'sexy' – and, according to Vietnamese men and international tourist men, the sight of this frail beauty in full virginal white, is one of the most erotic scenes in Asia – a daily scene all over Vietnam (Kelly and Jarvies 1997).

This is reinforced in the press. The following is an example in a business magazine 'culture' page with photographs:

> The *ao dai*'s lap's grace and elegance has made the wearer constantly careful, fearful of her own manners as she walks, stands, talks, smiles, thus the gentle, tender trait of an Eastern woman is enhanced.
>
> 'Laps of silk *ao dai* were lissome. Like white butterflies flying in the school yard' (butterflies have a sexual connotation, in such a statement it refers to female genitals). In films they may even mean that sexual intercourse is about to take place or is taking place.
>
> The *ao dai* has harmoniously combined delicate provocative traits, both modern and traditional, expressing the keen beauty conception of the Vietnamese in the world cultural exchange spirit: deeply, intimately concerned with people's character (Vietnam Business, August 1996).

Educational institutions also reinforce the sexuality of girls by making women teachers wear *ao dai*, which restrict their movements, and may certainly not be their own choice, while men teachers wear comfortable trousers and shirts. The messages to male youth must reinforce all that develops into a bulwark of gender inequality and reinforces the approval of women as decorative playthings. The status quo is maintained with the support of the Education Department.

HIV/AIDS AND MASCULINITY

Table 5.2 Official number of Persons Tested Seropositive for HIV as of January 2001

Person status	Total	Percentage	
		Men	Women
Persons infected with HIV virus	29,220	86%	14%
Person living with AIDS	4,830		
Persons who have died from AIDS related illnesses	2,443		

Source: NAC, Hanoi January 2001.

119

The number of HIV-seropositive persons has steadily increased since the first person, a woman, tested positive in 1991. The numbers of men and women show that the cases tested positive are predominantly men. This is probably more to do with the system of mandatory testing of drug-addicted people, who are predominantly men. Also the number of women found to be positive is predominantly amongst the sex workers because of the testing sample. The true picture can never really be discovered.

However, continued accepted behaviour of men, the result of society's construct of masculinity discussed in this paper, does not lead to great confidence that the HIV/AIDS epidemic will begin to subside. Men's power over women, their feelings of invincibility, 'I am strong, I know about these things' stand in the way of common sense. The situation is exacerbated by the assumed need for sexual gratification from more than one partner, 'Men need variety like eating "rice then cake" or "eat rice (wife) and eat *pho* (lover)",' coupled with a refusal to use condoms because of their 'reduced pleasure,' their poor communication skills, their submission to male group norms, and the need for freedom from any female control and from any responsibility for the consequences of their actions. This last is expressed in such excuses 'I go to prostitutes when she (the wife) nags me,' Over and above this is their inability to say 'no' when comfort is offered by a potential sex partner because a perceived physical need takes over from rational thinking: 'Men simply cannot refuse physically.'

HIV/AIDS programming has been directed mainly towards women, particularly women with multi partners. Trying to change the attitudes and behaviour of women and girls within the family and in the current patriarchal society is virtually impossible (e.g. trying to get them to take responsibility for safer sex when it is men who decide this) without some solid research on why men act as they do. Developing programmes to change the family and institutional settings in which current male dominated attitudes are developed and maintained remains too difficult an undertaking, unless they are based on the known data.

This cannot simply be attributed to the 'culture' – cultures are subject to continuous change. Vietnamese culture has reverted back to its 'traditional' style leaning more on Confucian values and mores. It can change again – other cultures have had to do this too in this era of HIV/AIDS.

Wolffers (2000) summed up the situation:

If researchers and authorities are about dealing appropriately with the AIDS threat in Asia, they will have to face these challenges. It is not useful to look at Asian societies from the point of view of cultural romanticism, but confront the realities and survival needs of populations that are living there at this moment in Asia. Culture is not a homogeneous and constant system that controls the lives of people.

Socialism today and the construct of masculinity
In a culture which can now be seen to be reverting to even stronger traditional roles, a change in attitudes and behaviour turning away from the dominant view would be very difficult for Vietnamese men. Even the statements by the leader of the ruling Communist Party in the April 2001 National Congress stated that the Party must 'fight individualism.'[5] The speech was very masculine using words and images drawn from revolutionary rhetoric. It is too difficult for men to not be 'men' as dictated by the norms, without a huge re-think from the top through to the grass-roots levels. However, it is a socialist system which could facilitate this far more easily than other forms of government. People in Vietnam look to the government for guidance, and are very comfortable with being directed by the government.

The socialist government has a philosophy of egalitarianism. Its political system ensures that the 150 representatives on the Communist Central Committee are, in fact, democratically elected from the grass-roots to the highest honour (unlike some democracies in which being wealthy enough to mount a campaign is an essential ingredient).

The laws on gender equality and the rights of women are in place and, in fact, women in Vietnam have greater opportunities to sit on decision-making bodies than women in any other neighbouring countries. Women generally agree that the situation is a direct result of socialist governance, albeit as a 'benevolent gift' (Oanh 1994).

There is little doubt that the construct of male sexuality could be questioned and changed by such a government. This could see the laws on equality and respect for others were followed and could ensure that men had less pressure on them to keep up the current and destructive 'male face.' Relationships in families could be more open and men and women could learn to communicate better about issues of power and sexuality. Boys growing up would not always be confronted by the role models and messages which (although there is no solid research as yet to know exactly what these are) mould 'men' into the current model of manhood. This is the one which brooks no deviation from the model set, causes injustices to women, supports rigid gender roles which keep them in power in families and society, and is responsible for the continuation of the HIV/AIDS and STD spread in Vietnam.

Cogently, it must be pointed out that only ten (fewer than before) out of the 150 members of the Central Committee are women as of the April 2001 National Congress of the Communist Party. This low number is criticized in that it is believed that there will be less chance of decisions being made which reflect women's attitudes. The fifteen members of the Politburo are all men.

The writer is concerned about whether this will really erode the gender equality balance even more in favour of men. Vietnam may well be different. It has been men who have developed the laws on equality since socialism was introduced. The women of Vietnam have not had to fight with men for their rights in some sort of Vietnam feminist uprising, they have been given them by the men through the due process of the law. The writer believes that it is the family itself whose values have reverted back to those based on old Confucian values, including feudalism, which opposes the changes in the population required to be able to follow the laws of equality. The return to the traditional cultural roles and attitudes towards sexuality of the population, not the government itself, is what currently dictates the rigid masculine and feminine roles. It is very hard to legislate in this regard and to implement the laws on equality already in place.

NOTES

1   The paper is a result of ten years work in Vietnam where only now the author feels she is asking the 'right' questions. The paper draws on research and experiences of the writer while with CARE International in Vietnam and then with other agencies, with Vietnamese and International organization partners and as a consultant. It also draws on research reports by a range of researchers and organizations.
2   Accepted when presented to the SCF (UK) team working on training packages on sex, sexuality, and rights, after the writer and the team debated the issues surrounding it.
3   Work published under the name of Le Thi.
4   The term 'different masculinities' is preferred to heterosexuality and homosexuality, the two most commonly discussed masculinities. This term is not a euphemism for homosexuality or other than heterosexuality but one which is now appearing in sexuality literature written by men to mean the range of masculinities in less defined extremes.
5   *Vietnam News* 20.04.01 'Nation to pursue further reform and remain firmly on the socialist path,' p. 3.

REFERENCES

Anh D. N., (1991) 'Position of Women in Two Rural Communes,' in: R. Liljestrom and T. Lai (eds) *Sociological Studies on the Vietnamese Family*. Hanoi: The Gioi.

Anh, T. and Le Hung (1997) *Women and Doi Moi*. Hanoi: Women's Publishing House.

Ballard, J. (1992) 'Sexuality and the State in Time of Epidemics,' in: R. Connell and G. Dowsett (eds) *Rethinking Sex, Social Theory and Sexuality Research*. Australia: Melbourne University Press.

Barry, K. (1996) 'Industrialization and Economic Development: The Cost to Women,' in: K. Barry (ed.) *Vietnam's Women in Transition*. London: Macmillan Press Ltd.

– (2001) 'Gender, Work and Sexual Sexual Exploitation in the Global Economy: Indo-China in Transition,' paper presented at the Conference on 'Gender in Indo-China,' 3–4 March 2001, Women's Action Resource Initiative, Bangkok.

Beesey, A. (1998) *The Crossroads of Risk and Responsibility – Truck Drivers and HIV/AIDS in Central Vietnam*. AusAID.

Caplan, P. (1987) *The Cultural Construction of Sexuality*. London: Routledge.

CARAM (1999) *Preliminary Results of Sex Workers* presented at the 5th ICAAP in Kuala Lumpur 1999.

CARE International in Vietnam (1994–8) Research findings (unpublished) 1994–8 and presented by Paula Kelly to conferences in 1995–8. Archival raw data (tapes and text) released for disposal (now with Paula Kelly).

– (2000) *Proceedings of Seminar in Domestic Violence: Addressing the Issue of Violence in the Home*. HCMC, 14.2.2000. CARE, NOVIB, Love Marriage Family, HCMC

Connell, R. (2000) *The Men and The Boys*. Australia: Allen and Unwin,.

– (1995) *Masculinities*. Australia: Allen and Unwin.

Connell, R. and G. Dowsett (eds) (1992) *Rethinking Sex: Social Theory and Sexuality Research*. Australia: Melbourne University Press.

De Bruin, L. and M. Starink (2001) *Mobility and Vulnerability: Sex Workers in Ho Chi Minh City*. Vietnam: MRSC.

Foreman, M. (1999) *AIDS and Men*. London: The Panos Institute/Zed Books.

Franklin, B. (1993) *The Risk of AIDS in Vietnam*. CARE, Hanoi.

Gammeltoft, T. (1999) *Women's Bodies, Women's Worries: Healthy and Family Planning in a Vietnamese Rural Community*. U.K.: Curzon/ Nordic Institute of Asian Studies.

Gioi T.M. and C. Esposito (1997) 'Facing the Entire HIV/AIDS Epidemic in Vietnam,' paper presented at 4th ICCAP Conference, Manila.

Hai L.N. (1996) *An Analysis of Gender Inequality in Vietnam's Patriarchal Society*. Thesis (MA) Mahidol University, (unpublished) Thailand.

Hanh, L.B. (2001) 'Women, Gender and Reproductive Health, HIV/AIDS,' paper presented at the Conference on 'Gender in Indo-China,' 3–4 March 2001, Women's Action Resource Initiative, Bangkok.

Harris, I. (1995) *Messages Men Hear: Constructing Masculinities*. London: Taylor and Francis.

– (1998) 'Incorporating Men into Vietnamese Gender Studies,' *Vietnam Social Science* 5(67), Hanoi: National Centre of Social Sciences and Humanities.

Hong, K.T. (1998) *Study on Sexuality in Vietnam: The Known and Unknown Issues*, South and East Asia Regional working papers 11, Hanoi: Population Council.

Jamieson, N. (1995) *Understanding Vietnam*. USA: University of California Press.

Kelly, P. and D. Jarvies (1997) ' The Construct of Sexuality for Women in Today's Vietnamese Culture,' paper presented at 'Beyond Boundaries: Sexuality Across Cultures' Conference, 29 July–1 August 1997, Amsterdam.

Kelly, P. and D. Le (1999) *Trafficking in Humans From and Within Vietnam: The Known From a Literature Review, Key Informant Interviews and Analysis*. IOM, Radda Barnen, SCF(UK), UNICEF.

Kelly, P. and D.T.N. Tam (2001) 'It's Time to Fill the Knowledge Void: Gender Knowledge in Vietnam,' paper presented at the Conference on 'Gender in Indo-China,' 3–4 March 2001, Bangkok: Women's Action Resource Imitative.

Khan, S. (1994) *Making the Visible the Invisible*. London: The Naz Foundation.

Le,Thi (ed.) (1995) *Vietnam Family: Responsibilities and Resources in the Changing of the Country*. Hanoi: Social Science Publishing House.

– (1996) 'The Women and The Family With Issues Posed to Ensure Happiness and Gender Equality Within The Family,' in: *Vietnam's Women Transition*. International Political Economy Series General Editor: Timothy M. Shaw.

– (1999) *The Role of the Family in the Formation of Vietnamese Personality*. Hanoi: The Gioi.

Le, T.N. and X. Vuong (1991) *Reproductive Culture in Vietnam*. Hanoi: The Gioi.

Liljestrom, R. and T. Lai (1991) *Sociological Studies on the Vietnamese Family*. Hanoi: The Gioi.

Mai, T.T. and T.N.T. Le (1978) *Women in Vietnam*. Hanoi: Foreign Languages Publishing House.

Nam, P.X. (1998) 'On the Identity of Vietnamese Culture in Regional and Global Cultural Exchange,' *Vietnam Social Sciences* 2(64), National Centre for Social Sciences and Humanities.

Ngan, N.T. (1995) *Role of Men and Grandparents in the Families in Viet Nam*. UNICEF.

Oanh, N.T. (1994) 'The Absence of Cultural Change and Gender Awareness,' paper presented at Gender and Development (GAD) Workshop, Vancouver 2–7 May 1994.

Plummer, D. (1999) *One of the Boys*. The Haworth Press, Inc

Population Council, Vietnam. (1997) *A Study of Vietnamese Youth's Decision. Making for Healthy and HIV/AIDS Prevention in Kien Giang and Quang Ninh Provinces*. UNAIDS/UNCEF and the Ministry of Education and Training.

Que, T.T. (1999) *Gender Basic Concepts and Gender Issues in Vietnam*. Hanoi: Nha Xuat Ban Thong Ke.

Quy, L.T. (1994a) *Reports*. Hanoi: Centre for Family and Women's Research.

– (1994b) 'Domestic Violence in Vietnam and Efforts to Curb it,' in: *Fire in the House: Determinants of Intra-familial Violence and Strategies for Its Elimination*. Thailand: UNICEF.

Rydstron, H. (1998) *Embodying Morality: Girls Socialization in a North Vietnamese Commune*. Sweden: Linkoping University.

Schunter, B. (2001) 'Where the Children Sit,' paper presented at the Conference on 'Gender in Indo-China,' 3–4 March 2001, Women's Action Resource Imitative, Bangkok.

Soucy, A. (2000) 'Masculinity and Reproductive Health: The Imperative and Integrated Approach to Gender,' paper presented at the Gender Donor Group Meeting, Hanoi. (Unpublished).

St Pierre, M. (1996) Unpublished papers on homosexual and bisexual men's knowledge attitude and behaviours regards HIV/AIDS

– (1998) Unpublished reports to SCF(UK) as part of PhD study into Vietnamese men who identify as outside the constructed male boundaries.

Stoltenberg, J. (1989) *Essays on Sex and Justice*. Meridian.

Tam, D.T.N. and P. Kelly (2001) 'Families Culture and Trafficking,' paper presented at the Conference on 'Gender in Indo-China,' 3–4 March 2001, Women's Action Resource Imitative, Bangkok.

Tam, D.T.N. (ed.) (2001) *Telling It Like It Is: The Action Research Project of CARAM in Vietnam*. Vietnam: MRSC.

Trang, N.N.N. (1999) *Vietnamese Migrant Workers and their Vulnerability to HIV/AIDS*. KIT thesis, Amsterdam (unpublished).

Vietnam News (2000), 20 April, Vietnam.

Vietnam Business (1996), August edition, Vietnam.

Vietnamese Studies 3(108) (1993) 'The Traditional Family in Transitional Period,' Xuhasaba, Hanoi, Vietnam.

Wolffers, I. (2000) 'La recherche sur les maladies sexuellement transmissibles en Asie face aux défis lancés par le VIH et le sida,' in: M.E. Blanc, L. Husson and E. Micollier (eds) *Sociétés asiatiques face au sida.* Paris L' Harmattan, coll. 'recherches asiatiques,' pp. 147–68.

Zeidenstein, S. and K. Moore (eds) (1996) *Learning About Sexuality: A Practical Beginning.* New York: Population Council/International Women's Health Coalition.

CHAPTER 6

THE BROKEN WOMEN OF CAMBODIA[1]

ANNUSKA DERKS

Sex work is not a universal or a-historical category (Kempadoo 1998:7), but involves a diversity of forms and actors, and it is subject to change and redefinition. An analysis of sex work should therefore consider the historical, political, economic, and cultural context in which it takes place. The context in which this paper on sex work is set is Cambodia. The unprecedented volume of the sex business in Cambodia is related to many different forces that have shaped the country after its opening up since the beginning of the 1990s. Yet, prostitution is not a new phenomenon in Cambodia. For a better understanding of the development of the sex industry in Cambodia, I will give a historical background to prostitution in Cambodia and will provide an overview of the diverse practices related to sex work in present-day Cambodia.

Pertinently I will pay attention to how sex work is perceived in the Cambodian context. Views on sex workers are closely related to ideals of what is proper behaviour for women and notions of sexuality as well as perceptions of ethnicity. The current attention paid to the trafficking of women and girls has raised the matter of the practice of prostitution in connection with the more common issues of choice and coercion in prostitution, which in the common perception are also related to the issue of ethnicity. Yet, individual experiences with sex work are more diverse and this aspect will be analysed through the various ways women and girls become involved in sex work, as well as by examining their working and living conditions.

A HISTORICAL OVERVIEW

Prostitution is not a recent phenomenon in Cambodia, although it has not always existed in the same forms or on a similar scale as it does nowadays. Lack of documentation regarding prostitution in the early history of Cambodia makes it difficult to delineate any clear picture. Although there is plenty of speculation about *apsaras* – the celestial beings adorning the walls of Angkor – as dancing girls in the Angkorian times, there is no concrete evidence about their specific role. According to the description of Chinese traveller Chou Ta-kuan, thousands of concubines and palace girls were 'serving' the King. Serving the King in this way was regarded as an honour, for 'when a beautiful girl is born in a family, no time is lost in sending her to the palace' (Chou 1993:13). This kind of court or temple prostitution is, however, very distinct from the secular prostitution, or sex work, practised at a later stage in Cambodian history.

Archival sources indicate that during the French colonial period, prostitution was practised in various urban centres within Cambodia. Concerned with public health and morals, the French administrators issued a number of decrees in order to regulate the *filles publiques*. According to these decrees all sex workers, whether working in *maisons de tolérance* – brothels – or independently were obliged to register with the police after which they received an identity card, which also had to be presented for the obligatory medical examinations. Special police and medical units were in charge of surveillance of sex workers. These measures were imposed on sex workers of all races and ages,[2] but the half-yearly taxation for brothels with Chinese or Japanese women was higher than for brothels with indigenous (Cambodian) or Vietnamese women. Sex workers were subject to certain behavioural codes, which denied them access to bars and forebade them to attract attention by employing inviting gestures or talk. When women wanted to stop working as a sex worker, they had to change their status at the police station and justify of their assured means of making a livelihood.

After independence sex work continued to be pursued in urban centres. There are, however, few records on the practice, except for those discussing the 'vices of prostitution' and its deleterious influence on Cambodian society. During the period under Lon Nol, from 1970 to 1975, sex work was more openly practised as various sex establishments opened up in urban areas. The sex business, thought to consist of predominantly Vietnamese women (Tarr 1996) also absorbed some of the refugees who filled the urban centres, most notably Phnom Penh, in order to escape the civil war and bombing then raging in the countryside (Shawcross 1991). This situation changed radically when the Khmer Rouge took power and emptied the cities, abolished money, markets or any kind of exchange relations. Prostitution was banned and all kinds of extramarital sex were punishable by death. During the 1980s sex work began to be practised again sporadically, though the Vietnamese-backed socialist regime imposed measures to control the practice. With a view to maintaining security and social order, sex workers were arrested and taken to an island in the Mekong for re-education and rehabilitation (Cambodian Women's Development Agency 1995).

Restrictions regarding the practice of sex work have undergone major changes since the beginning of the 1990s. After three decades of civil war, dictated ideology, and political instability, Cambodia had begun a transition from being a closed socialist system to becoming a capitalist open market system. The economic liberalization and the opening up of the country have created new economic possibilities and allowed for a freer movement of people. These processes have also been accompanied by an increase in the numbers of sex workers in the urban areas. This increase was initially stimulated by the arrival of approximately 20,000 civilian and military personnel during the United Nations Transitional Authority in Cambodia (UNTAC) in 1992 and 1993. Brothels, bars, and nightclubs flourished in Phnom Penh and the major provincial towns. Although the estimated number of sex workers somewhat decreased after UNTAC withdrew, studies have indicated that problems related to this military-inspired phenomenon, like the number of young girls in prostitution, the number of women trafficked, and HIV/AIDS infection rates among sex workers, have increased.

In an effort to deal with problems and immoral practices related to sex work, the government pursued a policy focusing on a crackdown of sex establishments. The policy, however, did not prove to be very effective. As critics pointed out brothels, which were closed in one location simply opened up again in another, often under the cover of a karaoke bar or massage parlour. Undoubtedly, corruption and the involvement of the police and military in the sex sector ensured that not all establishments were shut down. In 1999, after running a pilot project in Sihanoukville, the government decided to take a more pragmatic approach by implementing the so-called 100 per cent condom use strategy. The 100 per cent condom use strategy, copied from Thailand, is a campaign focused especially on countering a threatening HIV/AIDS epidemic and is simultaneously used to keep a check on sex establishments.

The problems associated with sex work have also prompted a large number of local and international organizations to work in the field. Their activities vary from HIV/AIDS education, medical services, and empowerment activities for sex workers to rescue operations of under-aged and trafficked sex workers.

BROKEN WOMEN AND VIRTUOUS WOMEN

The women in the Cambodian sex industry serve a demand for sexual services among different categories of customers, who are predominantly local Cambodians, but also overseas Chinese and other businessmen, expatriates, and international tourists. The women working in the sex industry are not all of them local Cambodian women. Most of the foreign women employed come from neighbouring Vietnam, while in some larger, more expensive establishments women of different nationalities, including some from the former Soviet Union, are catering for the richer niche customers. These women who work as sex workers contribute to the financial gains of those who control the sex business (brothel-owners and recruiters, as well as military and other officials protecting and supporting the business), but are also in a position to remit funds to their (usually rural-based) families of origin (Muecke 1992).

Though the scale of Cambodia's sex business is related to its economic profitability,[3] perceptions of sex work are determined much more by the socio-cultural context. Perceptions of sex workers are closely related to notions of ideal female behaviour and sexuality. In Cambodian society a range of legal and customary codes, Buddhist precepts and teachings, and traditions or norms of conduct guide various kinds of ideal or correct behaviour depending on status, age, and gender. The *srey krup leak* – perfect virtuous woman – is usually presented as industrious, sexually naïve, timid in the presence of males and is, when unmarried, always a virgin (Tarr and Aggleton 1996). The sexuality of a Cambodian woman is of utmost importance to her own reputation and to that of her family. For an unmarried woman to lose her virginity would lead to an enormous shame for the woman as well as for her family, and therefore her virginity needs to be protected (Ledgerwood 1990). This means that ideally a young woman should remain at or close to home, and preferably never leave the house without the company of a trusted relative. This control of female sexuality and of behaviour towards men are themes that can be found in various texts, folk-tales, and customary codes. A well-known monk remarked on this:

In our society, we have to take care that our daughters be good daughters. A good daughter, from the Khmer point of view, does not stray far from home. As the Khmer saying goes, 'Do not keep a good dessert for tomorrow; do not allow a woman to go far'...Our society places a value on the virginity of women. It is not like Europe or America, where they do not care about daughters who go away. Khmer men take care of virgins and, if parents do not allow their daughters to go [or work] far from home to study, we cannot blame them, because they know their daughters will lose their future if they lose their virginity.

Tarr and Aggleton (1996) have pointed out that contemporary social reality regarding female sexuality does not necessarily comply with such imaginary accounts of what it should be. Though the idea of Khmer tradition and traditional behaviour is highly cherished, after decades of war and dislocation Cambodian society is not isolated from the global flow of money, goods, ideas, culture, and people. These dynamics affect the possibilities, desires, and understandings of young Cambodians, including those related to sexuality (Tarr 1996).

The moral implications of these new possibilities, desires, and understandings are not the same for men as they are for women. Promiscuous behaviour by women is morally condemned, while men are not actively discouraged from having multiple sexual experiences before (or after) marriage. Visiting sex workers seems to be seen a 'perfectly normal form of entertainment' among many (especially urban) men (De Lind van Wijngaarden 2000). The disparaging term *kouc heay* – literally broken already – used to refer to a woman who has had sexual intercourse before marriage, is not applied to men in the same sense. The term *kouc* is also more generally used for disobedient children, but when used for women, i.e. *srey kouc*, the term refers specifically to women who have had multiple sexual partners and is most commonly used for prostitute. Literally *srey kouc* means 'broken' or 'damaged' woman, and refers to a woman who has gone bad and is considered to have been spoiled, physically or socially. Prostitutes are not only considered to be runned because of their sexual behaviour, but also because they use a language, are active at times, occupy spaces, and take liberties which are not open to 'virtuous' women.

Though *srey kouc* is the most common term used for a prostitute, many other terms exist, such as *srey sompheng* – sluggish woman; *srey pkar meas* or *srey peehsya* – golden flower girl; or *srey bon* – brothel girl. The negative connotation of the various words used for sex worker has induced NGO workers to use a less stigmatizing term, i.e. *srey rook sii plew peet*. The term *rook sii*, literally to find something to eat, means to do work to earn money, or to do business. A *srey rook sii plew peet* is thus a woman who is earning money by selling sex. This term comes closest to the English 'sex worker.' Sex workers, however, usually refer to themselves mostly as *srey kouc* or *srey luek kluen*, a woman who sells her body.

The various terms for sex workers are inextricably linked to moral ideas about the sexuality of women. Yet, as in any society or culture at any time, present-day Cambodia has to deal with many conflicting values and ideals. Ledgerwood has pointed out that 'on the one hand daughters are supposed to be protected, on the other, the teenage daughter must bicycle all the way to the city and sell her goods in order to support the family' (Ledgerwood 1992:5). Changing circumstances, opportunities, and practices have forced women to undertake all kinds of employment, even if this means moving far away from their own family. Young women, attracted by the thrills of modern-city life and by the idea of earning lots of money, are also tempted to exchange agricultural life in the village for work in the city. This explanation is, however far too facile. Very often, the need to support the family financially has left some young women with few other choices then to leave their home village and take up jobs that are not considered to be respectable but through which they can fulfil their obligation to support their family. This onus on familial obligations is thought to be especially strong for women. A sex worker elaborated on this:

> In general, in the case of Khmer children, the sons do not take care of their families very much. The main responsibility for the support of their family falls fairly and squarely on the shoulders of the girls. People think that all the responsibility which a boy might have for his family will finish after he gets married. Girls even if they become sex workers, they will always take care of their family.

SEX WORK AND ETHNICITY

Besides their link with notions of female behaviour and sexuality, perceptions of sex workers are commonly related to perceptions of ethnicity. For many Cambodians there is a clear link between prostitution and Vietnamese women. Not only are Vietnamese women considered to be very beautiful because of their fairer skin, they are also considered to be more sexually skilled than Khmer women. In her study about sexual behaviour among young Cambodians, Tarr quotes a 22-year old student who explained in detail how a Vietnamese sex worker actively seduced him and then noted:

'I would never expect a Khmer girl to behave this way. If she did I know that she would be like the Vietnamese… you know that Cambodian women must not initiate love-making or demonstrate they know how to suck your cock or do other things with you. It is not our custom to permit such things to occur…' (Tarr 1996:91)

Therefore, as Prasso wrote, prostitution is considered to be 'un-Khmer.' 'The rationalisation is, because all Khmer women are virtuous, all prostitutes must be Vietnamese'(Prasso 1995:22). One member of the local authority in Phnom Penh even argued that it is a cultural trait of Vietnamese families to put their daughters into prostitution.

> Nearly 100 per cent of the Vietnamese girls here are prostitutes. It is their tradition, even if the daughter is from a rich family. They usually sell their daughters themselves. For example, they sell the girl

to work with a *meebon* [brothel owner] for a while. Then she has to work for many months or years to repay her parent's loan.

Pertinently it is not only social, cultural, and somatic factors which feed the conviction among many Cambodians that most of the sex workers in Cambodia are ethnic Vietnamese. Compounding these factors comes the historico-political component that Vietnamese women have always been regarded as an important tool used by the Vietnamese to enter Cambodia. According to Cambodian chronicles, the first introduction of the Vietnamese to Cambodia took place at the beginning of the seventeenth century, with the marriage of King Chey Chestha II to a Vietnamese princess (Phnara 1974). In a popular version of this story, the Vietnamese king consciously used his daughter as a means to get a foothold on Cambodian territory, knowing that the Cambodian King would immediately fall in love with his beautiful daughter. Their marriage created the opportunity to send Vietnamese settlers to the Mekong Delta, with permission of King Chey Chesda, and 'enabled the Vietnamese king to lay the groundwork for overtaking the area' (Leonard 1996). The region in question is still known among Cambodians as Kampuchea Krom, or 'Lower Cambodia.' Thion refers to this particular story as a 'mixture of historical facts and legends' that is used as 'irrefutable proof of the "sordid use" of young girls' (Thion 1993:47) by the Vietnamese. This belief in the seductive powers of Vietnamese women forms a recurrent theme in various scenarios of how the Vietnamese will try to take over Cambodian territory. By blatantly wielding their seductive skills, Vietnamese women can easily cajole border police to let them cross over into Cambodia, and their overwhelming presence (especially as sex workers) could, some Cambodians claim, again lay the groundwork for a major Vietnamese take-over or at the very least pose a threat to Cambodian culture and society (Kim 1993).

Though statistical information on the number of sex workers and their ethnicity may not be very consistent, the data available do not give any support to such conspiracy theory or paranoid fantasy about an influx of Vietnamese women as spies for a greater power. In 1997, a National Assembly Commission on Human Rights and the Reception of Complaints recorded over 14,000 brothel-based sex workers throughout the country, of whom 18 per cent were Vietnamese. A 1998 PSI census of sex establishments in Phnom Penh (with Kampong Som the biggest centre for the sex industry) registered fewer than 1,500 sex workers, of whom 38 per cent were Vietnamese. Despite all evidence to the contrary, stereotypes regarding ethnic determinants have remained strong. There is a seemingly ineradicably strong belief that there are significant differences between Vietnamese and Cambodian sex workers. In most cases, the Vietnamese are considered to be

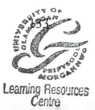

less prone to shame, smarter when it comes to earning money, and more hygienic. This argument can also be heard among Cambodian brothel-owners and among sex workers themselves, who feel disadvantaged in the competition for clients. A health worker explained that this is also related to the way Vietnamese and Cambodian women become involved in sex work.

> Generally speaking, the Vietnamese recruiters who bring Vietnamese women to work as prostitutes in Cambodia give some money to the parents of the women. If the women work in a brothel, the *meebon* takes a certain percentage for board and lodgings. The rest is for the women. This is 100 percent different for the Khmer women. They have all been deceived by the recruiters and by the *meebon*. When a Khmer woman comes to brothel, the *meebon* gives to the recruiter some money and provides her some clothes. After that she is not free to go. The money she earns goes to the *meebon*, and the woman herself does not receive any money. If she wants to leave for another brothel, she has to pay the *meebon* and sometimes she is simply sold to another *meebon*.

This view of the differences between Vietnamese and Cambodian prostitutes ties in nicely with the stereotype of Vietnamese being clever business people, whereas Cambodians are the simple farmers and casual labourers. A *meebon* in a southern province interpreted this in connection with different perceptions of honour.

> The Vietnamese women are not bothered about their honour, because they know that when they go back to Vietnam, they will still become wives. It is very interesting. They earn money for a motorbike, or a new house and when they get married they stop working here. The Khmer women can't earn money, while the Vietnamese women can earn plenty of money and after three or four months they go back to Vietnam. When they return again, they are reinvigorated and can receive a host of customers. They can receive ten customers per day. For them the most important thing is to earn money and they don't spend it. After receiving two or three customers the Khmer women are afraid and don't want to receive more. The Khmer women spend all their money. In the end, only their body remains.

These comparisons contribute greatly to the image that Vietnamese women will do anything for money. Their eyes are firmly fixed on a goal and they are unhampered by a sense of shame or a fear of losing their honour. This is explained by the idea that Vietnamese women who have worked as sex workers are still considered to be on the marriage market once they return to Vietnam. By contrast the Khmer women are described as victims of deception and exploitation who have no idea of how to make money out of a situation so dishonourable it renders them *srey kouc* forever. This point of view may be used by Khmer to confirm their negative image of Vietnamese and strengthen their ideal image of Cambodian women, but it fails to take account of the many similarities in the processes, attitudes, and reasons for entering sex work among both Vietnamese and Cambodian women.

GETTING INTO THE BUSINESS

As described above, in a picture of the calculating, dishonourable, money-hungry, voluntary Vietnamese sex worker is contrasted with that of the poor Khmer girl who has fallen victim to scrupulous and cruel gangsters who have forced her into prostitution. Such views regarding coercion as opposed to free choice in prostitution is not simply merely relevant in the Cambodian context, they form, in fact, the central point of the debate about the practice of prostitution. The fundamental difference in opinion in this debate is, Doezema argues, 'whether or not a person can choose prostitution as a profession' (Doezema 1998:37).

This issue of choice has been approached from various points of view focusing either on the individual characteristics of a woman or on structures and relationships in society (Holter 1994). Authors like Barry have argued that this issue of choice is essentially about 'non-choices.' Treating prostitution as a woman's choice is, in her view, a legitimization of the sexual objectification of women and in all instances prostitution should be seen as a form of male oppression of female sexuality. This assumes that, without such structures, no woman would ever chose to earn money through prostitution, because 'when the human being is reduced to a body, objectified to sexually serve another, whether or not there is a consent, violation of the human being has taken place' (Barry 1995:23).

Such an approach to the issue of choice has been strongly criticized by those who have chosen to emphasize female autonomy and the right to self-determination for women who voluntarily engage in prostitution. They examine a women's choice to enter in prostitution as either a rational, entrepreneurial choice that has to be respected or as a strategy for survival open to women who live in particular social, cultural, and economic structural conditions. Truong (1990) argued that prostitution should be seen as a category of sexual labour that is historically specific and encompasses class and race dimensions. In her discussion, she focuses on the social processes through which this category of labour is incorporated into the sphere of production and reproduction.

These analyses of the structural forces influencing women to enter prostitution should always be distinguished from individual experience concerning choice and the more direct forms of coercion in the recruitment and working conditions of prostitutes. The forms of coercion may vary from outright violence, abuse of authority, and debt bondage to outright deception (Wijers and Lin 1997), and they have been the major focus within the debate of trafficking of women and children for prostitution (and other purposes). The growth in the attention paid to the trafficking of women and children for prostitution is what has been the mainspring in the discussion about the division between forced and voluntary prostitution. Though a such distinction has now become a more widely accepted view, radical sex workers' groups have questioned the usefulness of making a distinction between free and forced prostitution, but for very different reasons to those which motivate authors like Barry. Such a free versus forced distinction, Doezema (1998) claims, puts the old division between the whore and the Madonna in a new light through a dichotomization between innocent victims who need protection and the free-wheeling whores who deserve what they get.

In the Cambodian context, this means distinguishing between those women whose nature, *saa rociet*, it is to be a sex worker, like the Vietnamese women, as opposed to the women or girls who have been forced, against their will, to become a sex worker. A social worker working in a shelter for 'rescued' sex workers also made such a distinction. She claimed that only the real victims of trafficking can be successfully educated to behave like a 'proper woman' and therefore are worth being helped. She quoted to a Khmer saying *kom put sroleuw, kom prodeuw srey kouc* – don't bend the *sroleuw* tree, don't advise a broken woman. The *sroleuw* is a kind of large tree with hard, dense wood. The implication is that prostitutes are as intractable as the *sroleuw* tree, indicating the uselessness of trying to convert a broken woman into a virtuous woman.

It is exactly this kind of dichotomization that sex workers' rights groups have dismissed out of hand. According to these sex workers' rights activists, the real harms stemming from prostitution are caused by moral attitudes and their legal consequences, which lead to the marginalization and victimisation of sex workers. This is also the (official) stance taken by several local and international NGOs in Cambodia which try to organize sex workers to give them a voice to 'speak out' and resolve problems arising from their individual situation as well as from their position as sex workers in Cambodian society.

Cogently, whether viewed as victims of male domination or agents who actively construct their own lives (Weitzer 2000), sex workers' experiences cannot be generalized. Economic, social, cultural, and historical structures as well as individualist characteristics and circumstances must all be examined in the context of the various forms and practices prevailing within the sex industry. In Cambodia the diversity of experiences among sex workers is related to various factors. Sex work is not limited to brothel-based sex workers, but is practised in various ways, some of them indirect. There are huge variations among sex workers regarding the degree and kind of choice they could express about their involvement in sex work. This variation also extends to the social and economic appreciation, control over working conditions, individual experiences, and adaptation to work among and within the various sex work categories. In earlier papers I have distinguished between voluntary, bonded or involuntary ways of entering sex work as a means to classify various experiences. Voluntary entry indicates that the woman, prostitute-to-be, approaches the owner/manager of a sex establishment herself; bonded entry implies the involvement of parents or guardians, who receive money from an agent or owner for giving away their daughter; and involuntary entry conveys the use of deception and coercion of the women by an agent or owner/manager (Hnin Hnin Pye in Asia Watch 1993:45).

I recognize that such distinction may lead to an unwanted dichotom-ization between so-called victims and true prostitutes and that such distinction is in reality not always easy to make. Nevertheless, I have argued that using such a tool in the context of Cambodian prostitution makes it possible to separate distinct ways of entering sex work experienced by individual women. Simultaneously, it leaves open the possibility to explore the underlying structures which cause women to enter sex work.

CHOOSING SEX WORK

A voluntary entry into prostitution assumes a rational choice by women who opt to use their sexuality as a means to earn an income. As such it is an entrepreneurial choice, which is often stimulated by the attraction of the amount of money that can be earned. Other factors like the attraction of a 'glamorous' life-style with beautiful clothes, make-up and jewellery also attract girls and young women to leave their hard agricultural life. A Vietnamese prostitute remarked that she was attracted by the wealth her friend earned in a brothel in Cambodia.

> I followed my friend in coming here. She lived in the same village and she had lived in Cambodia before. I saw that she had jewellery and that she brought money to her parents. So I asked her to take me to work in Cambodia with her.

After hearing about the (financial) advantages of working in sex work in urban centres like Phnom Penh, and even in Thailand, some girls or women do not need any 'guide' and decide to approach the owner of a sex establishment of their own accord. It is usually not difficult to get information from such people *motodup* (motor taxi-drivers) about how and where to find a brothel in which to work. *Motodup* are familiar with the people or places that employ prostitutes and are eager to share this information in return for some commission.

Although the term voluntary entry into prostitution suggests free will, it does not always mean a free choice among the economic alternatives for those women who make their own decision to enter sex work. Often these women took up the profession because they were driven by dire economic necessity within a specific social context. Many women said they ended up in sex work after they had been abandoned by a husband or a boyfriend. Economic alternatives to farming in the slowly modernizing economy of Cambodia are few and far between. It is all that more difficult for women with no or little education. A prostitute in a north-western province of Cambodia explained that for her prostitution seemed to be the only way to earn some money to feed her indigent mother and her five-year-old child, after her husband had left her for another woman.

> I heard that there was plenty of money to be earned in this job. I had no other way. I didn't tell my mother, stepmother, and sister that I came here to work. I just told them that I went to Poipet [on the border with Thailand] to sell fruit for two months. But I decided I wanted to do this work, because it is the only employment in which I can earn much money... I don't want people to say that I am a woman who can't find money. I just try to work hard to make a load of money and I will go back home to start some business, like other people.

BONDED PROSTITUTION

Bonded entry into prostitution entails parents or associates who sell a child or young woman to a person for promised employment in return for cash. Reynolds described this kind of entrance into sex work as a 'fairly consistent and quite distinct model of trafficking' (Reynolds 1996:2) in Cambodia. Reynolds continued that the use of bonded labour to repay a debt incurred either directly by the worker or by an associate of the worker was traditionally a common form of slavery in Cambodia. Osborne has written about the way in which the widespread presence of this practice throughout Southeast Asia is often misinterpreted by Western observers. 'Western observers to the traditional world of Southeast Asia seldom understood the difference, for instance, between "true" slaves, condemned to a life of servitude, and those who had voluntarily, but temporarily, given up their freedom in order to meet a debt or other unfulfilled obligation.' (Osborne 1995:59) He explains that, in theory at least, the condition of these debt slaves was subject to change once a debt had been covered, or an agreed period had elapsed (Osborne 1997:8). Muecke connects this practice to prostitution, referring to it as a 'historical practice of selling women,' which can be found throughout Southeast Asia. Pertinently it has provided an important precedent for the current practice in which adults sell family members, particularly daughters, for economic gain (Muecke 1992:892).

Many of the recent reports written on trafficking and prostitution in Cambodia focus on this involvement of parents, especially mothers, in the trafficking of young women for prostitution. Although it is hard to obtain reliable data on prostitution in Cambodia, some studies have claimed that half of the women and girls were 'sold' into prostitution by their parents or other relatives (UNICEF 1995). Yet, as Reynolds and Osborne have indicated, some care has to be taken in interpreting the concept of sale in these cases. A brothel madam argued that this practice should not be interpreted as parents selling their daughters, which would give her ownership rights over their daughter.

The parents bring their daughters here, but they do not sell them. They come to borrow my money, 40,000 or 50,000 or 60,000 riel[4]. The women have usually worked as a prostitute before. Their parents have taken them to different places. When other people come here to search for women, they want to buy from me but I do not dare to do that, because the parents of these women trust me.

Whether viewed as sale or as a loan, the practice has led many observers to question how it is possible for parents to be involved in introducing their own daughters into prostitution. Almost invariably, poverty is given as the main reason. A UNICEF report states that 'poor families are by definition more susceptible to promises of jobs for their young daughters, often desperate enough to sell their daughters or other relatives to pay of a debt.' (UNICEF 1995:17) Viewed in this light, the practice of debt bondage might be seen as a kind of household survival strategy. However, although important, economic reasons alone cannot explain the involvement of parents in this practice. Another, often mentioned reason is the male dominance in a patriarchal society which means that young women are more easily forced into 'degrading' work for the economic benefit of the family. The Minister of Women's Affairs has also argued that 'it is custom and tradition that allows men to think that women can be beaten, can be sold, can be bought. It is ingrained not just in men, but women also believe that it is their destiny, this is what we need to change' (AFP March 7, 2000). Although question marks may be set against speaking of a custom or traditional of selling and buying women, it has to be acknowledged that this practice is not purely and simply an issue of male mentality. Women play a major part in the practice of bonded prostitution as it us usually the mother (not father) who takes her daughters to a brothel and it is a woman who is managing the brothels.

In an attempt to find out the causes for and cultural background of the involvement of parents who introduce their daughters to prostitution, several authors have pointed at the economic responsibility women feel or are taught to feel towards their family of origin. Muecke has analysed this phenomenon in Northern Thailand and has written about the 'cultural continuity of prostitution.' She says that 'prostitution today is accomplishing what food vending did for the young women's mothers: both of these otherwise disparate endeavours have the effect of conserving norms by which women support the family, village and other basic institutions in Thai society' (Muecke 1992:892). As such, prostitution has become an important means through which young Thai women can fulfil certain cultural obligations towards their family and society.

As in the case of Thai women, prostitution has now opened up a possibility through which Cambodian daughters can also fulfil the cultural expectations of providing financial support for the family. Though the growing garment industry is now absorbing many more daughters, the short-term earnings in sex work can be much higher. A sex worker working in a southern province agreed with her parents to work as a prostitute in order to contribute to the household income that has to support the other nine children.

> I saw that the people who work here [in the brothel] have money and new clothes. They can help their parents... I don't save any money for myself, because my mother comes every month to take it.

With the growth of the sex business parents, often the mothers, are also well aware of the economic value of their daughters. A Vietnamese mother, living in an area of Phnom Penh, explained why she has taken her daughter to a brothel.

We had many debts, because we had to repay the loan we took out for buying a television. I had no money and was weighed down by debts. The owner came to disturb me every day asking for the money. But my husband could not earn enough money. That's why I decided to take my daughter to a shop [brothel]. I got 200 dollar because she was still a virgin.

This shows that the financial support that daughters manage to contribute to family income through sex work not only serves to cover dire economic necessities. In the wake of rising economic standards, the influx of 'modern' products and the media new expectations and desires are created. Under the influence of these rising expectations and desires, some parents will allow their daughters to work temporarily as sex workers to pay back the money borrowed from the *meebon* by which the family can relieve financial debts incurred to fulfil certain desires. This does not mean that bonded prostitution can be considered an accepted practice for the enrichment of families sanctioned by certain cultural norms. The practice may be related to certain cultural concepts and expectations of a daughter and to the obligations and responsibilities of a daughter toward the family, but it cannot be detached from the psychological dynamics between parents and children or from the diverse and sometimes contradictory values regarding acceptable behaviour for women.

TRAFFICKING FOR PROSTITUTION

In recent years the trafficking of women and girls for prostitution has become a major item on the agenda of national and international organizations as well as on that of the government in Cambodia. Trafficking can be defined in many ways, but I found the definition given by Wijers and Lin most useful. They defined trafficking as 'all acts involved in the recruitment and/or transportation of a person within and across national borders for work or services by means of violence or threat of violence, abuse of authority or dominant position, debt bondage, deception or other forms of coercion' (Wijers, and Lin 1997:36).

Though trafficking for prostitution (as well as other purposes) is a problem that requires serious attention, in the media and among some groups the topic has often been approached from a sensationalist point of view, indicating that girls and women are mostly lured, kidnapped, drugged or tricked into prostitution in some other dastardiy way. In my investigations, I found a more diverse picture of women and girls entering prostitution. In fact, many young women left their homes voluntarily and followed their trafficker in the hope of being able to earn a higher income elsewhere. A typical story is of recruiters, sometimes acquaintances, who make promises of a decent job with a high income somewhere in Phnom Penh or in Thailand, which is for many a metaphor for excitement, modernity, and pleasure. The attraction of such promises fosters wishful thinking that there is a way to escape poor living conditions in the countryside. A young woman working in a brothel commented on her recruitment in this vein:

> The woman did not persuade me to leave home. I just met her in the market-place, where the bus stops. She asked me where I was going and I told her that I had left home. She said that she could find me a job, so I followed her.

As in the case of this young woman who had left home because of a family conflict, several other factors combined with economic factors – which are more than simply outright poverty – put certain women and girls at risk of being deceived or forced into prostitution. Various studies have been conducted on the topic of trafficking for prostitution, yet the diverse results show that there are no reliable statistics on how many of the women and girls working in the sex business have been deceived or forced. While this aspect remains obscure, more is known about certain patterns of trafficking.

The persons who recruit the women, by convincing or deceiving them to enter prostitution, are called *meebon* – which is more commonly used for brothel-owner – *neak noam* – the person who takes away – or *meekcol* – a more general term for someone who organizes people for certain purposes. The recruiters are often female and come into a village or stand at entrances to schools or factories in order to pick out the attractive girls or young women. In order to convince the girls of the benefits of coming with her to work elsewhere, the recruiter often takes advantage of situations in which a woman or girl feels maltreated by her parents, other relatives, or their boy-friends. In her 'ignorance' and in her compulsion to escape her present situation, she will easily agree to go along with someone who promises a well-paid job, a new adventure in a big city or another country. A Vietnamese girl described how the recruiters operate to recruit young girls for sex work in Cambodia.

The people who persuade young girls to come to Cambodia are mostly women. They are like friends, but they sell their friends. They tell the girls that they can sell merchandise or work as a waitress...

For recruiters there are high profits to be earned as they often receive a recruitment fee, which the women will have to pay back, with interest, through their work in the brothel. It is difficult to tell how extended the network of recruiters and brothel-owners who employ these diverse kinds of recruitment of women for sex work is. It has become apparent that several layers of people are involved in the process. There are links between brothel-owners and the police, between different brothel-owners themselves, and between brothel-owners and recruiters. Research has shown that these links seemed to be based more on a personal, sometimes familial, set of relationships than being part of a well-established, organized crime syndicate: the system which is often believed to underlie the practice of trafficking.

The various facets and patterns involved in the recruitment of women and girls for prostitution indicate that neither structural changes and the patriarchal suppression of women as such, nor individual deviance or choice alone can explain the phenomenon of the trafficking of women for prostitution. Instead, macro or structural conditions underlying the practice of migration in general and trafficking in particular are closely linked to micro or individual circumstances. This complexity of the phenomenon raises questions regarding the various concepts of coercion. What does deception mean and where does free choice begin? There are no clear variables, but these ideas are obviously subject to different interpretations.

DOING SEX WORK

Sex work in Cambodia takes place in many different forms and places. At the upper end of the scale are the high-class sex workers, *srey kaliep*, in upmarket nightclubs and bars catering to rich businessmen, expatriates, and foreign tourists. At the lower end of the scale are the street hustlers who try to get some money for food by selling sex to cyclo drivers, construction workers, or day labourers. In between is a large area of practices covering a plethora of sex work, sometimes with very thin lines between what might be called direct or indirect sex work.

In the evenings, parks are populated with men interested in the young women sitting on benches stealing glances at them or in the, often a bit older, women carrying small bags of oranges to sell but offering potential for more. In restaurants and karaoke bars, beer promotion girls try to increase their monthly earnings by spending a night with a generous customer. Brothels also come in many different categories. To many observers, the brothel areas of Phnom Penh with fancily dressed women sitting in front of wooden shacks waiting for customers, make an impression of a 'gruesome' or immoral outlook on Cambodia's sex industry. The crackdown policy of the municipality tried to change this outlook albeit slightly, resulting in brothels functioning under the cover of karaoke bars, massage parlours, or *kokchol* (coin-rubbing) places. There are independent sex workers and not only in parks or in bars. There are some who rent a room from a brothel-owner. Though only a minority of the sex workers are working independently, brothel-owners do now turn more and more to renting out rooms since the police and other local officials cream off so much of the profit they get from running a 'regular' brothel.

The various ways in which sex work is practised are connected to the different categories in age or beauty of sex workers, hygiene practices, and working conditions. Cogently, though there are also young men and trans-genders working in bars, parks, or brothels, the majority of the sex workers are female. Most information on sex work in Cambodia relates to female sex workers and my own work has also focused on women in sex work. Normal payment for their sexual services varies between 4,000 riel for brothel-based sex to 20 dollars or more for a night with a dancing girl. The way in which women became involved in sex work and the length of time they have been in it as well as their connections and appearance have a great influence on the amount of money they can keep for themselves and their mobility.

In Cambodia, like in many other countries addressing prostitution by implementing an abolitionist approach, prostitution as such is not punishable by law. Yet, procuring, debauchery, benefiting from prostitution or the exploitation of prostitution of others, as well as child prostitution and forced prostitution are criminal offences. The active involvement of the police, military, and other government officials in the sex business has, however, led to major lapses in their sense of responsibility in addressing problems related to commercial sex. Every once in a while, the government has made efforts to close down brothels and raid the parks in order to crack down on prostitution and other immoral activities, and, in tandem with non-governmental organizations, organized raids to 'rescue' child prostitutes. Nevertheless, various actors continue to benefit greatly from the incomes, profits, and services on offer in Cambodia's sex business.

WORKING CONDITIONS

Contrary to most other kinds of work, sex work allows the possibility of obtaining money in advance, which has to be paid back later through work. The amount of money paid up front may vary from several tens to a thousand dollars, depending on the beauty of the woman and the kind of sex establishment. A contract is made to certify the loan and to ensure that the woman voluntarily agrees to remain and *rook luy* [find money] to pay the loan back. This indebtedness means that sex workers are kept under strict control. Some brothels with newly acquired women lock the door from the outside during the quiet noon hours. Brothel-owners also hire people, usually men, to hang around and keep an eye on the women to make sure that they will not run away.

It is difficult to generalize about the working conditions in sex work, as these vary from sex establishment to sex establishment. Included in any assessment are not only the degree of freedom and the percentage of the money a sex worker can receive, but it also covers the quality and quantity of food, hygiene and health care, degree of exposure to physical abuse, and protection from clients. Sex workers themselves make clear distinctions and rankings between the various categories of sex work, in which the amount of freedom of movement, regularity of and payment for sex are important criteria. A woman working in a nightclub noted:

> If we are dancing girls, we can go everywhere. But the prostitutes in a brothel are obliged to receive customers even when they are sick. Prostitutes also receive more customers than dancing girls. They are exploited more than the dancing girls. They cannot run away, because there are guards. If they do try to run away, these guards will beat them to death. But I also cannot go anywhere, because I have no money.

Women in the sex business make distinctions between the various forms of sex work, and such judgements influence the way they perceive themselves as sex workers (or not) and are perceived by clients. This has direct consequences for sexual behaviour. This has been recognized as an important issue in the light of HIV/AIDS. The high increase in HIV/AIDS rates in Cambodia, which are among the highest in Asia, has brought sex work into the spotlight of various initiatives of governmental departments, as well as drawing the attention of various local and international organizations. Heterosexual transmission is the predominant mode of infection and with 42.6 per cent HIV seroprevalence among brothel-based sex workers in 1998 (UNAIDS 2000), sex work has become associated more and more with an AIDS epidemic which, after Pol Pot and prolonged warfare, is now threatening Cambodia.

In an effort to interrupt the high levels of HIV transmission, a 100 per cent condom use policy is being implemented – initially in Sihanoukville and gradually extended to Phnom Penh, Battambang, and Kandal. The policy aims to regulate sex work by stimulating co-operation between brothel managers and health officials, and to introduce education and obligatory monthly STD check-up of sex workers.[5] The weak rule of law and the very involvement of police and local authorities in the sex business exacerbated by the tendency of brothel-owners to move into more indirect forms of sex work, thereby circumventing the regulations are presenting major obstacles to a proper implementation of this policy.

More concrete initiatives have been developed regarding HIV/AIDS awareness and condom distribution, reaching out directly to sex workers. In some brothel areas the multiple initiatives have been reaching out to the extent that a brothel-owner approached for an interview expressed outright frustration about the different groups and organizations coming to brothels, always asking the same questions about condom use, giving sex workers the feeling there is no longer anything to say. Though awareness about HIV prevention may have been increased, actual behavioural change is more difficult to accomplish when sex workers do not possess the negotiation skills and conditions necessary to convince customers to use a condom. Besides, it is widely known that sex workers do not (always) use condoms with regular customers or boyfriends. A Vietnamese prostitute illustrated this point:

> I have been afraid of catching diseases since I came to do this work in Cambodia. But I was more careful in Phnom Penh, because there are many girls. With my *sangsaa* (boy-friend) I don't use condoms, because I know him.

This shows, as Zalduondo (1999) has pointed out, that HIV/AIDS prevention measures focusing on sex workers will not be successful when they only take into account the frequency of sexual encounters, and not the meanings of sex within personal (and work) relationships.

VIRGIN PROSTITUTION

The fear for HIV/AIDS has also begun to influence certain practices in the sex industry of Cambodia, most pertinently child prostitution. Reliable statistics on child prostitution (as on sex work in general) are difficult to come by. According to a report of the National Assembly (1997), child prostitutes – according to its standards less than eighteen years old – constitute about 15.5 per cent of the total number of prostitutes in Cambodia. In the youngest age group, consisting of girls from nine to fifteen years old, about three-quarters were reported to be Vietnamese. Young, fresh, and healthy looking – i.e. not thin – girls are not only seen as being free from HIV, but 'deflowering' a young girl is believed by some (especially Chinese) men to have a rejuvenating effect. This is not only true of men seeking to deflower girls. During a group discussion, some sex workers noted that they believe that having sex with a virgin boy will give them strength and a fresh outlook.

The word used for deflowering is derived from the Vietnamese word *khui*. Literally, *khui* means to open a bottle, to uncork, or to make a hole. The term *khui* is also used figuratively to describe having sex with a girl or woman who is still a virgin. The first time a virgin – or more often the brothel-owner – can receive a few hundred up to a thousand dollars, depending on the age and beauty of the girl as well as the kind of customer. The second time, she is already worth a great deal less, after which her 'value' diminishes even further. These girls or women are so-called *khui haey* or *kouc haey* (deflowered already) and therefore have lost their special 'value.'

For the very young girls, forced defloration can be a traumatic experience, as they usually do not know what awaits them. A Vietnamese girl, who lived with her mother next to Svay Pak,[6] was taken to a brothel when she was fourteen years old. She remembered:

> My mother sold me for the first *khui* for 500 dollar. I did not know what to do, but she told me I had to stay in that place for four to ten days and that she would take me back home afterwards. Then the *meebon* ordered me to sleep with a guest. It hurt so much. I cried, I suffered heavy bleeding. I was so afraid.

The bleeding after deflowering is an important sign of the virginity of the girl for the *meebon* and especially for the client. In some cases, the *meebon* will have a doctor do a check-up in order to see whether a newly brought girl is really still a virgin. A client, who has agreed with the *meebon* to pay a high price for deflowering a virgin girl, expects the virgin girl to bleed. If not, the client can refuse paying anything at all. A sixteen-year-old girl interviewed in a shelter recounted how she 'devalued' after the *meebon* found out that she was no longer a virgin.

At that time we were very poor. Everyone looked down on us, even my sister. My mother told me to try to earn money, so that we did not need to be ashamed in front of our neighbours who had plenty of jewellery. My mother didn't know that I had been deflowered with my boyfriend. She thought that I was a virgin. She talked with a *meebon* about taking me to *khui*. They didn't know that I was *khui haey*. But after sleeping with a customer for the first time, I did not bleed. After this the *meebon* gave my mother only 50 dollar to take back home.

Some girls, who have already been deflowered, are made ready for a second time as a so-called *kromom pomme* (lit. apple virgin). Blood is taken from a vein in an arm and put on a cotton wool pad, which is put in the vagina, so that the customer will see blood on his penis after having sex. The entrance to the vagina entrance is also made smaller by using some *tnam* (medicine)[7] and the girl is then told to scream, even when it is not painful in order to make the customer believe she is a virgin.

Although some girls are (made) aware of their worth as a virgin and therefore agree to be deflowered, others are deceived and do not receive any financial compensation for losing their virginity. There are more or less specialized middlemen or -women, who recruit virgin girls for the sex business in Thailand and Cambodia. A Vietnamese girl in a massage parlour in Sihanoukville recalled how she was deceived when she was seventeen years old and deflowered in a brothel in Phnom Penh.

A woman told me that if I were to work in Cambodia as a cook for other people and I could earn one *chi*[8] of gold a month. So I followed her and the man who was working with her. They ordered me not to tell my mother, because she would not allow me to go with them and then I would not find a good job in Cambodia. When we came in Phnom Penh, they took me to a shop. I saw many prostitutes of my age. I saw that the *meebon* gave 7 *chi* to the people who had brought me there and then they left. Later the *meebon* told me that these people had brought me to his shop to sell me for seven *chi* of gold so that I could be deflowered. The same day I was deflowered. At first I didn't agree, but they hit me and they used electricity shocks to force me.

Like this girl, those who have been recruited as virgin prostitutes often continue to work as prostitutes after being deflowered. In many cases they are held by brothel-owners who claim that they need to pay back the initial loan or recruitment fee. Other girls continue as prostitutes or re-enter the business at a later age as they feel humiliated by the fact that they feel spoiled or they are attracted by the money they can earn, especially when they can work under less restrictive conditions. As long as the girls are young, they can earn a fair amount of money for the *meebon* and, therefore, their freedom of movement is greatly restricted. One reason they are kept fairly hidden away is that their appearance might alarm police or NGO workers, who could come to rescue them and arrest the *meebon*. A fifteen-year old girl recounted:

> We were not allowed to sit outside and gesture to the guests with our hands. This was done by the *meebon*. The *meebon* only let us receive Taiwanese and foreign guests. If Khmer guests came, the *meebon* had the other prostitutes receive them.

Freedom of movement as well as adaptation to the kind of work often seem to increase the longer a young woman stays in the sex business. Also the length of time and the number of brothels in which the woman or girl has been working as a prostitute is related to the degree to which she is working 'voluntarily' for a *meebon*. These factors again determine the financial relationship with and degree of dependency on the brothel-owner.

MATRON–CLIENT RELATIONS

The relationship between the *meebon* and prostitutes is very much based on a mutual dependency. The *meebon* cannot earn money without the girls and women, and therefore in many different ways they are made dependent on the *meebon*. The dependency of the women and girls is explicitly announced in the term used for employing sex workers. *Meebon* prefer to use the term *ceñcem*, or to nourish, which implies an almost parent–child relationship. It means that the *meebon* provides food and shelter for the women who work in her brothel. Also, the *meebon* will provide money for medicine, clothes, and police protection, which are all expenses that add to the financial obligations of the women and girls to the *meebon*.

In the case of those women and girls who are taken from Cambodia to Thailand or from Vietnam to Cambodia without knowing the language, people, and other places to go, the financial bonds of dependency are easily created by the *meebon*. The *meebon* can end up as a kind of 'rescuer' for those who have been deceived by other *meebon*, or who fall into the hands of police. Therefore, for many of these girls and women, the *meebon* becomes a kind of matronly figure who expects services in exchange for food, shelter, and protection. This kind of protection is not only necessary for those who are residing illegally in Cambodia or Thailand, it is also required for the brothel-owners themselves. Many of the brothel-owners interviewed were married to police, military, or border officials, or were otherwise on good terms with them. They are expected to pay for being allowed to run a brothel, either in cash or in kind, i.e. a box of beer or sleeping with 'her' women without paying. This is not only a 'loss' the *meebon* can suffer, but it means that the women have to work longer to repay their loan. One *meebon* noted that women have to work longer in order to compensate the 'taxes' she has to pay the police.

> Most of the girls here were brought by their mothers ... I give them a loan of 500 dollars or 700 dollars, depending on the beauty of the girl. The girl can go back home, when she has repaid the loan. In general they work for three months, but if the police come often to cause trouble, they have to work for five months.

They are not allowed to go before fulfilling their financial obligations, most notably the loan that is given as an advance or the high recruitment fee which was paid to the recruiter. In these cases the *meebon* will keep all the money earned. In the best cases, the *meebon* takes half of the money earned. Some keep a strict account for the money, like a *meebon* in Svay Pak

> I receive the money from the customers, but the girls know how much they can earn per customer. They know how often they have sex per night. They have their own book and so do I. I note it all myself, because I don't trust anybody. I also pity the girls, because they must suffer so much. They have to work for 300, 400 or 500 dollars, whatever they took out first [as a loan]. When they earn money, I deduct this from the loan. If their parents come to borrow more money, I have to add it. The customers sometimes give money to the girls to buy some cake. When they have used all of this, I lend them more money. At the end of the month, I verify how much their income was and how much they still owe me in my notebook. Then I call them in to set the account straight, so as to make clear how much money still needs to be earned in the coming months.

In cases where young women are brought to a brothel by their mother, the mother makes the financial arrangements concerning the loan that commits her daughter to be bonded to the *meebon*. These bonds are extended when the mother requests additional loans. In such a situation, the daughter is temporarily put on loan with the brothel-owner, who then has the responsibility to *cencem* the girl. The connivance of parents in bringing their daughter into prostitution therefore also involves a special relationship between the parent and the brothel-owner. A brothel-owner in a southern province explained how she sees her responsibility towards the families of the women working in her brothel.

> Sometimes other *meebon* also ask me to bring girls to their premises. But to do that is against the law. If I took these girls to other *meebon*, and if they mistreated the girls, the girls will say that I took them there. So I will be in trouble...I keep the girls in my house and I am responsible for them. Everybody knows me, so I don't dare take them to other places.

The shades of morality and responsibility and 'legal obligation' as formulated by this *meebon,* and she is by no means alone, are interesting. What seems important is that the girls are working under a known and trusted brothel-owner, not that the girls are going to work as prostitutes. Several brothel-owners interviewed stressed the importance of having some kind of contract or relationship of trust with the parents, especially the mothers, who have sent their daughters to work in their brothel. This is in contrast with those brothel-owners who are involved in re-selling a girl to an unknown third party, which runs counter to the 'rules' of morality, responsibility and legal obligation of the brothel-owner.

Brothel-owners claim that issues of morality also concern the sex workers themselves. The loan given in advance puts the brothel-owner at risk of losing money should a sex worker run away to (the protection of) another brothel-owner. This concern is not unfounded, as the mobility of sex workers is known to be high, especially among more experienced sex workers who have developed useful contacts among peers, befriended customers, and other brothel-owners.

Researching sex work gives a picture of the contradictions that exist between oppression and exploitation on the one hand and power and freedom on the other. Indubitably, sex work is fraught with practices of sexual exploitation, trafficking, bondage systems as well as health dangers. Opposed to this, sex workers undeniably show the strength of women who, by Khmer standards, display extremely outspoken behaviour and allow themselves certain freedoms which belie the image of the shy, fearful and submissive Cambodian woman. Therefore, it is also interesting to look at what kind of power sex workers have within their working and living situation. Though the economic gains are maybe most obvious, I found that mobility is an important theme to be explored further here. This mobility does not encompass the regular changes of sex establishments, it covers the relationships sex workers maintain within their working and home situations, requiring mobility of place as well as conduct.

In order to analyse sex work and sex workers' experiences comprehensively, it is essential to include the historical, economic, political, and socio-cultural structures, values, and influences within society, which also influence gender relations and sexual behaviour. Within the Cambodian context, gender and sexuality cannot be detached from the concepts of the broken woman and the virtuous woman. At this moment in a changing society in which contradictory moralities regarding individual responsibilities and ideals for proper behaviour compete, these cannot be considered clear-cut categories. Sex workers 'do not constitute a single, unified, social group even within a single country, but rather...mirror in their own differentiation many of the other groups in the wider society' (Davidson 1998:205).

NOTES

1 This paper is a revised version of paper 'Ideals and Attractions: Commercial Sex Work in Cambodia,' presented at the Conference on Health, Sexuality and Civil Society in East Asia, IIAS, 6–7 July 2000, Amsterdam. It is predominantly based on research conducted in 1997/1998 (see References).
2 Prostitution of girls below the age of fifteen was prohibited by law.
3 See also Lin (1998) for a more general analysis of the economic significance of the 'sex sector' in Southeast Asia.
4 At the time of this survey one dollar equalled 2,700 riel.
5 Some resemblance to the contagious disease policies implemented in the nineteenth century cannot be ignored.
6 The brothel area 11 kilometres north of Phnom Penh.
7 This is how it was described by a sex worker who had undergone this treatment several times, but did not know what kind of medicine was used to constrict the entrance to her vagina.
8 One *chi* of gold is worth about 37 dollars.

REFERENCES

AFP (2000) 'Plight of Cambodia's Women amongst Worst in Southeast Asia,' 7 March 2000, (from Camnews).

Asia Watch and the Women's Rights Project (1993) *A Modern Form of Slavery: Trafficking of Burmese Women and Girls into Brothels in Thailand*. New York: Human Rights Watch.

Barry, Kathleen (1995) *The Prostitution of Sexuality*. New York and London: New York University Press.

Bullough, Vern, and Bonnie Bullough (1987) *Women and Prostitution: A Social History*. New York: Prometheus Books.

Cambodian Women's Development Agency (CWDA) (1995) 'The Prostitution and Traffic of Women and Children: A Dialogue on the Cambodian Situation,' paper presented at the Workshop-Conference on Prostitution and Traffic of Women and Children, 4–5 May 1995, Phnom Penh.

Chapkis, Wendy (1997) *Live Sex Acts: Women Performing Erotic Labor*. New York: Routledge.

Chommie, Michael (1999) *Census of Commercial Sex Establishments in Phnom Penh, Kampong Cham and Kandal 1998*. PSI: Phnom Penh.

Chou, Ta-Kuan (1993) *The Customs of Cambodia*. Translated into English by J. Gilman d'Arcy, Paul Bangkok: The Siam Society.

Davidson, Julia O'Connell (1998) *Prostitution, Power and Freedom*. Ann Arbor: University of Michigan Press.

De Lind van Wijngaarden, W. Jan (2000) 'Broken Women, Virgins and Housewives: Reviewing the Socio-Cultural Contexts of Sex Work and AIDS in Cambodia,' FHI-Impact: Phnom Penh.

Derks, Annuska (1996) 'Diversity in Ethnicity: A Picture of Ethnic Vietnamese in Cambodia,' in: *Final Draft Reports Interdisciplinary Research on Ethnic Groups in Cambodia*. Phnom Penh: Center for Advanced Study, pp. 251–75.

– (1997) *Trafficking of Cambodian Women and Children to Thailand*. Phnom Penh: IOM/CAS.

– (1998), *Trafficking of Vietnamese Women and Children to Cambodia*. Phnom Penh: IOM/CAS.

– (1998), *Reintegration of Victims of Trafficking in Cambodia*. Phnom Penh: IOM/CAS.

– (2000), 'From White Slaves to Trafficking Survivors,' paper presented at the Conference on Migration and Development, 4–6 May, Princeton University, Princeton.

Doezema, Jo (1998) 'Forced to Choose: Beyond the Voluntary v. Forced Prostitution Dichotomy,' in: Kempadoo, and Doezema (eds) *Global Sex Workers: Rights, Resistance and Redefinition*. New York/London: Routledge, pp.34–50.

Holter, Uta (1994) *Bezahlt, geliebt, verstossen. Prostitution und andere Sonderformen institutionalierter Sexualität in verschiedene Kulturen.* Bonn: Honos Verlag.

Journal Officiel de l'Indochine Française, Résidence Supérieure au Cambodge, Arrêté du 11 Février 1933, Phnom Penh.

Kempadoo, Kamala (1998) 'Introduction: Globalizing Sex Workers' Rights,' in: Kempadoo and Doezema (eds) *Global Sex Workers: Rights, Resistance and Redefinition.* New York and London: Routledge, pp. 1–28.

Kim, Chou (1993) 'The Problem of Prostitution in Cambodia: Is it normal for the Khmer Society?,' *Khmer Conscience* VII(2), pp. 17–20.

Ledgerwood, Judy (1990) *Changing Khmer Conceptions of Gender: Women, Stories and the Social Order*, Ph.D. Dissertation: Cornell University.

– (1992) *Analysis of the Situation of Women in Cambodia: Research on Women in Khmer Society.* Phnom Penh: UNICEF.

Leonard, Christine S. (1996) 'Becoming Cambodian: Ethnic Identity and the Vietnamese in Kampuchea,' in: *Final Draft Reports Interdisciplinary Research on Ethnic Groups in Cambodia.* Phnom Penh: Center for Advanced Study, pp. 277–305.

Lin, Lean Lim (1998) *The Sex Sector: The Economic and Social Bases of Prostitution in Asia.* Geneva: International Labour Office.

Muecke, Marjorie (1992) 'Mother Sold Food, Daughter Sells her Body: The Cultural Continuity of Prostitution,' *Social Science & Medicine* 7, pp. 891–901.

National Assembly, Commission on Human Rights & Reception of Complaints (1997) *Report on the Problem of Sexual Exploitation and Trafficking in Cambodia.* Phnom Penh.

Ong, Aihwa, and Michael Peletz (eds) (1995) *Bewitching Women, Pious Men. Gender and Body Politics in Southeast Asia.* Berkeley and Los Angeles: University of California Press.

Osborne, Milton (1995) *Southeast Asia: An Introductory History.* St Leonards: Allen & Unwin.

(1997) *The French Presence in Cochinchina and Cambodia.* Bangkok: White Lotus Press (first published in 1969).

Phnara, Khy (1974) *La communaute vietnamienne au Cambodge á l'époque du protectorat français (1863–1953)*, thèse, tome I, Université de la Sorbonne nouvelle, Paris III.

Prasso, Sherri (1995) *Violence, Ethnicity and Ethnic Cleansing: Cambodia and the Khmer Rouge.* Cambridge: Department of Sociology: University of Cambridge (unpublished paper).

Protectorat du Cambodge, Cabinet du Résident-Maire, Arrêté du 29 Mai 1906, Phnom Penh.

Reynolds, Rocque (1996) *Trafficking and Prostitution: The Law of Cambodia*. University of New South Wales, Sydney (unpublished paper).

Shawcross, William (1991) *Sideshow: Kissinger Nixon and the Destruction of Cambodia*. London: Hogarth Press (first published in 1979).

Tarr, Chou Meng, and Peter Aggleton (1996) 'Sexualising the Culture(s) of Young Cambodians Dominant Discourse and Social Reality,' Paper presented at First International Conference on Khmer Studies, University of Phnom Penh, Phnom Penh.

Tarr, Chou Meng (1996) *People in Cambodia Don't Talk About Sex, They Simply do it: A Study of the Social and Contextual Factors Affecting Risk-Related Sexual Behaviour among Young Cambodians*. Phnom Penh: UNAIDS.

Thion, Serge (1993) *Watching Cambodia*. Bangkok: White Lotus Press.

Truong, Thanh-Dam (1990) *Sex Money and Morality. Prostitution and Tourism in Southeast Asia*. London: Zed Books Ltd.

UNAIDS (2000) *The HIV/AIDS/STD Situation and the National Response in the Kingdom of Cambodia: Country Profile*. Third Edition, Phnom Penh.

UNICEF (1995) *The Trafficking and Prostitution of Children in Cambodia. A Situation Report 1995*. Phnom Penh.

Weitzer, Ronald (2000) *Sex for Sale: Prostitution, Pornography, and the Sex Industry*. New York and London: Routledge.

Wijers, Marjan, and Lap-Chew Lin (1997) *Trafficking in Women, Forced Labour and Slavery-like Practices in Marriage, Domestic Labour and Prostitution*. Utrecht: Foundation Against Trafficking in Women.

Zalduondo, Barbara O. (1999) 'Prostitution Viewed Cross-culturally: Toward Recontextualizing Sex Work in AIDS Prevention Research,' in: Parker and Aggleton (eds) *Culture, Society and Sexuality*. London: UCL Press, pp. 307–24.

Part Two
The Social Construction of Sexual Risk in the light of STDs/AIDS Control

CHAPTER 7

PUBLIC HEALTH POLICY VS. COLONIAL LAISSEZ-FAIRE: STDS AND PROSTITUTION IN REPUBLICAN SHANGHAI

CHRISTIAN HENRIOT

STDs are inseparably related to prostitution. Yet the nature of this relationship is far more complex than is generally assumed because the issue is as much about actual medical problems as about social representations of the diseases. In Shanghai, the fear of the dangers of STDs in the late nineteenth century led a group of Western physicians in the foreign settlements to call for strict regulatory measures and for the medical control of the prostitutes by the authorities. Similarly, in the 1920s the transmission of STDs by prostitutes was a central element in the abolitionist campaign launched by the Moral Welfare League.[1] Finally, the Chinese authorities themselves adopted the same discourse after World War II to legitimize their attempt to establish a regulationist system in order to control prostitution and reduce the spread of STDs among the population. Chinese sources for the nineteenth century are almost completely silent on this topic, especially as they deal only with courtesans. The few references that exist are to be found in the medical journals published by missionaries. Because of their strong religious and moral tone and the lack of precise scientific techniques and instruments by which to identify STDs, however, these early testimonies can hardly be relied on. The following paper, therefore, will deal only with the period after the 1911 revolution. I shall briefly present the general position of prostitution and public health in China to avoid giving an unduly biased view of the Shanghai case. In this the measures adopted by the foreign and Chinese authorities in their more or less determined fight against STDs will feature prominently. The second part will examine the issue of STDs in relation to the role of physicians among the population and the prostitutes.

COMING TO TERMS WITH STDS: LAISSEZ-FAIRE AND PREJUDICE

This is not the place for me to attempt to reconstruct a history of STDs in China. This would be an uphill battle as the history of diseases, epidemics, and health issues in this country is still *terra incognita* for the most part.[2] In a previous study, I relied on medical journals and various testimonies by foreign missionaries and physicians to assess the extent of STDs in China and analyse what discourse, if any, such a phenomenon had generated within the medical profession (Henriot 1992). What the examination of these sources revealed, however, was the high prevalence of STDs throughout the country as early as the mid-nineteenth century. This is something that struck all the foreign physicians who worked in China, whatever their location, even if they were far from being able to detect all the cases that came to them.[3] As new techniques were invented, especially blood tests, the physicians who carried out surveys confirmed the high prevalence of the STDs in China.[4] They also noted that there was an acceleration in their diffusion because of the greater mobility of the population thanks to the modern means of transportation, and also as a result of the migrations caused by wars and the movement of troops throughout many parts of China. In the middle of the 1920s – most of my data relate to this period – all the provinces were affected, even the most peripheral ones. STDs had by then become a major public health problem at a time when the health system in China was barely struggling to emerge as it was hampered by the weakness and lack of interest by the state.[5]

In this context, the case of Shanghai, is therefore not exceptional, even if, as in all the large metropolises, especially as an international harbour city, the prevalence of STDs was particularly high there. What distinguishes this city from the rest of the country are the efforts that were made in the field of public health, especially with regard to prostitution, and the high concentration of physicians and hospitals.[6] Elsewhere in China, the authorities generally refrained from establishing any regulated system of prostitution. The few examples that I came across were concentrated in Manchuria, where such measures were imposed by the Japanese army (Wu 1927:30). Among the large cities, only Peking imposed a medical examination of prostitutes and measures of seclusion until a diseased prostitute was fully cured. Such rules, however, were never seriously implemented.[7]

In Shanghai, the Shanghai Municipal Council (SMC) of the International Settlement implemented an ambiguous and contradictory policy that focused exclusively on the foreign residents and sojourners. The adoption of concrete measures for the benefit of the foreign community dates back to the 1920s. It followed the debate on the abolition of prostitution and the visit by a delegation of the NCCVD, the association in charge of fighting STDs in Great Britain, in 1920.[8] The SMC organized a series of meetings between the delegates and various local organizations and benefited from the conclusions of these exchanges (SB, 9 Dec. 1920; 17 Dec. 1920). Among other measures, the NCCVD delegates recommended the circulation of medical information to teenagers and adults, the establishment of cost-free institutions for the treatment of foreigners and the employees of the SMC suffering from STDs, and the creation of STD clinics in Chinese hospitals.[9] Two years later, in reply to a letter of inquiry by the NCCVD about the outcome of its recommendations, the SMC stated that it had appointed a medical officer to tackle the problem of STDs. Because of other more pressing issues, however, the new appointee could not devote much time to this task. The SMC added that this was an extremely controversial topic, especially in Great Britain where the Board of Health had appointed a commission of inquiry to study the most appropriate means of fighting STDs. The Council was in the opinion it was better to wait for the conclusions of the commission before undertaking any particular policy.[10]

In 1923, the authorities of the International Settlement eventually decided to open an evening anti-VD clinic, the General Hospital. Announcements were published in the press in English, Japanese, and Russian to inform the foreign residents of the existence of the new establishment. Patients flocked there in large numbers almost immediately. During the first six months after its inauguration, the clinic received 1170 visits (for 191 patients). Afterwards the number of patients remained fairly stable, in spite of a drop related to the hostilities of 1937–8 in Shanghai. Patients suffering from syphilis were treated with six-weekly injections of N.A.B., the famous '606', followed by nine injections of mercurial salt. A control test was done three months later. If it proved positive, the treatment was repeated following the same schedule over a period of two months.[11] Very rapidly, the demand exceeded the capacity of the clinic. Fifty to sixty patients used to come every evening. Although the director of the establishment pointed out the services were provided for short-term sojourners, especially seamen, the statistics showed that most of the patients were locals, most notably Russians.[12] The SMC also planned the opening of a clinic exclusively for women, but it lacked the gumption to overcome the hostile reactions this project generated among one segment of foreign public opinion.[13]

The surveys made among the patients on the place of origin of their disease, with the view of determining the main zones on infection in the city, laid the burden of responsibility on the prostitutes located in the Chinese municipality or in the French settlement.[14] Although the method was itself questionable, the SMC complained about this situation and blamed the authorities in the neighboring districts. In 1926, it also led the Council to ask for a financial contribution from the French concession, as a compensation to the expenses incurred by the clinic. The French municipal council rejected the demand, to the great displeasure of the SMC.[15] In 1928, 20 per cent of the patients were resident in the French Concession and another 17 per cent declared they had been infected by a prostitute in the Concession.[16] This was not, however, the major issue at stake. With the passing of time the physicians of the clinic realized that their establishment could not cope with the whole issue of STDs, because the sources of infection were multiple and largely beyond the control of the authorities.[17] In 1934, the same physicians acknowledged that the work of the clinic was no more than palliative. The annual report of the SMC in 1937 even announced its closure after the outbreak of the hostilities between Japan and China, but it must have reopened afterwards since my data go up to 1940.[18] The authorities in the International Settlement cared only about the health of the foreign residents. In 1933, they were preparing a new version of the instruction booklet about STDs in ... Hindi.[19]

In the French Concession, the municipal council did not adopt any particular policy until very late, despite the long tradition of the passing of regulations both in France and in the Concession itself. In the nineteenth century, the Health officer had taken the initiative to ask for a regulation of prostitution and the medical examination of those prostitutes patronized by foreigners (Henriot 2001, Chapter 11). His suggestion, however, had actually been implemented in the International Settlement, under the pressure of Edward Henderson, the SMC health officer. After much debate among the foreign ratepayers and a dispute with the French authorities – the French insisted on the seclusion of diseased prostitutes, not just medical control – a lock hospital was established in January 1877 under the auspices of the two settlements. It closed its doors with the advent of the abolitionist campaign in 1920. Afterwards, no other institution ever took its place.[20]

In 1931, the municipal council inaugurated a new municipal dispensary, a facility was designed to provide free medical treatment to the poor. It did not specifically take care of STDs.[21] Dr Rabaute, the head of the *Service d'hygiène et d'assistance*, was not satisfied with this arrangement. He was keenly aware of the prevalence of STDs, not only among the patients who came to the dispensary, but also among the general population of the Concession. He was also receptive to the criticisms levelled by the SMC, which attributed the majority of the cases treated in the anti-VD clinic to the French concession. In November 1934, he presented a long report in which he emphasized the dissemination of STDs in Shanghai and the impossibility of relying on the Chinese state or on simple education to wipe out this scourge: '*Il n'existe qu'un moyen de prophylaxie [...] c'est la lutte par le traitement de ces affections, de beaucoup le plus efficace [...] il nous faut accepter ici ce que nous ne pouvons pas empêcher'* [There is but one means of prophylaxis...[...] it is the battling of these infections through the treatment, this is by far the most efficacious way [...] we must accept here what we cannot prevent]. Rabaute recommended the creation of an anti-VD clinic that would be part of the municipal dispensary. It should be open outside of the normal working hours so that the largest number of people could have access to it. The establishment would provide medical care on a cost-free or paying basis, depending on the financial circumstances of the patient. Rabaute also urged the creation of similar clinics in all the hospitals in the Concession. The recommendations of Dr. Rabaute do not seem to have been implemented by the *Conseil municipal.*[22]

In the districts under Chinese jurisdiction, no initiative to combat the diseases was ever taken during the same period. At the outbreak of the Sino-Japanese war, the bureau of health was actually abolished and it was not re-established before 1941. Because access to the archives is at present not possible, I am not in a position to elaborate on its actual operation. Initially it planned to get in touch with the French Concession in order to adopt measures about STDs, but the annual report of the following year did not even mention this matter.[23] A major change occurred with the return to the city of the Nationalist authorities in 1945. For the first time in the history of Shanghai, the city came under the jurisdiction of a single municipal government. The regulatory policy that was carried out in the following years included an important dimension to the fight against STDs, especially among prostitutes. One of the instruments of this policy was the anti-VD dispensary, established in February 1946.[24] Two years later, its staff was composed of twenty-five persons, including six physicians and six nurses.[25] To facilitate the access to medical care to the population at large, the Bureau of Health ordered Shanghai hospitals to open special departments for the treatment of STDs. By 1948, sixteen establishments had already complied.[26]

The prostitutes were subject to monthly examinations and, if they were infected, they had the choice between receiving treatment at the dispensary or from one of the private physicians registered with the authorities.[27] The police station in the *Tilanqiao* district even provided medicine for the diseased prostitutes, either free or at a price that varied according to their income. It seems that this was an isolated initiative of which I have not found any mention elsewhere.[28] The prostitutes were not allowed to resume their activities for two years if they contracted syphilis. Since such a severe prohibition had negative counter-effects, the Bureau of Health suggested lifting the two-year time limit as soon as the blood tests proved negative. The Bureau hoped that this less stringent policy would entice more prostitutes who were diseased to come forward for medical treatment without the fear of losing their source of income.[29] Realizing the magnitude of the task, the municipal government oriented its policy toward a self-responsibility system of health care by the prostitutes themselves.[30]

The original project foresaw the medical examination of 200 women per day.[31] In fact, the number of prostitutes received in the dispensary fell short of this objective. The documents kept by the dispensary do not allow a correct assessment of the number of prostitutes who were examined since only the visits were counted. Moreover, the dispensary made a distinction between visits which served to provide treatment and examination which corresponded to the regular medical examinations of the prostitutes. Table 7.1 gives an idea of the number of visits to the establishment from 1946 to 1948. There was a clear increase over the whole period, but it is almost impossible to determine whether this relates to a greater number of women examined or to a larger number of examinations per prostitute. A paper by the director of the dispensary did cast some light on the number of prostitutes concerned. In the two years 1946 and 1947, the dispensary examined respectively 1,420 and 3,550 women (cf. Table 7.2), a figure which was below the number of officially registered prostitutes (8,000 in 1946, 3,000 in 1947, 10,000 in 1948).[32] The police archives confirm the lack of respect shown to the regulations by the prostitutes, even in the largest establishments for prostitution. In January 1948, an inspection at the *Taotao* revealed that fifty-five women out of a total of 117 had not attended the medical examination as required by the prescribed schedule. At the *Meixing*, twenty prostitutes out of fifty-three did not have the card issued by the dispensary. Finally, of the thirty-three inmates of the *Haishang*, eighteen were diseased and had outdated cards.[33]

Table 7.1

Number of medical visits and examinations at the municipal dispensary
(1946–1948)

Year	Prostitutes First visit	Prostitutes Follow-ups	Number of cards issued by the dispensary		Total number examinations
			First examination	Renewed examination	
1946	1 310	6 988	1 022	2 096	9 749
1947	1 439	9 426	1 639	6 689	17 865
1948	1 955	12 382	1 192	11 170	26 502

Source: *Shanghai shi weishengju san nian lai gongzuo gaikuang*, 1949, p. 9.

In spite of the facilities provided the prostitutes, especially low-cost medical treatment, the dispensary observed that it failed to attract more than a quarter of the registered prostitutes. Most of them belonged to the lower categories and were often diseased.[34] The Bureau of Health planned the creation of mobile teams that would visit the registered houses to accelerate the process of medical examination and the treatment. In the face of financial difficulties, the municipal government forced the bureau to give up this project and to postpone it to more favourable times.[35] One of the major difficulties in the implementation of the medical examination was the problem of co-ordination between the various services involved in health administration. During the first year of its existence, the Bureau of Health had to secure the assistance of a private laboratory to perform the blood tests. This procedure resulted in a ten-day delay between the medical examination and the transmission of the results. Later, with the establishment of a laboratory on its own premises, the dispensary reduced the delay to three or four days (Yu 1948:18). The most serious problem was the lack of efficient liaison with the police. The latter was responsible for the administration of prostitution, but it was unable to forward the required documents on time. The Bureau of Health repeatedly wrote to complain about the delays that stretched up to one month. The time lapses that resulted from this inability made the regular medical examination simply impossible. The women who were summoned after such a delay often used the pretext of their menstrual period to avoid examination.[36]

The ambassador of the United States in China as well as the American military medical officers exerted strong pressure on the Chinese municipal government to impose strict medical control on the prostitutes.[37] The Chinese authorities frequently received official queries about women who were suspected of having infected an American soldier (who had since returned home). When the Chinese police eventually managed to trace the prostitute a few months later on the basis of the very imprecise information provided by the US army, she was generally no longer in the establishment concerned or the latter had closed.[38] The foreign military authorities also asked the municipal government to ban prostitutes in the vicinity of the quarters where their troops were stationed.[39]

PEOPLE, MEDICINE, AND STDS: ANXIETIES AND PROFITS

One of the major causes of the spread of STDs in China was without any doubt the lack of treatment or the taking of totally inadequate medicine. In 1925, a gynaecologist noted that at least a quarter of the 2837 patients she had seen over eight years were or had been affected with STDs. Seventy per cent of the cases of sterility she had come across had their origin in untreated gonorrhoea.[40] Two years later, another medical survey on 2500 persons showed that 90 per cent of those suffering from syphilis had received no modern treatment.[41] According to what these physicians recorded and to the scattered evidence gathered in the press or from the archives, it seems that the population, especially the prostitutes, availed themselves of the services of traditional native physicians rather than those of Western-trained doctors.[42] We cannot generalize this attitude to the whole Republican period or to all social groups. Probably, economics often dictated such a choice. The treatments prescribed by native physicians were much less expensive than the medicines imported from the West. The traditional treatment consisted in inhalations or absorption of mercury or calomel.[43] An author noted that when the first treatment had failed, the dissatisfied patients turned toward Western medicine (Heimburger 1927:548).

The spread of STDs created a profitable market for all kinds of physicians and medicines. The Shanghai press is strewn with advertisements placed by medical practitioners specializing in these diseases (*hualiuke*) or in medicines with miraculous curative properties. Similar advertisements have reappeared in the streets of Chinese cities since the early 1980s in the form of small posters pasted on walls. In the Republic, some physicians made a living from just performing injections of '606' or '914', the two main products for the treatment of syphilis before the introduction of antibiotics.[44] Wu Lien-teh, a respected physician, indicated that in Harbin, a city of 300,000 inhabitants, there were more than 200 private 'anti-VD clinics.' By 1927, physicians charged 20 to 30 Yuan per injection, which was much more profitable than providing advice on prophylaxis (Wu 1927:34). In Shanghai, a physician was said to have hired a few jobless fellows who sat in his waiting room to convey the idea that his talent was much in demand, and attract more customers.[45] Medicines were relatively expensive. In 1928, the *Heisidian* – a new product imported from Germany according to an advertisement – cost 3 Yuan for one box. A full treatment required three boxes. A bottle of '606'– two injections – was sold for 7 Yuan.[46] At the beginning of the 1940s, the cost of a full treatment ranged from 70 to several hundred Yuan.[47]

There is some evidence that what happened in Shanghai may have been particular. One Chinese historian has demonstrated this in a study of the medical advertisements published in the *Shen Bao*, the main Shanghai daily, between 1912 and 1927.[48] Although sex was omitted or hidden, or even repressed, in the public arena or in social contacts, it was expressed under various guises through pressures exerted on the individual, especially men. There was a latent male anxiety towards all that was related to sex, which merchants were apt to play on by making sex the central factor of diseases. Consequently, a large number of ordinary illnesses were attributed to a weakness of genital organs or to excessive sexual activity.[49] The profusion of advertisements for medicines designed to treat STDs, which represented the buck of medical advertisements, was only one element in a more general craze for sexual revitalization. The period chosen by this historian is arbitrary as it takes two dates in political history as its limits. The chronological scope of such a study needs to be expanded. As early as the end of the 1890s, the *Shen Bao* ran announcements on pills designed to cure gonorrhoea (*baizhuowan*). The same brand was still on sale in the 1920s (*SB*, 12 Sept. 1899). Through their message (text or image), these advertisements exploited the feelings of anxiety STDs generated. They explicitly associated these diseases with prostitution, juxtaposing, for instance, the face of a beautiful woman and a skull.

The authorities made some attempts to control the trade in these medicines. In the police archives, several times I have come across a bunch of small newspapers (the so-called mosquito newspapers) of the same day. All the advertisements for such medicines had been carefully circled with a red pen.[50] The police used to carry out investigations of the producers of such medicine. An analysis of the content of these newspapers showed that they carried a high number of advertisements for anti-VD medicines. For instance, on April 27, 1930, my reading of various newspapers produced the following figures:[51]

Xinwenbao (The News): 46
Shishi xinwen (China Times): 7
Shen Bao: 16

The large number of advertisements certainly reflected the extent of the demand for such products. Many patients preferred to treat their disease themselves, for the sake of either discretion or economy. Some companies even promoted their products by correspondence.[52] The sufferers had a large choice of medicines, but they also ran the risk of falling victims to their credulity. Charlatans were not rare among physicians, in spite of the control by the authorities, and a 1942 Shanghai guide recommended newcomers seek the advice of reliable friends before going to see a 'flower and willow' doctor (*hualiu yisheng*).[53] Nevertheless, these advertisements did not necessarily convey a negative image of prostitution. Patronizing prostitutes was considered a normal act of life, but this habit could sometimes have undesirable consequences that customers would have to face. Yet, indubitably prostitutes were indeed singled out for a key role in the transmission of STDs.

What does seem surprising is the complete absence of any recommendations about the use of condoms before 1945. This may be related to the fact that I had no access to the small booklets that were distributed to seamen upon their arrival in Shanghai or to similar literature distributed to the foreign population by the Shanghai Municipal Council. Nevertheless, unless self-censorship excluded the public mention of such recommendations, none of the papers published in the two main medical journals ever referred to this possibility, even when the author dealt with STDs. In 1927, Wu Lien-teh proposed the sale of cheap prophylactic products, but it seems he intended them to be used by prostitutes only (Wu 1927:34). In a less technical genre, no guide to Shanghai, nor any 'gallant's compass' (*piaojie zhinan*) advocated the use of condoms even though they warned their readers about the high risk of getting infected if they were to patronize the lower classes of prostitutes.[54] It was only in 1945 that the police explicitly ordered the houses of prostitution to purchase prophylactic products and instruments for the inmates and the use of condoms by customers. In 94 per cent of the cases checked by the police, these instructions were not followed (Yu 1948b:13).

The more prevalent STDs at that time were syphilis, gonorrhoea, and soft chancre. Gonorrhoea represented the highest number of cases in all the statistical samples I have found. At the Shantung Hospital, it made up 48.5 per cent of all the new cases of STDs in 1923. Syphilis and soft chancre shared the rest with 33.8 and 17.7 per cent respectively.[55] Data provided by the anti-VD clinic of the Shanghai Municipal Council from 1923 to 1940.[56] Gonorrhoea always ranks first with an average of 40 per cent of all cases, followed by syphilis (18.8 per cent) and soft chancre (18.5 per cent). It is difficult to assess the extent of the spread of STDs among the population at large. The registers of the General Hospital for the period 1875–1922 give an average rate of 9.9 per cent of STD infections among its patients. The Shantung Road Hospital registered a lower rate of 6.6 per cent from 1870 to 1922. These figures were probably underestimated because of the absence of blood tests for the most part of the period of the reference.[57] The director of the municipal dispensary, Yu Wei, put the number of syphilitics at 10 per cent of the population in 1938 and 15 per cent in 1945. In his opinion, gonorrhoea affected one half of the population. He drew these figures from a study of the statistics held by the various hospitals of the city (Yu 1948a:17). His view may have been too gloomy as the blood test campaigns carried out after 1949 did not produce such alarming results.[58] Among the 31,861 persons examined in three hospitals from 1945 to 1950, only nine per cent showed a positive reaction to STD detection tests.[59] These data raise the same problem. Even if the conclusions of the pre-war physicians were, as I think, biased by the prevailing social imagery constructed around the issue of prostitution, the prevalence of STDs in Shanghai must have been higher than rates computed from the hospital registers.

PROSTITUTES AND STDS

This leads to the question of the prostitutes being stigmatized as the 'source of all evils.' The data I have collected are all partial and certainly open to discussion. In order to achieve some balance, I shall compare them with surveys made among various groups of prostitutes in other Chinese cities. The overall image is undoubtedly disturbing. According to the declarations made by the patients at the SMC anti-VD clinic, in most cases, they had contracted their infection from Chinese prostitutes (Table 2). Given the Chinese social context of the strict separation of men and women, they could hardly have been infected from any other source.

Table 7.2
Sources of infection according to the declarations of patients (1926–1929)

Source of infection	1926	1927	1929
Chinese prostitutes	64	70	75
Russian prostitutes	27	20	12
Japanese prostitutes	5	**	**
Other prostitutes	4	10	13

Sources: Shanghai Municipal Council, *Report for the Year 1926, op. cit.*, p. 195; *Report for the Year 1927, op. cit.*, p. 183; *Report for the Year 1929, op. cit.*, p. 150

The articles published in medical journals confirm beyond any reasonable doubt the poor state of health of the prostitutes. A Chinese physician, Daniel Lai, wrote several papers on syphilis in China. In 1930, he published the results of a survey carried out among 137 prostitutes from Shanghai (104), Nanjing (22), and Suzhou (11). These women had quit prostitution and were living in refuges. On average, 49 per cent had syphilis, those from Shanghai having the lowest rate with 40.4 per cent (Lai, Dr 1930:559–60). It has to be admitted that this sample was small and random. Besides this, there are two supplementary statistical series on the health of Shanghai prostitutes. The first, presented in Table 7.3, was collected by the municipal dispensary for 1946 and 1947. It reveals that more than 80 per cent of the women had a venereal infection. The distribution of the diseases is different from that observed among the patients of the SMC anti-VD clinic. Syphilis accounted for 80 per cent of all infections, but the director thought that the smear method used to detect the diseases could not be relied on.[60] Furthermore, he claimed that 95 per cent of the prostitutes had contracted gonorrhoea (Yu 1948b:13).

Table 7.3

The prevalence of STDs among the prostitutes
examined at the municipal dispensary (1946–1947)

	1946	1946	1947	1947
Number of women examined	1 420		3 550	
Total number of infections	1 062		2 611	
Number of women infected	*931*	*87.7%*	*2 205*	*84.5%*
Syphilis	885	83.3%	2069	79.2%
Gonorrhoea	174	16.4%	533	20.4%
Soft chancre	1	0.1%	5	0.2%
Others	2	0.2%	4	0.2%
Primary syphilis	32	4%	24	1%
Secondary syphilis	21	2%	46	2%
Tertiary syphilis	832	94%	1 999	97%

Source : Yu Wei, 'Shanghai changji wu bai ge an diaocha,' p. 13

In this table the total number of infections was higher than the number of women, which means that some prostitutes suffered from two or more diseases at the same time.[61] Moreover, most of the syphilitic prostitutes had reached the third stage of the disease. These data may be biased since the dispensary mostly received prostitutes from the lower categories, who had been in the trade for a long time and had been more exposed to the risk of infection.[62] The second series of statistics come from the first group of 501 prostitutes arrested by the police in 1951. Healthy women represented only 10.9 per cent of the whole group. The others had syphilis (11.5 per cent), gonorrhoea (30 per cent), or both at the same time (47.6 per cent). As in the previous sample, a large number (73.7 per cent) had reached the third stage of syphilis (He, Yang 1988:73).[63]

The various forms of surveys carried out in other Chinese cities before 1949 also confirm the prevalence of STDs among prostitutes. A 1948 medical survey among 576 prostitutes and ninety-five taxi dancers[64] in Qingdao (Shandong) showed that 80 and 60 per cent of them respectively had syphilis (Lai, Daniel 1948: 389–90). In the same year, two physicians carried out a survey among the prostitutes registered with the Beijing municipal dispensary. They selected 876 women they followed over a period of forty-one days.[65] This unusual procedure demonstrated that 89 per cent of the prostitutes caught an infection during the time of the survey.[66] In 1950, 96 per cent of the 1303 Beijing prostitutes interned by the authorities were diseased, of whom 1107 had syphilis.[67] It is not necessary to multiply the examples. The vast majority of Chinese prostitutes suffered from venereal infections that in most cases went unnoticed, untreated, or at best they were treated with inadequate medicines. The consequences of this sad reality were dreadful when the prostitutes left the trade and went back to their villages.

The practices of the Chinese prostitutes partly explain the high degree of infection they presented, even if some establishments at least did take precautionary measures. At the *Taotao*, a physician was employed full time to treat the inmates. Cogently, his honorarium and the cost of medicines were borne by the prostitutes themselves. The latter complained about the high tariff was imposed on them (80,000 Yuan per month including laundry service).[68] Health regulations were very rudimentary. The prostitutes were required to wash their genitalia only once a day and apparently did not use condoms.[69] In most houses, such minimal care was not even guaranteed. To protect themselves against STDs, especially syphilis, some women took regular injections of Salvarsan (the famous '606'). In 1947, a prostitute stated that she received two injections per month at a cost of 20 US dollars (200,000 Yuan) each. The same medicine cost only one dollar at the municipal dispensary. The price of the injections of Salvarsan followed the curve of inflation. One year earlier, it had cost only 50,000 Yuan per injection. When the prostitutes did not have enough money, the madam lent them the required amount and received the reimbursement the following day or when the women had made some more income.[70] A diseased woman who was treated in 1948 by a physician introduced to her by her madam paid 80 US dollars (800,000 Yuan) for the first injection of Neosalvarsan. She was charged 40 dollars each for the next two.[71] A document issued by the Bureau of Health noted that more than 60 per cent of the general practitioners and hospitals did not use the most efficient medicines to treat STDs. Although antibiotics were then available, they still prescribed the older arsenic-based products.[72] The municipal dispensary itself lacked the funds to purchase the most efficient treatments that could cure a person in a few hours in the case of gonorrhoea or in a few days for syphilis. Instead, months of treatment were required and this procrastination discouraged the prostitutes from coming as they knew their licences would be withdrawn (Yu 1948a:18).

The fate of the diseased women could sometimes take a tragic turn. The inconvenience or even the pain caused by their infections during sexual intercourse forced the prostitutes to refuse customers. Some madams did not have the least consideration for the health of the women. They denied them the possibility to seek a treatment and forced them to continue with their work. Those who became seriously ill had to give up at a certain point, having an enforced break until they were cured. Frustratingly, the lack of data means it is impossible to say to what extent the prostitutes had the freedom to make such a choice and to undergo a treatment. This depended very much on the status under which they had become involved into prostitution (sold, pawned, or free-choice).[73] The press provides examples of women who were exploited to the very end, whatever the period. In 1899, a prostitute (*yeji*) who was in the last stage of syphilis was sent to a private clinic in the French Concession. After ten days, as her state of health was becoming critical, the director refused to keep her any longer because of the other patients and had her sent over to the brothel. The madam did not want her either and threw her out in the street, where a policeman picked her up some time later (*SB*, 14 Oct. 1899). In 1909, during a visit of inspection the police discovered the unregistered corpse of a prostitute who had succumbed to her diseases (*SB*, 29 Sept. 1909). In 1921, in another brothel the *Garde Municipale* found a woman who was seriously ill and to whom the madam had refused all medical treatment *(SB*, 2 April 1921).[74] Three years later, a diseased *huayanjian*[75] who had been abandoned in the street by the owner of the establishment where she had worked died in a small lodging house *(SB*, 20 April 1924). These cases reported in the press are isolated incidents, but how many other women suffered the same or a similar fate? Although these may not have been the majority of them, these extreme cases reveal the degree of indifference, egoism, and cynicism that could prevail in the relations between the madams and the prostitutes.

CONCLUSION

The patronizing of prostitutes by customers who scarcely bothered to take care of their own health condition greatly contributed to the widespread diffusion of STDs in China. By 1937, there were around 30 to 35 millions syphilitics, a figure that continued to increase in the following decade (Henriot 1992:105). It is no accident that the new regime launched a vigorous campaign of eradication after 1949. STDs had become a public scourge (Horn 1971). This situation resulted first from the lack of sanitary infrastructures that could accommodate the needs of either the prostitutes or the population at large. Public health, a concept imported at a later stage from the West, was never on top of the list of priorities of the successive Chinese governments. In Shanghai, the establishment of a full-fledged public health administration only took place in 1927. In spite of its accomplishments during the following decade, its main field of action was not directed toward the issue of STDs (Henriot 1993, Chapter 8). In the foreign settlements, the authorities made a weak attempt to rein in the spread of these diseases. Their efforts were pretty futile as they focused only on very small segments of the population, namely the permanent or transient foreign communities, and on the prostitutes who catered to their needs. A mere drop in the ocean, these efforts were fundamentally useless since they tackled only a small part of the problem.

Although some voices raised the issue of prevention through education as early as the 1920s – this was the dominant position among Shanghai physicians as expressed by the Shanghai Medical Association – no steps were even taken in this direction by the Shanghai Municipal Council, the authorities in the French Concession, or the Chinese municipal government. What prevailed was a logic of control and repression that targeted those who were considered to be the source of all problems: the prostitutes. It is true that the vast majority of prostitutes carried diseases. It is equally true that they hardly ever availed themselves of the services of a doctor, even after the introduction of antibiotics in 1945, although most of them were infected with STDs that must have had severe sequels a long time after they had retired from prostitution. Pertinently, their attitude was not so much the consequence of a lack of consciousness about the 'perils of the trade', about hygiene standards, or indeed about the existence of medical treatments. It was above all the result of a mixture of circumstances that conspired to inhibit any such possibility. This mixture included the conditions under which these women had been recruited and worked, their economic situation, and the policies implemented by the foreign and Chinese authorities. The last ran counter to their intended purpose simply because they were designed on the basis of prejudiced ideas about prostitution and prostitutes, without any direct contact with them or any attempt to acquire a proper knowledge of this milieu.

For almost a quarter of a century, the Chinese government was able to eradicate prostitution from its cities.[76] The return to a more open economic and social system, with increased exchanges and mobility both within and outside the domestic realm, has again created conditions for the forceful re-emergence of prostitution throughout the country. While no direct parallel with the Republican period can be traced, the dominant mode of intervention by the present Chinese authorities has still been stigmatization and repression.[77] As in the past, the approach to the problem of prostitution and STDs – a problem made more sensitive by the advent of HIV and AIDS – is derived from prejudiced views rather than from any genuine attempt to confront the social dynamics that underlie prostitution and from a deliberate policy to impose a blackout on these issues, especially the extent of HIV-infection in China, both internally and externally. Demonizing HIV and AIDS can only contribute to driving further 'underground' those who are infected, especially prostitutes, thereby stimulating the spread of the pandemics in China.

NOTES

1 The Moral Welfare League was an organization established in 1918 by a group of Protestant missionaries and activists to put an end the policy of medical control of the prostitutes by the Shanghai Municipal Council in the International Settlement and to eliminate prostitution from the settlement. See Henriot (2001).

2 The major studies of diseases in China have focused on the plague, see for instance Benedict (1996).

3 A woman physician wrote: 'Syphilology was not so widely disseminated in those days [mid-1890s] as it is now, not even among practicing physicians. In many cases, we did not recognize syphilis when we met it and in others, we did not know exactly how to treat it.' Fearn (1939: 59)

4 Pasteur's work opened the way to the discovery of transmissible diseases. Gonococcus, the pathogenic agent of gonorrhoea, was identified in 1879, but it was not before 1905 that *Treponema pallidum*, the microbe of syphilis, was discovered. The following year saw the invention of the first blood test (Wassermann) that could reliably detect a syphilitic infection. Quetel (1990:140–1).

5 See the summary made by Frazier in 1937 (1937:1043–6). On the development of public health in Nationalist China, see Yip Ka-che (1995).

6 Health issues were a major source of concern to Westerners from the outset. They were one of the major driving motives that led to the establishment and development of a municipal administration in the International Settlement. The reference on this topic is MacPherson (1987). On public health in a Chinese city, see Rogaski (1996).

7 'Commercialized Vice in China' (1922) *National Medical Journal* 8:3, p. 397

8 In 1913, the British government instituted the Royal Commission on Venereal Diseases which presented its conclusions three years later. To implement the measures proposed by the Commission, a National Council for Combating Venereal Diseases (NCCVD) was established. It was an organization of volunteers recognized by the ministry of Health as the agent of propaganda in the fight against venereal diseases throughout the country. The members of the Royal Commission were appointed to the executive board of the Council (Peter 1921:62, 64).

9 Shanghai Municipal Council *Report for the Year 1920*, Shanghai, Kelly and Walsh, pp. 262–5A.

10 Shanghai Municipal Council *Report for the Year 1922, op. cit.*, pp. 308–9A. The Shanghai Municipal Council also emphasized STDs were only one of the contagious diseases against which its Board of Health was battling.

11 Shanghai Municipal Council *Report for the Year 1923, op. cit.*, pp. 123–4. On average, the number of visits per patient rose to thirty after 1925 when the clinic was well established. This is an indication of the serious follow-up that was held on patients. This figure is computed from the data in Table 7.1.

12 Many seamen preferred to go to the dispensary rather than declaring their disease to their own medical officer. Besides the lack of appropriate treatment on board, they feared the financial penalties that would result from their being put on sick leave. Shanghai Municipal Council, *Report for the Year 1924, op. cit.*, pp. 148–9; *Report for the Year 1926, op. cit.*, p. 195; *Report for the Year 1927, op. cit.*, p. 182.

13 Shanghai Municipal Council, *Report for the Year 1924, op. cit.*, p. 148; *Report for the Year 1925, op. cit.*, p. 134.

14 Shanghai Municipal Council, *Report for the Year 1926, op. cit.*, p. 195; *Report for the Year 1927, op. cit.*, p. 183.

15 Minutes of the *Commission d'administration municipale*, 29 Dec. 1926, Ordonnances consulaires (Jul. 1926–Dec. 1928), Archives diplomatiques, Nantes. The Shanghai Municipal Council publicly expressed its disappointment in its 1927 annual report: 'It is very much to be regretted that the administration of the French Concession have declined to contribute toward the cost of maintaining the clinic.' Shanghai Municipal Council, *Report for the Year 1927, op. cit.*, p. 183.

16 Shanghai Municipal Council, *Report for the Year 1928, op. cit.*, p. 160

17 Shanghai Municipal Council, *Report for the Year 1931, op. cit.*, p. 175.

18 Shanghai Municipal Council, *Report for the Year 1934, op. cit.*, p. 137; *Report for the Year 1937, op. cit.*, p. 153

19 Shanghai Municipal Council, *Report for the Year 1933, op. cit.*, p. 170.

20 On the establishment of the lock hospital and the adoption of various control measures in the nineteenth century, see the excellent chapter in Kerrie L. MacPherson, (1987:213–58).

21 *Le Journal de Shanghai*, 4 June 1931

22 Report dated 23 November 1934, Archives diplomatiques, Nantes, Box No 39.

23 *Yewu baogao* (Annual report) (1941: 1, 19); *Yewu baogao* (Annual report) (1942).

24 The dispensary was officially inaugurated on 1 December, 1945, but because of problems of organization it did not receive prostitutes before February 1946. Letters of the Bureau of Health, 14 Feb. 1946, Police Archives (1945–9), file 011-4-269; 19 Feb. 1946, Police Archives (1945–9), File 011-4-261.

25 Organizational regulations of the dispensary, 5 Feb. 1948, Police Archives. (1945–9), File 011-4-269.

26 Instruction of the Bureau of Health, Oct. 1946; letter of the Bureau of Health, 1 May, 1948, Police Archives (1945–9), File 011-4-269.

27 *Changji jianyan buzou shuoming* (Instructions on the procedure for the examination of prostitutes), Police Archives (1945–9), File 011-4-269.

28 Document of the Bureau of Police, Oct. 1946, Police Archives (1945–9), file 011-4-269.

29 Letter from the Bureau of Health, 2 Dec., 1946, Police Archives (1945–9), File 1-10-246 (May 1946–Jan. 1949).

30 Letter from the mayor, 8 Dec., 1947, Police Archives (1945–9), File 6-19-666.

31 Document of the Bureau of Police, 18 Feb., 1946, Police Archives (1945–9), File 011-4-269.

32 Yu Wei (1948:10). Those prostitutes arrested who did not possess a card from the dispensary were fined or sent to jail for two or three days. Police Archives (1945–9), file 011-4-171: *Jinü bu zhao guiding jianyan shenti an* (Cases of breaches of regulation on the sanitary control of prostitutes), Dec. 1947–May 1948. On the Nationalist policy toward prostitution, see Henriot (2001, Chapter 13).

33 Police report, 30 Jan., 1948, Police Archives (1945–9), File 011-4-161: Aug. 1947–July 1949.

34 Letter from the Bureau of Health, 30 Oct., 1946, Police Archives (1945–9), File 011-4-269.

35 Letters from the mayor, 15 June, 1946; 12 Aug., 1946; undated project of the Bureau of Health; Letter of the bureau, 6 Aug., 1946, Police Archives (1945–9), File 011-4-261.

36 Letters from the Bureau of Health, 27 Sept., 1946; 22 Oct., 1946, Police Archives (1945–9), File 011-4-269.

37 Letter from the Bureau of Health, 8 June, 1946; report of the medical service of the U.S. army in a file of the Bureau of Health, 22 June, 1946, Police Archives (1945–9), File 011-4-269.

38 Two letters from military medical services in the United States, 2 Dec., 1946; 9 Sept., 1947; Two letters from the headquarters of the US Navy in Shanghai, 2 Jan., 1946; 3 Oct., 1946, Police Archives (1945–9), File 011-4-269; survey report, March 1948, Police Archives (1945–9), File 011-4-269.

39 Letter from Edwin W. Weissman, Area Provost Marshall, 17 June, 1946, Police Archives (1945–9), File 011-4-175: Dec. 1946-Nov. 1948; undated letter from the Italian ambassador, Police Archives (1945-9), File 011-4-174

40 Heath (1925:701-3).

41 According to the author, 53.4 per cent had received no treatment while 36.9 per cent had taken Chinese oral medicine. Only 5.9 per cent had been treated with Salvarsan and 1.6 per cent with mercury. Heimburger (1927:548).

42 Statistics are self-explanatory. From 1927 to 1933, there were 4,681 traditional native physicians and 596 Western-trained doctors in Shanghai. The proportion among hospitals was just the opposite. Among the thirty-one registered establishments, twenty-eight practised Western medicine and only three offered traditional medicine. Huang Kewu (1988) 'Cong Shen Bao yiyao guanggao kan min chu Shanghai de yiliao wenhua yu shehui shenghuo,' 1912–26 (The Medical Culture and Social Life in Shanghai: A Study Based on the Medicine Advertisements in *Shen Pao*, 1912–26), *Jindaishi yanjiusuo jikan* (Bulletin of the Institute of Modern History, Academia Sinica) XVII, part II, p. 149.

43 The use of mercury in the treatment of syphilis since the Ming dynasty (1368–1644), or even since the eighth century, is borne out by a treatise on the history of medicine in China. However, it is generally considered that syphilis was not introduced into China before the fourteenth century (Wong, Wu 1932:218–19).

44 The rather strange names of these medicines have their origin in the number of experiments made by its inventor, Dr Ehrlich, of Frankfurt. Salvarsan was born on the 606th attempt, although it was improved afterward through renewed experiments. The 914th one produced Neosalvarsan. Other treatments based on bismuth were also introduced after 1921 (Quetel 1990:142–3).

45 Ji Longsheng (1942 *Da Shanghai* (Greater Shanghai), Taibei, Nanfang zazhi chubanshe p. 111.

46 *SB*, advertisement, 15 Aug. 1928

47 Ji Longsheng, *Da Shanghai, op. cit.,* p. 111.

48 Huang Kewu, 'Cong Shen Bao yiyao guanggao kan min chu Shanghai de yiliao wenhua yu shehui shenghuo, 1912–26,' *op. cit.*, pp. 141–94.

49 Huang Kewu, 'Cong Shen Bao yiyao guanggao kan min chu Shanghai de yiliao wenhua yu shehui shenghuo, 1912–26,' *op. cit.*, p. 162–3, p. 168 and p. 180.

50 Archives of the Secretariat. International settlement (Secretariat, Shanghai Municipal Council) (1920–4), Shanghai Municipal Archives: 3-00445: File 1486, part 3, Secretariat (SMC), 'Prostitution: Brothels: Withdrawal of licenses, 1920–4.'

51 The other titles of newspapers that were collected (undated, [April 1930]) are: *Xiaoxiao da mimi* (Big and Small Secrets), *Liyuan gongbao* (The Player), *Qiongbao* (Jade), *Xiaoribao* (The Little Daily), *Shanghaitan* (The Shanghai Bund), *Que'ersideng* (The Cherleston), *Da shanghai* (Greater Shanghai), *Qingsi* (The Thread of Feeling), *Lingbao* (The Bell), *Shangsheng* (The Voice of Commerce), *Fu'ermosi* (?).

52 Huang Kewu, 'Cong Shen Bao yiyao guanggao kan min chu Shanghai de yiliao wenhua yu shehui shenghuo, 1912–26,' *op. cit.*, p. 162, 173 and pp. 182–3.

53 Ji Longsheng, *Da Shanghai, op. cit.*, p. 111.

54 Cf. *Shanghai zhinan* (1919) (Guide to Shanghai: A Chinese Directory of the Port), Shanghai, Shangwu yinshuguan, (1st ed., 1909), V, p. 19.

55 Shanghai Municipal Council, *Report for the Year 1923, op. cit.*, p. 125.

56 Shanghai Municipal Council, *Report for the Year 1923*, p. 123; *1924*, p. 148; *1925*, p. 134; *1926*, p. 196; *1927*, p. 182; *1929*, p. 150; *1930*, p. 166; *1931*, p. 148; *1932*, p. 175, *1933*, p. 170; *1934*, p. 137; *1935*, p. 116; *1936*, p. 144; *1937*, p. 153; *1938*, p. 174; *1939*, p. 152; *1940*, p. 178.

57 'Report on the Control and Treatment of Venereal Disease in Shanghai' (1924) *China Medical Journal,* Supplement, 38, pp. 19–21.

58 In Shanghai, the whole population was subject to quick blood samples (ear) to detect syphilis. Around 3,600 persons were mobilized to carry out this campaign over a short period of time. Horn (1971:92); Banister (1987:53–4).

59 'Xingbing he jiyuan'(STDs and brothels), *Wenhuibao*.

60 To detect syphilis, the dispensary used the Wasserman test. For gonorrhoea, the physicians resorted to cervical smear. Unfortunately, they kept no statistics of this infection (Yu 1948b:13).

61 In 1946, of the 931 diseased prostitutes treated in the dispensary, 233 contracted another venereal infection during the time of their treatment. This is an indication of the fact that the prostitutes, although they were diseased, did not stop practising their trade in violation of the regulation (Yu 1948a:18).

62 Letter from the Bureau of Health, 30 Oct., 1946, Police Archives (1945–9), File 011-4-269.

63 It must also be borne in mind that the new communist authorities were eager to show the extent of the damage and may have exaggerated the results.

64 Taxi dancers were professional female dancers who could be hired for dancing in the dance halls that flourished in Chinese cities after World War I, see Henriot (2001, Chapter 4).

65 This was an experiment aimed at testing a new medicine against gonorrhoea on a group of prostitutes through a comparison with a similar sample that did not take the medicine. The experiment was a failure in terms of medical protection.

66 This is an average number. The higher the number of visits, the higher the probability that a woman would be found to have an infection. Those who came more than five times during the time of the survey all tested positive. An age group analysis revealed that those between twenty and twenty-nine years had the highest rates of infection (Chu and Huang 1948:312–18).

67 *Xing bing zai Zhongguo* (STDs in China) (1990:4).

68 At this time, a visit to the dispensary cost only 20,000 Yuan. In July 1948, this fee was raised to 60,000 Yuan because of inflation. Letters of the Bureau of Health, 22 Nov., 1947; 2 July, 1948, Police Archives (1945–9), File 011-4-269.

69 Police report, undated, Police Archives (1945–9), File 011-4-263: Oct. 1947.

70 Statement by a prostitute, 18 Oct., 1947, Police Archives (1945–9), File 011-4-263: Oct. 1947.

71 Statement by a prostitute, 15 June, 1948, Police Archives (1945–9), File 011-4-269.

72 Letter of the Bureau of Health, 2 Dec., 1946, Police Archives (1945–9), file 1-10-246: May 1946–Jan. 1949

73 This, in turn, also varied over time. After the mid-1930s, the state of virtual slavery which had characterized the situation of a very large segment of the prostitutes virtually disappeared. Before that, however, many prostitutes were completely deprived of their freedom during the

time they served in a brothel. On the condition of prostitutes, see Henriot (2001, Chapter 9).

74 It is true that the madams were afraid that the prostitutes would take the opportunity to go out or stay in a hospital to run away, as many actually did. *SB*, 17 May 1920; 2 April 1921.

75 At the end of the century, the walled city in Shanghai had a large number of opium dens where customers were attended by young women who also provided sexual services. Originally, these places were just opium dens which, in order to compete with each other and attract customers, recruited or simply purchased young girls to replace male waiters. Very soon, these girls would be coerced into prostitution, whence the name of their establishments *huayanjian* or *yanhuajian* (literally 'chambers of smoke and flowers'). See Henriot, Christian (2001, chapter 3).

76 Henriot (1995:148–67); *Beijing fengbi jiyuan jishi* (The True Story of the Closure of the Houses of Prostitution in Peking) (1988); He, Yang (1988).

77 For a genuine attempt to understand prostitution in China, see Pan's study (1999).

REFERENCES

Archives diplomatiques, Nantes. Minutes of the Commission d'administration municipale, 29 Dec. 1926, Ordonnances consulaires (Jul. 1926–Dec. 1928), Box No 39.

Archives of the police (*jingchaju*) (1945-1949). File 011-4-269; file 011-4-261; file 1-10-246; file 6-19-666; file 011-4-171; file 011-4-161; file 011-4-174; file 011-4-263.

Archives of the Secretariat. International settlement (Secretariat, Shanghai Municipal Council) (1920–4), Shanghai Municipal Archives: 3-00445: File 1486.

Banister, Judith (1987) *China's Changing Population.* Stanford: Stanford University Press.

Beijing fengbi jiyuan jishi (1988) (The True Story of the Closure of the Houses of Prostitution in Peking). Beijing: Zhongguo heping chubanshe.

Benedict, Carol (1996) *Bubonic Plague in Nineteenth-Century China.* Stanford: Stanford University Press.

Chu L.W. and C.H. Huang (1948) 'Gonorrhea Among Prostitutes' [Peking], *Chinese Medical Journal* 66, pp. 312–8.

'Commercialized Vice in China' (1922) *National Medical Journal* 8(3), pp. 396–7.

Fearn, Anne W. (1939) *My Days of Strength: An American Woman Doctor's Forty Years in China.* New York: Harper & Brothers Publishers.

Frazier, Chester N. (1937) 'The Prevention and Control of Syphilis,' *Chinese Medical Journal* 51: January, pp. 1043–6.

He Wannan and Jiezeng Yang (1988) *Shanghai changji gaizao shihua* (A Short History of the Re-Education of Prostitutes in Shanghai), Shanghai: Sanlian shudian.

Heath, Frances J. (1925) 'Review of Eight Years' Work in China in a Gynecologic Out-patient Clinic,' *China Medical Journal* 39, pp. 701–5.

Heimburger, L.F. (1927) 'The Incidence of Syphilis at the Shantung Christian University Dispensary,' *China Medical Journal* 41, pp. 541–50.

Henriot, Christian (1992) 'Medicine, V.D., and Prostitution in Pre-Revolutionary China,' *Social History of Medicine* V:1, pp. 95–120.

– (1993) *Shanghai, 1927–1937. Elites, locality, and municipal power in Nationalist China.* Berkeley: University of California Press.

– (1995) ' "La Fermeture": The Abolition of Prostitution in Shanghai, 1949–1958,' *The China Quarterly*, December, pp. 148–67.

– (2001) *Prostitution and Sexuality in Shanghai. A Social History (1849–1949).* New York: Cambridge University Press.

Horn, Joshua S. (1971) *Away With All Pests. An English Surgeon in People's China: 1954–1969.* London/New York: Monthly Review Press.

Huang Kewu (1988) 'Cong Shen Bao yiyao guanggao kan min chu Shanghai de yiliao wenhua yu shehui shenghuo, 1912–1926' (The Medical Culture and Social Life in Shanghai: A Study Based on the Medicine Advertisements in *Shen Pao*, 1912–1926), *Jindaishi yanjiusuo jikan* (Bulletin of the Institute of Modern History, Academia Sinica) XVII, part II, pp. 141–94.

Ji Longsheng (1942) *Da Shanghai* (Greater Shanghai). Taibei, Nanfang zazhi chubanshe.

Lai, Daniel (1948) 'Incidence of Syphilis among Prostitutes and Cabaret Hostesses in Tsingtao,' *Chinese Medical Journal* 66, pp. 389–90.

Lai, Dr. (1930) 'Syphilis and Prostitution in Kiangsu,' *China Medical Journal* 44, pp. 558–63.

Le Journal de Shanghai, 1931.

MacPherson, Kerrie L. (1987) *A Wilderness of Marshes. The Origins of Public Health in Shanghai, 1843–1893.* Oxford: Oxford University Press.

Pan Suiming (1999) *Zhongguo hongdengqu jishi* (A True Record of China's Red Light Districts). Beijing: Qunyan chubanshe.

Peter, W.W. (1921) 'Fighting Venereal Disease Openly,' *China Medical Journal* 35: January, pp. 61–6.

Quetel, Claude (1990) *History of syphilis*. Baltimore: The Johns Hopkins University Press.

'Report on the Control and Treatment of Venereal Disease in Shanghai' (1924) *China Medical Journal,* Supplement 38, pp. 19–21.

Rogaski, Ruth (1996) *From protecting life to protecting the nation: The emergence of public health in Tianjin, 1859–1953.* Doctoral dissertation, Yale University.

Shanghai Municipal Council (1920–1940) *Report for the Year ...*, Shanghai: Kelly and Walsh.

Shanghai zhinan (1919) (Guide to Shanghai: A Chinese Directory of the Port). Shanghai: Shangwu yinshuguan, (1st ed., 1909).

Shen Bao, Shanghai, daily, 1920–1925.

Wong K.C., and Lien-teh Wu (1932) *History of Chinese Medicine*. Tientsin, Tientsin Press Ltd., pp. 218–9.

Wu, Lien-teh (1927) 'The Problem of Venereal Diseases in China,' *China Medical Journal* 41, January, pp. 28–36.

'Xingbing he jiyuan' (STDs and brothel houses), *Wenhuibao*, 25 Nov. 1951, p. 72.

Xing bing zai Zhongguo, (STDs in China) (1990) Beijing: Beijing shiyue wenyi chubanshe.

Yewu baogao (Annual report) (1941) Shanghai: Shanghai tebie shi weishengju bian.

– (1942) Shanghai, Shanghai tebie shi weishengju bian.

Yip, Ka-che (1995) *Health and National Reconstruction in Nationalist China. The Development of Modern Health Services, 1928–1937*. Ann Arbor: Association for Asian Studies.

Yu, Wei (1948) 'Jin chang yu xingbing fangzhi' (The prohibition of prostitution and the prevention of venereal diseases), *Shizheng pinglun* (The Municipal affairs weekly) 9(9/10), pp. 17–18.

– (1948) 'Shanghai changji wu bai ge an diaocha' (A survey of five hundred Shanghai prostitutes), *Shizheng pinglun* (The Municipal affairs weekly) 10:9/10, pp. 10–14.

CHAPTER 8

REPRESENTATIONS OF 'US' AND 'OTHERS' IN THE AIDS NEWS DISCOURSE: A TAIWANESE EXPERIENCE[1]

MEI-LING HSU, WEN-CHI LIN AND TSUI-SUNG WU

WHY STUDY NEWS MEDIA?

For years, the mass media have been a major conduit through which public perceptions of and attitudes towards AIDS have been formed and influenced. Large-scale media campaigns around the world have played a critical role in instilling intended effects of AIDS awareness and prevention, but the unintended effects of the news coverage about AIDS cannot be overlooked. At a more general level, research has shown that news media are important sources of health information for both private individuals (Freimuth *et al.* 1984; Simpkins and Brenner 1984; Wallack 1990) and for policy makers (Weiss 1974). Given their predominance in modern society, news media sometimes have a stronger impact on public cognition, attitudes, and preventive behaviour than planned media campaigns do. For the population at large, those who have no direct contact with AIDS or its sufferers, the awareness of the disease is mostly media related. Therefore, it is to these media portrayals that we must turn to, if we are to achieve a better understanding of how and why stigmatization of AIDS-related groups occurs.

In addressing the functions of the mass media, Watney (1987) maintained that the mass media use a mode of address which constructs recipients of the messages as a unified 'general public' with shared values and characteristics. Deviant or marginalized groups are excised and made to stand outside the general public, inevitably assuming the appearance of a threat to its internal cohesion. Newspapers in particular tend to construct an ideal audience of national family units, surrounded by the threatening spectacle of the deviants. In other words, the ideal audience addressed by the newspapers can be seen as the implicit 'us' group in the mainstream society. Those who are considered to threaten the norms or welfare of the ideal audience are thus categorized as 'Others.' An issue worth addressing here is: Who are the members of these 'Us' and 'Other' groups formed in the news discourse? How have they been changed over time?

Indeed, moralistic overtones in disease discourse tend to posit a clear boundary between 'healthy Us' and 'diseased Others' (Gilman 1988). Believing that AIDS affects 'them' not 'Us' means people of the 'Us' category can deny they are at risk. Such textual tactics enables the 'Us' group to exercise control over the reality of the 'Others,' and deny its own vulnerability to the disease. Therefore, discourses on sexually transmitted diseases such as AIDS tend to show a greater propensity towards stigmatization of the disease and the diseased (Bardhan 1996).

In a content analysis of 1996–1997 news coverage about AIDS in Taiwan, Hsu (1998) found that the most commonly occurring themes were AIDS prevention efforts and campaign activities, individuals or groups involved in the AIDS epidemic, and AIDS research. An analysis of the AIDS-related individuals or groups represented in the news discourse since the first AIDS case identified in 1984 can help us understand what the patterns and changes are when addressing the 'Us' vs. 'Other' categorization. Thus, through a textual analysis of the AIDS coverage in the Taiwanese news media, we attempt to sort out and summarize those shared characteristics that distinguish between the groups of 'Us' and 'Others' in the discourse. Moreover, the stigmatizing conditions and features vary in the extent to which they elicit stigmatization. That is, some groups socially labelled as 'Others' may be more stigmatized. Similarly, within the big umbrella of the 'Us' groups, being in a position of power, for example, may enable certain sub-groups to be more privileged than the others. This being so, we will further explore the discourse patterns in the AIDS news, which contributed to these levels of differences in forming 'Us' and 'Other' sub-groups, respectively in more detail.

The study comprises five parts. In addition to the preceding introduction highlighting the significance of studying news media as a site, the second part consists of an outline of the theoretical framework that will be used in our analysis. Following this in the third section is a brief outline of the AIDS epidemic in Taiwan. The fourth part will introduce the method and then analyse the results found in the AIDS discourse. The study will conclude with a discussion of the findings and their implications for future research.

THEORETICAL CONCEPTS TO BE USED

The social construction of AIDS-related groups or individuals as 'Us' vs. 'Others' is closely linked to the human psychology of stigma formation as well as to the social process of deviance and marginalization. In this section, we shall give an explication of these concepts and then see how they can be applied to our analysis of the AIDS discourse.

Stigma

The epidemic of stigma that accompanies AIDS has perhaps exerted much greater impact on society and the general population than the contagion of HIV itself has (Goldin 1994). A stigmatized reaction towards people with AIDS or HIV (PWA/HIVs) may jeopardize the well-being of most of the individuals involved, because it may well discourage attempts to go for an HIV test, and lead to abrasive relations among members of a society (Blendon and Donelan 1988). The term 'stigma' originally referred to a sign or mark, cut or burned into the body, that designated the bearer as a person who was morally defective and to be avoided (Goffman 1963). In a modern society, stigma can be seen as an identity that is socially constructed (Archer 1985). It can also be perceived as a type of social identity that is devalued in a particular context (Crocker, Major and Steele 1998).

Nevertheless, stigmatization cannot simply be explained by single or even sets of clearly defining features. Some social psychologists (e.g., Cantor and Michel 1979; Rosch 1978) prefer to think of conditions that stigmatize as a 'fuzzy' set in which stigmatized groups are likely to share several features. Goffman (1963) offered the first organization scheme to categorize stigmatizing conditions into three types:

(1) Tribal stigmas, which are passed down from generation to generation, and include membership in devalued racial, ethnic, or religious groups;
(2) Abominations of the body, which are un-inherited physical characteristics that convey a devalued social identity, such as being physically disadvantaged; and
(3) Blemishes of individual character, which are devalued social identities related to one's personality or behaviour, such as prostitutes or homosexuals.

It should be noted that some stigmatizing conditions might fit into two or more types. In relation to the AIDS epidemic, Albert (1986) explained that underlying and fuelling the stigmatization of AIDS risk groups is the fear that the social distinctions which serve as protection will be breached, leaving the general population open to the onslaught of the fatal infections that infection with AIDS permits. Consequently, the maintenance of social distance is crucial, which results in laying the blame for one's disability on an individual who is seen as responsible. In the Western nations, this has been well manifested in accusations in news reports that gay men are justifiable objects of the righteous punishment of God for sinful behaviour.

In this study, we can observe which of the stigmatizing conditions sketched by Goffman are the predominant types. We can also analyse the language mechanisms used in the news discourse which facilitate the forming of these categorizations.

DEVIANCE

Deviance is another term used to exclude certain groups, transforming them into 'Others.' It is a quality that implies hostility, stigma, and condemnation; it is intrinsically negative, invidious, a quality that attracts scorn (Watney 1987). During times of crisis or panic such as the AIDS epidemic, those considered to be deviants may serve as scapegoats, secondary targets to deflect attention away from some of society's most pressing but insoluble problems (Best 1990).

Like stigma, deviance is not an either-or proposition. It is a matter of degree. Plummer (1979) distinguished between societal and situational deviance. Societal deviance is made up of widely condemned classes or categories of behaviour; situational deviance ignores such broad, society-wide judgments and examines only concrete negative judgments of behaviour and individuals in specific contexts. Similarly, Sarbin (1967) noted that sanctions against deviance and their intensity vary on a continuum related to performance of ascribed and achieved role expectations. Toward the achieved role expectation pole, negative labelling is relatively minimal whereas meritorious performance is highly rewarded. Conversely, no positive reward is attached to ascribed role performance, whereas negative performance elicits strong sanctions.

In the context of AIDS, it can be seen that certain groups or communities are labelled deviants mainly because of their failure to fulfil their role expectations. Pertinently, the extent to which these groups deviate from the mainstream society differs, depending on whether their association with AIDS is situational, stemming from a lack of personal control (namely, haemophiliacs, mother-to-child transmission), or normative/societal, stemming from an individual choice (namely, gay men, sex workers, intravenous drug users). Following this line, we will distinguish between these groups in our analysis of the AIDS discourse in the news.

MARGINALIZATION

In a similar vein, Cohen (1999: 54–76) sketched four general patterns of marginalization, which function to exaggerate and manipulate differences within marginal groups:

(1)   Categorical strategies of marginalization include practices that seek to exclude an entire class or group of people from any central control over dominant resources and institutions. Such strategies are mobilized when some belief, characteristics, or behaviour shared by all targeted group members (namely race, gender, religion, or sexual preference) is used to signal the 'inherent' inferiority or 'natural' deviance of a group, promoting the idea that these individuals are somehow deserving of their marginal status.

(2)   Integrative marginalization provides control by unequivocally regulating the majority of marginal community members while allowing a chosen few to have limited access to dominant institutions and resources. Nevertheless, those privileged marginal group members are not viewed as equals within the dominant communities.

(3)   Advanced marginalization focuses on the heightened stratification of marginal communities. Those marginal group members who conform to dominant norms and behaviour are included and legitimized in the 'Us' groups.

(4)   Secondary processes of marginalization can be exercised by the more privileged members of the marginal groups as attempts to demonstrate their 'just as good as you' qualities to the mainstream communities. Those members of marginal communities reportedly extreme in their 'nonconformist behaviour' are defined as standing outside the norms and behaviour agreed upon by the community.

According to Cohen (1999), the above patterns of marginalization may overlap and may change over time in response to both the resistance on the part of excluded groups and the evolving and diversified interests of both marginal and dominant group members. Cohen went on to identify three kinds of practices that facilitate the processes of marginalization: ideologies, institutions, and social relationships. Ideology takes on a more neutral or progressive definition than that which has been recognized by social philosophers such as Marx and Gramsci (Cohen 1999). A group's physical environment, material sources, and social position all help to shape the local manifestations of commonly held ideologies. In the case of AIDS, ideologies and definitions of deviance and abnormality have been used to position PWA/HIVs outside not only the traditional health-care system, but also have pushed them beyond the bounds of the larger moral fabric of the society.

Institutional practices have been useful in implementing measures of social control of the 'Others.' These include public laws and organizational rules, plus the application of less formal mechanisms such as informal networks of recruiting and hiring, unspoken job segregation, and a hostile work or living environment (Cohen 1999). Through the control of

187

institutions, the 'Us' groups not only restrict access to the dominant resources, they also disseminate ideologies of stigmatization that justifies the exclusion of certain groups. Abundant examples have been documented in Western history to prove this point. Whether the institution is the prison or the mental hospital, as detailed by Foucault (1979), or the educational system, as explored by Paulo Freire (1972), such structures embody the ability to monitor and restrict the behaviour of the less powerful, resource-poor marginal group members.

In the absence of state-sponsored institutional marginalization, individuals and groups often continue to judge marginal groups as inferior and deviant. Informal interactions or social relationships provide the basis for such lasting exclusion. Cohen (1999) noted that they are harder to identify than formal laws, rules, or institutional structures.

This suggests that who or what constitutes 'Us' vs. 'Others' may follow the same patterns, motivated by economic profit, social positioning, or political power. In this study, we expect to be able to locate the patterns of marginalization in the AIDS discourse. We also expect to be able to identify those mechanisms that contributed to the processes of marginalization.

From the foregoing, we learn that terms such as stigma, deviance, and marginalization approximate the present use of 'Other.' We prefer to use the term 'Other' because we are attracted by its vagueness, which can refer to practically anything, depending on the context or situation. How, then, do the news media represent certain groups or individuals in order to marginalize or stigmatize them into the 'Other' category? Watney (1987) noted that scandal serves the purpose of exemplary exclusion in the newspaper discourse, and is the dominant means by which readers find themselves reassured and reconciled as 'normal' law-abiding citizens. For example, homosexuality is constructed in the press as an exemplary and admonitory sign of Otherness in order to unite sexual and national identification among readers prevailing over all divisions and distinctions of class, race and gender.

In contrast to research on 'Others,' fewer studies have been conducted to address the formation of the 'Us' category specifically. This would seem to demonstrate that the formation of 'Us' depends on what constitutes 'Others.' Therefore, a comparison of the terms 'Self' vs. 'Other' is helpful in conceptualizing the 'Us' group formation in the study. Todorov (1982) identified three dimensions in the relationship between 'Self' and 'Other': (1) value judgment, e.g., the 'Other' may be deemed good or bad, equal or inferior to the 'Self'; (2) social distance, i.e., the physical and psychological distance the 'Self' maintains from the 'Other'; and (3) knowledge, meaning the extent to which the history and culture of the 'Other' is known to the

'Self.' Positive value judgments, low social distance, and a sophisticated knowledge of the 'Other' are generally associated with each other.

Specifically, Bradley (1998) found three 'innocent victim' categories of people at risk as appearing in the AIDS research: female partners of male drug users; recipients of blood transfusions (apart from haemophiliacs); and children born to women with AIDS. She also found that in the US AIDS news coverage, the public was categorized into three types: (1) high risk groups composed of male homosexuals, bisexuals, intravenous drug users, and haemophiliacs; (2) low-to-medium risk groups, composed of promiscuous heterosexuals, recipients of blood transfusions, and spouses of haemophiliacs; and (3) no risk groups, composed of the monogamous and people who had received no blood products. The same distinction may not be the same in other cultures when identifying the 'Us' vs. 'Others.' Yet the extent to which those groups are considered to be at risk reflects to the extent to which they have deviated from the 'normal' and healthy values in the society.

Furthermore, to name one's 'Self' is a fundamental human right that frequently is denied to 'Others.' Members of an 'Us' group may be identified by personal name more often than others outside the group, who are identified anonymously according to occupation, age, or some other social status. Expressions that are the most revealing of the boundaries separating 'Self' and 'Other' are inclusive and exclusive pronouns and possessives such as we and they, us and them, and ours and theirs (Riggins 1997). In this study, we shall also identify members of the 'Us' group as it is formed in relation to the 'Others' group in the AIDS discourse in the Taiwanese news media.

AIDS IN TAIWAN: STATE OF THE ART

Taiwan is located off the eastern coast of Asia, separated from the Chinese mainland by the Taiwan Strait. With a total area of nearly 36,000 square kilometres, Taiwan has a population of roughly 23 million, with the population density ranking the second highest in the world after Bangladesh. Longer education, delayed marriages, the rise of nuclear families and comparatively fewer potential mothers between the ages of twenty and thirty-four have reduced the birth rate. The classical conception of family-based support has been challenged by the emergence of a modern, post-agricultural economy in Taiwan. Many young people have left the farming households in which they grew up and established nuclear families in urban areas (50 per cent of the population lives in either Taipei, Taichung, Tainan, or Kaohsiung) (Government Information Office 2000).

Like in most parts of the world, during its initial years the issue of AIDS had not received enormous medical, social and, thus, media attention in Taiwan. The first AIDS case (a foreigner in transit) was identified in late December 1984. The first non-foreigner, HIV-seropositive was reported in 1986. Since then, the number of PWA/HIVs has increased steadily. By June 2001, Taiwan had documented 3,552 people infected with HIV (Department of Health 2001). Nevertheless, the exact number of HIV cases in Taiwan could be as much as four or five times the official statistics. By the definition of the World Health Organization, Taiwan can be classified as a 'Pattern I' country where heterosexual contact is the main form of HIV transmission (Bloor 1995). Of the 3,552 HIV positives, 3,252 (92.6 per cent) are locals, and 300 foreigners. According to the categorization of the Department of Health (DOH), of the 3,252 HIV positive locals, 1,383 (42.5 per cent) are heterosexuals; 1,091 (32.5 per cent), male homosexuals; 437 (13.4 per cent), male bisexuals; 53 (1.6 per cent), haemophiliacs; 57 (1.8 per cent), intravenous drug (IVD) users; 13 (0.4 per cent), blood receivers; 7 (0.2 per cent), babies through vertical transmission; and 211 (6.5 per cent), unknown. In addition, most of them are male (3,004 cases, 92.4 per cent), aged 20–29 years (1,180 cases, 36.3 per cent), followed by those in age groups 30–39 years (1,078 cases, 33.1 per cent).

Note that like in many other regions, the line between male homosexual, bisexual, and even heterosexual may not be clear in Taiwan. These distinctions, however, are used by the DOH in Taiwan in reporting local AIDS epidemic.

In May 1985, an AIDS prevention task force was established within the DOH, the highest health authority in Taiwan, to address the public health issues associated with AIDS. In November 1990, the Legislative Yuan, the major law-making body in Taiwan, passed a law on AIDS prevention. Nevertheless, it was not until January 1994 that a programme for the prevention and control of AIDS was approved for implementation. Perhaps because of the relatively mild epidemiological profile of the disease compared to other countries in the world, particularly South and Southeast Asian countries, AIDS was recognized as a category of catastrophic diseases. This meant that medical care services, outpatient, and hospitalization used to be free for AIDS patients until January 1998, when HIV/AIDS was included in the coverage of National Health Insurance.

In 1985, the DOH began to screen the so-called high-risk groups. Since 1988, general screenings of blood for transfusion and blood products have been conducted to protect the blood users. In 1989, screening of the military draftees; in 1990, screening of the prison inmates; and in 1991, screening of foreign labourers began. To prevent individuals with high-risk behaviour from using blood tests for the testing of HIV infection, blood donors are not to be notified of the test findings. Requirements for blood donors have also been revised and the recipients of blood are to be followed up. Since 1 July 1995, blood centres have been asked to conduct HIV-1/2 testing. A set of compensation measures for up to approximately $60,000 for any person infected accidentally with HIV through blood transfusion has been decided (Department of Health 2000).

The DOH also formulated health education programmes in which employees of sanitary establishments and special occupations, gay men, tour guides, factory workers, prison inmates, students, military draftees, sailors, women, and the general public have been classified as priority groups for education about AIDS and other sexually transmitted diseases. Despite these measures, AIDS prevention campaigns in Taiwan were not initiated until 1992, when the DOH started sponsoring campaigns and forming patient support groups. The DOH also asked several local non-governmental organizations (NGOs) to organize health education programmes for prostitutes, gay men, and adolescents in custody (Department of Health 2000).

In fact, over the years, it has been these NGOs which have been dedicated to changing the public's negative responses to AIDS and its victims. For example, *Light of Friendship AIDS Control Association* (LOFAA), established by a group of concerned citizens in the summer of 1992, aims to train voluntary workers and to stop the spread of HIV/AIDS before it assumes epidemic proportions. *Living with Hope*, which concentrates on providing support to PWA/HIVs, first brought the *NAME Memorial Quilt Project* from the United States to Taiwan in 1995 in memory of those who are infected with or had died of the AIDS virus. *Persons with HIV/AIDS Rights Advocacy Association*, the first voluntary group focusing on the legal rights of people with AIDS and HIV, was organized in November 1997. In January 1999, a group named *Floating Wood Helping Association* was formed to promote the rights of the PWA/HIVs infected by blood products, and more importantly, to demand national compensation through legal channels (Hsu 1998).

AIDS DISCOURSE IN TAIWANESE NEWS MEDIA

The study will analyse the AIDS discourse as represented in the Taiwanese news media. Specifically, we shall examine how the groups of 'Us' and 'Others' have been constructed in the news texts and structures informing the public about AIDS epidemic and prevention. In this section, we shall begin by introducing the method used, and then we shall proceed with analyses of the results found in the news discourse.

METHOD

We conducted a textual analysis of the AIDS discourse in the news from the first reported AIDS case in 1984 up to the end of 1999. A specific sample was selected based on the AIDS key events or issues within this time frame. Specifically, we selected three mainstream newspapers for this purpose, including *China Times, United Daily News* and *Min Seng Bao*. The first two papers have the largest circulation, and the last one is the only paper in Taiwan that has a full-page health section targeted at medical care workers. As the major purpose of our study is to examine the patterns of and changes in AIDS discourse in the mainstream news media as a whole, we shall not compare the differences in news reporting among the three newspapers in any greater detail.

By using 'AIDS' as the keyword for our news search, we first conducted a headline search on two on-line database systems: One from the *Central News Agency,* and the other from *Sino21* information net. A list of thousands of AIDS articles was generated by compiling the news headlines from the two systems. We then narrowed down the number of the articles by focusing on those that dealt with PWA/HIVs or AIDS-related persons and groups. After collecting the relevant news articles from the library, we looked into the texts across a time span of fifteen years to identify the patterns and changes in the AIDS discourse in relation to our research questions.

ANALYSIS OF REPRESENTATIONS

To facilitate a better understanding of the patterns and changes found in our analysis of the news texts, we categorized the fifteen years of AIDS discourse into six periods, based mainly on the predominant features of the AIDS-related groups during that specific time period. These periods include: (1) AIDS as an imported product from the West (late-1984-mid-1985); (2) AIDS as a gay man's disease (mid-1985-late-1988); (3) AIDS as an intruder in the family units (late-1988-mid-1991); (4) AIDS as an imported product from South and Southeast Asia (mid-1991-early-1993); (5) AIDS as a site of identity change (early-1993-late-1996); and (6) AIDS as a public forum for human rights (late-1996-late-1999).

AIDS AS AN IMPORTED PRODUCT FROM THE WEST (LATE-1984-MID-1985)

Before 1984, when no AIDS cases had been reported in Taiwan, AIDS was considered a disease occurring only in the West. Occasionally, stories translated from the Western news agencies regarding the exoticness of the disease could be found in the local press.

When the first AIDS case was identified in December 1984 and then leaked to the press two months later, the patient's identity as 'an American physician visiting Taiwan' was emphasized (*Min Seng Bao, United Daily, China Times* 8 March 1985). He was also identified as a gay man with an 'abnormal' lifestyle. Therefore, AIDS was said to infect people through some 'special' channels, such as anal sex (*Min Seng Bao* 8 March 1985). The patient was also described as having an eight-year history of homosexuality (*United Daily, China Times* 8 March 1985). Being an alien and deviant 'Other,' he was deprived of his privacy. Like a criminal at large, his full name and a clear photograph of him were published (e.g., *Min Seng Bao*). Among all of his identities: medical professional, gay man, and foreigner, the patient's identity as a foreigner seemed to have raised the greatest concern in the news discourse. Therefore, public health officials and local medical sources reassured the public not to worry about getting the disease. The DOH did not intend to implement the testing policy because no local cases had been found. Also quoting an American medical professional, the press emphasized, 'Taiwan was not a high-risk area of AIDS'(*Min Seng Bao* 13 March 1985).

The foreign connection of AIDS prevailed in the news reports during this period. An AIDS 'suspect,' though later tested negative, was made to admit that he was a gay and had had 'abnormal' sex abroad (*Min Seng Bao* 13 May 1985). The press went into details about his sex life, emphasizing that he had had one hundred or so sex partners, of whom at least ten were foreigners (*Min Seng Bao* 27 June 1985). When the first local AIDS case was reported, the press still stressed the foreign connection by stating that the patient had lived abroad for a long time and that half of his sex partners had been foreigners. Therefore, he may have contracted AIDS from those foreigners (*United Daily, China Times, Min Seng Bao* 30 August 1985). In fact, as can be found in other AIDS-related reports, tracking AIDS patients' sex histories was a routine pattern in the news reporting.

At this initial stage of the AIDS epidemic, gay men and foreigners were the two major groups identified and consequently stigmatized as 'Others' in the news discourse. It is worth noting that although all PWA/HIVs mentioned in the AIDS news were gay men, the fact that they were foreigners seemed to outweigh their sexual orientation in the news discourse. By applying Goffman's (1963) categorization, we observed a predominant pattern of using tribal stigmas in labelling AIDS patients. The metaphor of the decadent West was also salient in the news discourse. The health authority's decision not to take any policy initiative served as an institutional force in marginalizing the groups concerned. People other than foreigners and gay men implicitly assumed to be the 'Us' category in the discourse. In particular, Taiwanese locals were the priority 'Us' group to be protected from the disease.

AIDS AS A GAY MAN'S DISEASE (MID-1985–LATE-1988)

Gay men and foreigners were still blamed as AIDS carriers in this period, but the issue of homosexuality appeared to raise greater concerns in the news discourse as well as in the campaign pamphlets after August 1985. In addition to the routine reports of AIDS cases as related to gay men, expert sources and public forums attacking homosexuality were evident. Therefore, a DOH official indicated that promiscuous gay men should be seriously concerned, particularly if half of them engage in such a lifestyle (*Min Seng Bao* 4 September 1985). *Min Seng Bao* (16 September 1985) even ran an editorial on homosexual behaviour:

'Because of their deviant behaviour, gay men are more likely to contract AIDS than the general public. As they change their sex partners very often, the spread of the virus is greater. Gay men can transmit the virus to their wives and children. I am not greatly concerned about the *bo li chuan*,[2] but if they transmit the virus to the general public, they become the enemies of the people. If you know of any gay men, please advise them to be tested. If you are a gay man, I hope you can be tested to protect yourself and your loved ones. You should be discreet in the future too.'

Although gay men as a whole were regarded as deviants, the distinctions between societal and situational deviance, as proposed by Plummer (1979), can be found in the discourse. Citing a physician, *Min Seng Bao* (4 September 1985) indicated 'the public should not confuse gay men with people with occasional homosexual behaviour, which may occur among curious teenagers or in all-male environments such as the prison and the military (*Min Seng Bao, China Times* 28 February 1986). In the health authority there was still a belief that homosexuality could be corrected and be restrained to some extent. This latter category was considered situational, and consequently less deviant than those born homosexual.

At first sight, representations of gay men in the news seemed to suggest a use of categorical strategies of marginalization (Cohen 1999) to exclude the entire group. For example, when the first local AIDS patient died, his identity as a gay man having sexual contacts with foreigners was stated again in the news. An emphasis on having no heterosexual relationship and having never donated blood were other strategies to enable the risk group to be labelled exclusively homosexual. Therefore, the health authority urged that gay men, who were at high risk, should go for testing as soon as possible. At this time, AIDS was still not considered serious in Taiwan (*Min Seng Bao* 2 October 1985). The authority indicated, 'AIDS should not be a legalized infectious disease, for it only affects certain high-risk groups, through special channels. The general public will not easily contract the disease' (*United Daily* 8 March 1986).

A further analysis of the AIDS news shows that the patterns of integrative marginalization and secondary processes of marginalization were also evident. As far as the integrative marginalization is concerned, gay men who denounced their promiscuity and took the blood tests were included, but not necessarily legitimized in the 'Us' group. Therefore, one leading medical centre announced that as long as gay men tested negative, 'innocent' ID cards would be issued to them (*Min Seng Bao* 4 September 1985). The same pattern of marginalization can be found in coverage of an HIV-positive gay man, masked and regretful at a news conference, admitting that he had casual sex with five strangers. Contritely, he warned the public not to engage in one-night-stand relationships and urged gay men to come out for testing (*China Times, United Daily* 26 June 1987). It should be noted that although the masked young man urged the government to pay attention to the rights and privileges of the PWA/HIVs (*Min Seng Bao* 26 June 1987), this issue did not seem to reach the news agenda until 1994.

Secondary processes of marginalization often occurred when privileged members of the gay community had come to redefine themselves to the non-gay public. During an interview, a gay activist mentioned that most gay men used to have multiple partners, but had begun to establish one-to-one relationships because of the widespread appearance of AIDS (*Min Seng Bao* 15 September 1985). Another then opinion leader of the gay community, Chi Jia-Wei, also a voluntary worker for the DOH, explained to the press how a gay man could contract AIDS, 'He may have played the "female" role without wearing condoms during man-to-man sex' (*United Daily* 8 May 1988).

Attempts to locate the 'dangerous' gay men served as another marginalizing apparatus. Locations where male homosexuality could be spotted, such as Taipei New Park, Tainan Park, Kaohsiung Love River, underground shopping streets in Kaohsiung, and bathhouses in downtown Taipei were all stigmatized as paradises of promiscuity in the news discourse (*United Daily* 5 May, 10 July, 6 August 1988; *Min Seng Bao* 19 July 1988).

The gay-bashing came to a climax when a male student from a teacher's training college was tested HIV positive at a military training camp.[3] Stories about the threat he posed to the campus, the once pure place for the young and the teachers-to-be, were run in the press for two summers (July 1987–September 1988). Typical patterns of stigmatizing gay men were again

195

found: the student had led a promiscuous sex life, including having sex with men and female prostitutes (*Min Seng Bao* 24, 25 July 1987); his homosexual behaviour began when he was at junior high school; and he had had more than a thousand sex partners (*United Daily* 25 July 1987). Anecdotal narratives of the student's personal life, clothed by an implied heterosexual perspective in the press, served as ideological practices to marginalize gay men. Therefore, the student was said to have tried to begin relationships with the opposite sex in recent years but had failed (*United Daily* 25 July 1987). The press emphasized that learning from his example, we should 'prevent teenagers from having engaged in homosexuality in their young age' (*United Daily* 26 July 1987).

Institutional practices of marginalization also came into play under the pretext of controlling the 'guilty' and protecting the 'innocent.' The AIDS student, who was seen as a deviant, was expelled from his college (*Min Seng Bao* 12 September 1987). The Ministry of Defence also decided to enforce mandatory testing policy in the army. PWA/HIVs can therefore be exempted from the compulsory military service (*Min Seng Bao* 1 August 1987).

Nevertheless, whether this student with AIDS was a member of 'Us' or 'Others' remained controversial. There is plenty of evidence to show that the DOH claimed that the student's rights should not be jeopardized, for AIDS cannot be transmitted in daily campus contacts (*Min Seng Bao* 12 September 1987). A year later, a DOH official urged the school to resume the student's right to education (*Min Seng Bao* 17 August 1988). A newspaper editorial even criticized the school for having demonstrated such negative lessons to the public (*Min Seng Bao* 21 August 1988). This was, however contradicted by the school authority which claimed that gay men were not suitable to be teachers. The president of another university said: 'Gay men with multiple partners are filthy. They should maintain permanent relationships as heterosexuals do' (*United Daily* 20 August 1988). While this controversy raged, press stories looking for new members of the 'Others' continued. A news headline reads, 'If students contracting AIDS should be punished, what about faculty with homosexual relationships?' (*United Daily* 20 August 1988) Fear about AIDS seemed to be being spread among campuses. The link between homosexuality and AIDS was unequivocal.

This above controversy eventually resolved itself. The student resumed school after having confessed that he had made a mistake in starting homosexual behaviour as a teenager, not at college. He was also deprived of the privileges of living in the dormitory and going swimming as well as being required to have minimum contact with his fellow students as far as this was possible (*United Daily, Min Seng Bao* 6 September 1988). There seemed to be an inclusion of the student as part of 'Us,' but the afore-mentioned institutional practices of control still marginalized him as an

'Other.' In addition, more institutional control was enforced in order to protect the innocent on campus, of which mandatory testing on the freshmen in several colleges was one (*Min Seng Bao* 8 September 1988).

During this period when gay men were stigmatized as the extreme other, occasional reports on how blood products could transmit AIDS virus were to be found. However, connections between 'dangerous' blood and 'foreignness' and homosexuality were predominant. For example, a story in *Min Seng Bao* on 17 September 1986 indicated that 15 per cent of gay men have donated blood at least once. The first PWA/HIV via blood transfusions was found and it was discovered that the blood product was imported (*Min Seng Bao* 5 September 1987). As a consequence, haemophiliacs became worried about being labelled a high-risk group, but a physician was soon quoted, reassuring them that they were still members of the 'Us' group: 'Haemophiliacs are innocent. The general public should not exclude them, for they have suffered enough because of their disease. It is unfair to them' (*Min Seng Bao* 12 September 1987).

AIDS AS AN INTRUDER IN THE FAMILY UNITS (LATE-1988–MID-1991)

Before 1989, male homosexuality virtually seemed to be a synonym to AIDS in Taiwan. The social as well as physical distance created between gay men and the heterosexual population served as a shield to protect family units and normative values from being intruded upon. When the first mother-to-child transmission was found in late 1988, an alarm bell was sounded claiming that AIDS had started to invade the family units in the news. A search for the new 'Others' was initiated. Cogently we can also observe patterns of redefining the 'Us' groups in the discourse.

Generally, women were categorized and stereotyped by a good/bad dichotomy during this period. The bipolar division such as home/street, controlled/loose, day/night, light/dark, as was well documented in the Western literature (Kitzinger 1994) was widely used in the news. In the first case of the vertical transmission, the infected baby undoubtedly belonged to the group of the innocent victims. As the mother's German husband did not contract AIDS, she was blamed for having many foreign sex partners before marriage (*China Times*, *Min Seng Bao* 29 December 1988; *United Daily* 5 May 1989; *China Times* 6 May 1989). The old connection between AIDS and 'foreignness' still existed, but the 'loose woman' label marginalized the mother even further into a bad-woman Other. Advisory quotes from the health authority and expert sources functioned as an ideological vehicle to define what abnormality and deviance were. In a story headlined: 'AIDS has endangered the next generation,' the DOH urged that 'women who have sex contacts with many people and are at high risk should take the blood tests before they get married or plan to become pregnant' (*China Times* 29 December 1988). The DOH also suggested that pregnant women who were HIV positive should consider a Caesarean section (*Min Seng Bao* 15 May 1989). Besides this, an AIDS researcher was quoted as saying, 'We should prevent families from being intruded upon by the AIDS virus. In particular, people should be careful when making friends with foreigners' (*Min Seng Bao* 31 December 1988).

Nevertheless, HIV-positive women were still members of the 'Us' group, if they were indeed proved 'innocent' because they had contracted AIDS from their lawful husbands. In contrast, the bipolar good/bad label did not seem to apply to HIV-positive men, be they married or single. They could be haemophiliacs who had received contaminated blood products (*United Daily, Min Seng Bao* 21 April 1989), bisexuals (*Min Seng Bao* 21 April 1989), clients of prostitutes (*United Daily, Min Seng Bao* 7 May 1989),[4] sailors who had had sex with foreign women (*Min Seng Bao* 4 November 1989), or even prisoners who had prostitute girl friends (*United Daily, Min Seng Bao* 7 September 1989). Whoever they were, the old connections with foreignness and homosexuality, plus the new one with 'bad women,' reprieved these men from being stigmatized categorically. In other words, there were always 'Others' to blame for the victimization of the HIV-positive men, whose deviance, if they were any at all, was basically seen as situational rather than normal or societal.

Within this context, female sex workers, and occasionally 'loose' foreign women, were described as reservoirs of infection or an index to the spread of heterosexual AIDS. As a consequence, the following warnings were quite common in the news discourse: 'Don't have sex with prostitutes' (*United Daily, Min Seng Bao* 5 May 1989); 'The best way to prevent AIDS is not to visit the porn-related places' (*China Times* 5 May 1989); 'Prostitutes are the main source of venereal diseases and AIDS' (*United Daily* 6 November 1989); 'There are a few foreign female prostitutes in Taiwan... men should have more self control' (*United Daily* 7 February 1990). Statistics showing how seriously AIDS can damage family members were also reported to reinforce the ideological control (*Min Seng Bao* 21 April 1989). Institutional practices too were implemented to prevent the 'Others' from spreading the virus to the 'Us' group. For example, the DOH started to require the short-term foreign visitors to prove they were HIV-negative upon entering Taiwan (*Min Seng Bao* 7 February 1990). Condom use was emphasized for marital sex for the first time (*Min Seng Bao* 21 April 1989).

The attention to the heterosexual others during this period did not take the old blame away from gay men. Quotes from the health authorities and medical sources again functioned ideologically to distinguish between 'Us' and 'Others.' Therefore, the DOH warned the public, 'Gay men with AIDS are hidden everywhere and they are just like time bombs, which can explode at any time' (*China Times* 2 November 1990). A physician was also quoted as saying, 'Quite a number of bisexuals who are HIV-positive have married. They should be educated and they should not have sex with their wives' (*Min Seng Bao* 21 April 1989). A recurring pattern of discourse is highly significant: When being interrogated in detail about their heterosexual promiscuity (e.g., having sex with female prostitutes or foreign women), some HIV-positive men would strongly deny their homosexual connection (*United Daily, Min Seng Bao* 7 May 1989; *United Daily, China Times* 9 August 1989). An indication that homosexuality is considered more deviant than heterosexual promiscuity is patent in the news discourse.

AIDS AS AN IMPORTED PRODUCT FROM SOUTH AND SOUTHEAST ASIA (MID-1991–EARLY-1993)

In addition to the continuous blaming of sex workers for endangering family cohesion, after 1991 the AIDS discourse created a new deviant group: foreigners from South and Southeast Asia. Note that before 1991, the term 'foreigner' often connoted Westerners in the AIDS news in Taiwan. In 1990, Taiwan's society entered its 'post-industrial' era, in which the high-tech industry and the service industry are the two pillars of its economic performance. Because of a shortage in the labour force in Taiwan since the late 1980s, in December 1990 the Council of Labour Affairs decided to allow local construction and manufacturing industries to employ foreign workers. Therefore, in the early 1990s, the Taiwanese labour force underwent a structural change in which a relatively large number of blue-collar workers from South and Southeast Asia were employed by the local industries. Furthermore, the rapid growth of the AIDS cases in South and Southeast Asia, particularly Thailand, started to trouble the Taiwanese health authority, which feared that any association with people from those regions might mean bringing in the fatal disease. Therefore, ideological and institutional practices were both widely used to marginalize South and Southeast Asians, whether they were workers in Taiwan or sex workers in the so-called sex tourism industry in their home countries.

A recurring news pattern about foreign workers who were HIV positive can be found: they came from the geographical areas where AIDS was rampant, and the Taiwanese government will soon repatriate them (*United Daily* 10 July 1991; *China Times, Min Seng Bao, United Daily* 16 October 1991). In fact, in the news samples we analysed during this period, all of these HIV-positive workers came from Thailand. The DOH reminded the foreign workers that they must be discreet sexually so that they would not introduce the AIDS virus to increase the public burden of this country (*United Daily* 21 September 1991). The government also admitted that no policy could regulate these foreign workers effectively. Therefore, in the wards of an official of the Council of Labour Affairs, 'Foreign workers in Taiwan should show reports of their medical examinations to prove they are not infected.' The 'time bomb' metaphor was again used to describe people hiring illegal foreign workers, because such an act could be 'dangerous' (*China Times, Min Seng Bao, United Daily* 16 October 1991).

Indeed, during this period, the DOH considered foreign labourers and sex workers to be the highest risk category in passing the AIDS virus to the 'innocent' locals (*United Daily* 27 October 1991). Female sex workers from South and Southeast Asia, either working in Taiwan illegally or in their own home countries, were particularly marginalized as societal/normal deviants. Unlike Western sex workers or 'loose women,' who were previously stigmatized as merely having individual character blemishes, female sex workers from South and Southeast Asia were seen as carrying tribal stigmas, tantamount to saying that they were genetically inferior. Through its efforts to find a scapegoat, the DOH played a major role in facilitating ideological and institutional practices. The health authority first targeted Thailand. By citing scientific figures related to the AIDS epidemic (*China Times, United Daily* 8 October 1991; *China Times* 4 September 1992; *China Times* 15 February 1993), the DOH warned Taiwanese tourists, particularly men, that 'they will surely bring back dangerous "souvenirs" (i.e., AIDS virus) if they visit the Thai brothels' (*Min Seng Bao* 6 August 1991; *China Times* 10 October 1991). Unlicensed Thai sex workers found in Taiwan and later tested HIV positive were also reported in the news to work on the fears of the locals (*China Times* 21 November 1991; *China Times* 26 May 1992).

After Thailand, Vietnam (*China Times* 12 December 1991; *United Daily* 4 July 1992), India (*China Times* 26 August 1992), Myanmar (*China Times* 7 December 1992), and even China (*United Daily* 9 October 1991), were the targets to be marginalized. Statistics of the AIDS epidemic and the DOH warnings were again used to mobilize and shape ideological consensus among the public.

Trying another line of attack as well, the health authority, medical experts and even the Tourism Bureau stressed family values and personal responsibility in efforts to discourage Taiwanese men from visiting sex workers (*Min Seng Bao* 15 May 1992). The message was that a responsible husband was one who 'will think twice before visiting prostitutes' (*Min Seng Bao* 8 October 1991), and 'won't hurt the family members' (*Min Seng Bao* 20 June 1991; *Min Seng Bao* 9 October 1991). Suggestions such as wearing condoms and taking the blood tests were made (*China Times,*

United Daily 8 October 1991; *China Times* 23 December 1992) as institutional practices to protect the 'Us' groups.

Following the same line of thinking, wives and mothers were seen as targets for control to protect the next generation. A physician was quoted as warning, 'If the mother is HIV positive, then the possibility that she will pass the virus to her child is half. And the possibility that a husband will pass the virus to the wife is only one-quarter. Therefore, women should also be tested before they get pregnant' (*China Times* 3 December 1991). This leads to HIV testing being suggested as part of the prenatal examination (*Min Seng Bao* 16 May 1992). In the news discourse, AIDS was not just framed as a threat to individuals and families. There was a stress on the fact it could cause serious social problems in the form of an increasing number of AIDS orphans and the mounting burden of medical care (*Min Seng Bao* 22 November 1992).

The foregoing clearly shows that members of the heterosexual family, including husbands, wives and children, were the predominant 'Us' group members framed in the AIDS discourse. Ethnic aliens such as South and Southeast Asians were seen as the major carriers of the disease. But this was not the only process afoot. The formation of the 'Us' sub-groups in this period is worth noting. These sub-groups included health-care workers, who might have direct contact with the AIDS patients (*Min Seng Bao* 14 July 1991), students, who were then not seen at high risk and were exempt from the mandatory testing (*China Times, Min Seng Bao* 2 December 1992), and more interestingly, Taiwanese AIDS scientists who received awards in Western societies (*United Daily* 19 February 1993).

The formation of the Taiwanese AIDS scientists as an 'Us' sub-group went beyond the victim/guilty dichotomy found in the previous discourse. A story of a Harvard graduate, Chou Yung-Kuan, born in Taiwan and said to have made great academic achievements in AIDS research, is a typical example of this type. As quoted in the news, Chou's father claimed that 'Chou will do his best to help more people and thus to honour Taiwan.' Chou himself was also quoted as saying, 'Although I have a US citizenship, I'll never forget where I come from. If Taiwan needs me, I will go back to do short-term research' (*United Daily* 19 February 1993). Specifically, we will name people like Chou as members of the 'honoured Us' who not only protect the general 'Us' from being invaded by the AIDS virus, but also honour their mother culture by their excellent performance in the West. Since Dr David Ho, an AIDS scientist who invented the combination therapy, was chosen as *Person of the Year* by *Time* magazine in late 1996, representations of the 'honoured Us' have gained more attention in the news discourse. We will discuss this in more detail later.

AIDS AS A SITE OF IDENTITY CHANGE (EARLY-1993–LATE-1996)

AIDS-related discourse in the news was more diversified during this period than it had been in the previous years. In addition to the unremitting blaming of gay men and bisexuals (*China Times* 31 December 1993; *United Daily* 11 October 1994), female sex workers, local (*China Times, Min Seng Bao* 13 April 1993; *China Times* 4 August 1993; *China Times* 29 November 1994; *China Times* 7 June 1995; *China Times* 30 March 1996), and foreign sex workers (*China Times* 23 July 1993; *China Times* 7 August 1993; *Min Seng Bao* 26 November 1993; *China Times* 21 July 1994; *China Times* 26 June 1995); 'loose' women (*China Times* 4 August 1993; *China Times, United Daily* 13 February 1996); foreign labour (*Min Seng Bao* 12 October 1993; *China Times, United Daily* 15 January 1994; *United Daily, Min Seng Bao* 18 January 1994), plus a number of other dubious categories, meant that new groups of 'Us' and 'Others' were created. Several highly publicized issues or events during this period marked as points of departure for some groups and individuals to transform their social identities. Among these one of the most interesting is the changing roles of women as a result of several events. The boycott from the gay community regarding Chi Jia-Wei's role as an AIDS activist, a news leak about a schoolboy contracting AIDS through blood transfusions, and the government's refusal to allow Magic Johnson to enter Taiwan have also raised great attention.

Changing roles of women

Unlike heterosexual men who were generally perceived as members of the 'Us' group in the AIDS discourse, HIV-positive women have been subjected to various sorts of treatment, depending on how they became infected. Sex workers and 'loose' women, either adults or underage, local or foreign, were basically represented as 'Others' who might endanger the family units. For a lawfully married woman, the receipt of contaminated blood products, either by the woman herself or by her husband, marked her as innocent victim. Infection from her husband whose own infection was attributed to promiscuity of which the woman remained ignorant also enabled her to claim innocent victim status. This was another shift in emphasis when children came into the picture. Concern for the baby seemed to outweigh concern for the mother. The growing number of babies infected during pregnancy or breast-feeding by HIV-positive mothers were dubbed the 'innocent victims,' implying that the others were guilty. That is, a mother who transmitted AIDS virus to her baby during pregnancy or birth was subject to blame for the unhappy consequences of her, presumably, reprehensible actions.

Therefore, the following warnings appeared quite commonly in the AIDS news during this period: the DOH urged the public that 'it is wrong to think that underage prostitutes are safe' (*China Times* 1, 2 March 1993); doctors hoped that pregnant women who had had 'abnormal' sex or sex contacts with many people should take the blood tests so as to avoid the birth of the innocent AIDS babies (*Min Seng Bao, United Daily, China Times* 3 March 1993). Discourse such as 'don't hurt the next generation' and 'AIDS babies will be a social burden' clearly categorized the 'Us' vs. 'Other' groups.

Representations of women as an 'endangering other' appeared not only in the mainstream news media, they also figured prominently in the government's AIDS campaign material. In the latter, the female body was represented as personifying sexual danger, a theme which had resonated through the propaganda against venereal disease during the First and Second World Wars in Western countries (Kitzinger 1994). This, again, raised heated discussions in the Taiwanese public forums. Specifically, six women's groups protested and claimed that the campaign materials distorted information and thus stigmatized women as the source of the AIDS virus (*Min Seng Bao* 1 December 1993). These groups, together with an AIDS NGO, demanded that the government eliminate the use of women as objects of fear in the AIDS campaign material. They also asked for more attention to be paid to the issue of women and AIDS, in which women should be treated as potential victims instead of being blamed for the disease (*Min Seng Bao* 1, 2 December 1993).

The protest from the women's groups and the AIDS NGOs, though slow in changing the government's campaign strategies, did exert certain influences on the representations of women in the news discourse and later again, on the legal perspective of women's rights. Months later and in the following years, women were emphasized as the next target to be assailed by AIDS. They were also said to be more vulnerable biologically to infection than were men (*United Daily* 8 September 1993; *Min Seng Bao* 1 December 1995). More importantly, HIV-positive women infected by their husbands were given the right to file for divorce and ask for compensation from their husbands (*United Daily* 31 March 1996). A change of women from the 'Others' to the 'Us' group started to emerge.

Controversial role of an AIDS activist

As mentioned earlier, Chi Jia-Wei, a gay activist and a DOH voluntary worker, played an important role in facilitating communication between the gay community and the health authority during the time when AIDS was still seen as a gay men's disease. He often spared no efforts to explain gay men's lifestyle to the public and tried to sort out the 'good/conforming' gay members from the 'bad/deviant' ones. In a sense, Chi exercised secondary processes of marginalization in his attempt to redefine the gay community. However, after examining the news representations of his image, we found that Chi was still not treated as an equal to the dominant 'Us' communities. For example, reports on Chi's participation in AIDS prevention activities tended to centre on his odd outfits when he was distributing condoms to the young students, not on what he was doing or why (*Min Seng Bao* 15 May 1992, *United Daily* 22 October 1993, see cover picture). That is, integrative marginalization was thrust upon him, which meant he had limited access to the dominant resources, but he was never really considered to be a true 'Us' member.

Chi later lost the trust of the gay community and consequently his voluntary work from the DOH. Two events contributed to this change. First, Chi revealed the address of an AIDS halfway house to the press. The gay community was disappointed in his behaviour (*United Daily* 21 March 1993). Worse than that, Chi went to sue an AIDS patient who was said to have sex with others without wearing condoms (*China Times* 21 July 1994). According to the AIDS Prevention Law in Taiwan, those PWA/HIVs who intentionally pass the virus to others without informing them they are infected, can be sentenced to a maximum of seven years in prison. By publicizing the name to the press, Chi was blamed by the patient's family, the medical community, as well as the health authorities for having intruded on the patient's privacy and for acting in an unethical way as a voluntary worker (*Min Seng Bao* 23 July 1994; *China Times* 22, 23 July 1994). Chi was then excluded from both the mainstream heterosexual society and from the marginal gay community (*Min Seng Bao* 27 July 1994).

News leak of an HIV-positive schoolboy

The news leak of a nine-year-old schoolboy who had contracted AIDS through blood transfusions occurred in August 1994. It caused twenty-two of the boy's classmates to transfer to other primary schools. Parents of the students who transferred and local councillors also protested about the boy's continuing study at the school (*China Times, United Daily* 14 December 1994). Even schoolteachers were worried that the boy's saliva and blood might infect the other students (*China Times* 7 September 1994).

At first glance, the boy was perceived as an 'Other,' threatening the school community. Nevertheless, unlike previous blood product-related AIDS patients, he was later transformed into an 'innocent Us' member. Doctors in his neighbourhood were quoted as saying, 'It is unfortunate and unfair for the boy to contract AIDS' (*United Daily* 24 August 1994). In this case, institutional practices were strongly enforced by the health authority. Schoolteachers were asked to acquire an accurate knowledge of AIDS transmission and promise not to reveal information about the boy to the public (*United Daily* 2 September 1994). The staff of the hospital where the boy received his medical treatment were also told to protect the boy's privacy (*United Daily* 25 August 1994). As stated by Chang Bo-Ya, the then head of the DOH, 'The "innocent" boy should be protected, and we should avoid hurting him again' (*China Times* 26 August 1994). The DOH even warned that penalties would be doled out to people who deprived AIDS patients of their rights to medical treatment, work, and education (*Min Seng Bao* 19 October 1994).

It should be noted that although issues about patients' civil rights had been widely debated in this case, the final judgement basically rested on the schoolboy being categorized as an 'innocent Us' member. To judge from reactions to other AIDS cases in which the patients were infected through sexual transmission, the era of true human rights was yet to come.

Magic Johnson refused entry to Taiwan

This highly publicized event sprang from the Taiwanese government's decision to deny Magic Johnson entry to Taiwan in October 1995. Although invited by a local basketball team to promote both the sport and AIDS prevention, Johnson was eventually not allowed to visit Taiwan because of his HIV-positive status. Topics of debate about Johnson included misinformation about AIDS transmission, civil rights of patients, plus the attitudes of the health authority and thus the pitfalls of the AIDS policies. Chang Bo-Ya again played a critical role in enforcing ideological and institutional practices of marginalization. She not only stated that foreigners who tested HIV-positive would be repatriated, but also revealed frankly that AIDS is a sexually transmitted disease and she did not want Johnson to pass the virus on to Taiwanese locals (*United Daily* 6, 7 October 1995). In fact, Chang was quite a controversial AIDS spokesperson during this period. She was later criticized by the medical community for discriminating against AIDS patients, an assessment made on the basis of her remarks made in the public (*China Times* 9 December 1995; *Min Seng Bao* 7 December 1995).

The DOH decision on the Johnson case was heavily criticized by speakers of the Democratic Progressive Party, the then opposition political party in Taiwan. They accused the DOH of having violated the human rights of PWA/HIVs, and demanded the DOH to apologize to the patients and their families (*China Times* 7 October 1995). The denial of Johnson's entry to Taiwan was also criticized as a negative lesson in AIDS prevention. It was even said to be 'a shame of our country' (*United Daily* 7 October 1995). Johnson did not succeed in visiting Taiwan, despite the fact that he is a celebrity and a popular spokesperson for the AIDS prevention in the US. That is, although he is accepted as an 'Us' member in the West, he was still perceived as a member of the alien 'Others' by the Taiwanese health authority. The metaphor of the decadent West was again in the ascendant.

AIDS AS A PUBLIC FORUM FOR HUMAN RIGHTS (LATE-1996–LATE-1999)[5]

Controversies surrounding PWA/HIVs had not necessarily been resolved in the previous period, but they had given rise to more voices striving for human rights in Taiwanese society. Discriminatory statements by the DOH head, Chang Bo-Ya, helped speed up the institutionalization of several AIDS advocacy groups. In an attempt to reduce the costs for AIDS medical care, Chang continued to insist on distinguishing between 'innocent' victims and those who deserved the fatal disease. In her eyes, we should sympathize with those infected with the virus through blood products and sexually through their lawful spouses. But, as for those who got the disease because of their 'abnormal' personal behaviour, they themselves should take responsibility for it. On the basis of this distinction, Chang argued that all PWA/HIVs' rights to education and work would be guaranteed, but only 'innocent' victims qualified for free medical care. She even proposed a revision of the AIDS policy to prevent the 'guilty' PWA/HIVs from receiving the free treatment ((*Min Seng Bao* 29 November 1996).

Chang's moral conservatism on AIDS policy did not stop the AIDS activists and individual PWA/HIVs from demanding more social equality and justice. An AIDS patient accused a blood donation centre of leaking the test results to his health insurance company, which then terminated the patient's insurance policy. The patient demanded his rights to insurance be restored (*Min Seng Bao, China Times, United Daily* 31 May 1997).

In November 1997, the first voluntary group focusing on the legal rights of the PWA/HIVs, *Persons with HIV/AIDS Rights Advocacy Association,* was established. A month later, a 1995 anti-discrimination law was revised to guarantee the rights of PWA/HIVs to a certain degree at least (*Min Seng Bao* 17 December 1997). Although this has been characterized a mostly symbolic rather than a practical measure, such institutionalization has played a critical role in transforming the once 'Others' into 'Us' members in order to gain protection.

A more influential change came from a group of HIV-positive haemophiliacs who claimed that they had been infected by contaminated blood products and asked for indemnity from the government and the medical corporations (*China Times, United Daily, Min Seng Bao* 13 February 1998). While denying any legal responsibility, the DOH was willing to negotiate between the haemophiliac PWA/HIVs and the pharmaceutics companies (*Min Seng Bao, United Daily, China Times* 8, 15 November 1997). The issue was debated in the news discourse for about a year, highlighted by demands from the PWA/HIVs involved for legal sanctions and reparations. The controversy resulted in Bayer's offer of US $1.06 billion (*Min Seng Bao* 20 February 1998), and the government's approval for establishing a fund for national indemnity (*Min Seng Bao* 20 May, 14 October, 11 December 1998). In January 1999, these victims organized a group named *Floating Wood Helping Association,* of which the purpose was to promote the rights of the PWA/HIVs infected by blood products.

As mentioned previously, AIDS scientists with a Taiwanese, or even a Chinese, ethnic link, had been perceived as members of the 'honoured Us.' Since the early 1990s, occasional reports of these scientists' achievements and sometimes, stories of their lives, have become typical patterns of representing this group. Nevertheless, it was not until the end of 1996, when Dr David Ho was chosen *Man of the Year* by *Time* magazine that the 'honoured Us' was able to exert any strong practical influence on the AIDS policy and the rights of the PWA/HIVs.

When Ho was invited to visit his motherland in January 1997, he was treated almost like a national hero (*Min Seng Bao* 30 January 1997). He was said to be one of Magic Johnson's AIDS doctors in fact the one who has saved the basketball celebrity from death. Praise from the academic community, his parents (*United Daily* 25 December 1996), and his former teachers (*United Daily* 23 December 1996), all proved that Ho was a credit to Taiwan. The following message was repeatedly emphasized in the news discourse, 'Ho would like to share all his achievements with people in Taiwan' (*United Daily* 24 December 1996). In the wake of Ho's international popularity, news reports on AIDS research, including his combination therapy for AIDS patients, started to boom. This prompted the government to decide to adopt Ho's therapy as part of the medical care to PWA/HIVs. A similar discourse occurred when another Taiwan-born AIDS scientist won academic awards in the United States (*Min Seng Bao, United Daily* 18 March 1999).

Concerns about human rights were extended to the care for AIDS patients. Several halfway houses were established in 1999 (*Min Seng Bao, China Times* 1 July 1999; *Min Seng Bao* 18 December 1999). Nevertheless, an incident involving two lifeguards using mouth-to-mouth artificial respiration on a drowning AIDS patient brought up another controversial issue concerning the rights and responsibilities of the PWA/HIVs and their families. The patient eventually died in the hospital but his family was accused of not notifying the lifeguards about the patient's AIDS status. Without knowing whether the two lifeguards had contracted AIDS, their employer discharged them and attempted to pledge national indemnity. This event highlighted a general misconception about AIDS infection through saliva, regardless of the fact that local AIDS prevention campaigns have tried to dismiss the myth (*Min Seng Bao, United Daily, China Times* 7 August 1998).

In the meantime, new groups of 'Others' emerged in which HIV-positive brides from Southeast Asia and China created the most discussion in the news. Cases of infected wives transmitting the virus to their Taiwanese husbands were reported. Old warnings from the DOH, which functioned as ideological and institutional marginalization, reappeared in the discourse, 'Be careful when having sex with foreigners, including your spouses,' and 'You'd better be tested before marrying a foreigner' (*Min Seng Bao, China Times* 24 May 1997; *Min Seng Bao* 21 March, 5 December 1998). Foreign spouses were also requested to show their medical examination reports upon entering Taiwan (*Min Seng Bao, China Times* 9 October 1998). Once again, men were being represented again as the AIDS victims and their foreign brides were to blame (*Min Seng Bao* 24 May 1997).

Youngsters, who may engage in high-risk sexual behaviour, were seen as a major target for AIDS prevention and interventions during this period. The Ministry of Education, the highest educational authority in Taiwan, even incorporated on-campus AIDS prevention into students' college-life projects (*China Times* 15 December 1998). Generally, they were perceived as members of the 'Us' groups.

It should be noted that clients of the unlicensed sex workers, while previously perceived as being part of 'Us,' were represented as 'Others' during this period. Once they had been caught, they were required to attend classes of sex education. A fine of approximately $ 900 was also imposed on them (*United Daily* 17 December 1997).

DISCUSSION AND CONCLUSION

Representations of the disease encompassed major cultural, social, political and scientific changes. Like other causes of epidemics, AIDS is more than a medical phenomenon. Particularly, constructions of AIDS as a disease of high-risk groups have been shaped by prevailing ideologies of health and sexuality (Frankenberg 1994). As reviewed in the research literature and analysed in our study, the major function of marginalization, stigmatization, or deviance naming in the AIDS discourse is to maintain the social distance between the more powerful mainstream groups and the less powerful minority ones. By doing that, the mainstream 'Us' group members can be protected not only from the disease, but also from people devalued by the society. In our study, these people, or who were categorized as 'Others,' had been devalued based on the basis of their sexual orientation (e.g., gay men), personal behaviour (e.g., promiscuous lifestyle), social status (e.g., sex workers, foreign labourers, women), or cultural backgrounds (e.g., Westerners, South or Southeast Asians). Once having been labelled as members of 'Other' groups, they were further deprived of their rights to health and other social resources.

From our analysis of the news discourse on AIDS between 1984 and 1999, we found that AIDS has been a site of struggle not only over the disease itself, but becoming a focus of what can go wrong in Taiwan. With official documented HIV cases at around 3,000, comparatively speaking Taiwan is not an area of serious AIDS epidemic. Nevertheless, negative reactions to and representations of the disease and of its victims have been no less serious than those found in regions where AIDS has presented a catastrophe. Specifically, denial, scapegoating, and blame were common reactions from the establishments, and, of course, the news media. There has been a ready recognition that it is behaviour and not individuals that must be avoided, and sexual behaviour rather than sexual identity should be used as a criterion for risk. Still, being reinforced by the health authorities and medical community, the AIDS discourse in the news presented a reality which indicated that most uninfected people could distance themselves from the identified high-risk groups, leaving their own behaviour and notions of risk unchallenged.

To conclude the study, we will highlight the following two issues generated by our analyses of the news texts in Taiwan. The first has to do with the construction of groups, including various sub-groups of 'Others' and 'Us'; the other focal point of discussion concerns those agents participating in the processes of marginalization. We shall also compare these findings with relevant research literature addressing the same issues in various cultures whenever necessary.

CONSTRUCTION OF GROUPS IN THE AIDS DISCOURSE

In the AIDS discourse, it is the natural property of the 'Other,' be this person foreigner, gay man, female, to be diseased and dangerous as it is the natural property of the 'Not Other' to be clean, healthy and safe (Wilton 1997). In the study, we identified the formation of the following groups, including their patterns and changes, worth further elaboration.

FOREIGNERS AS A RISK GROUP

As in many cultures, AIDS was introduced to Taiwan as a foreign or an imported product. The foreign connection of AIDS excluded the locals from a fear of contagion. Foreigners, Westerners in particular, were represented as more sexually promiscuous during the early years of AIDS epidemic in Taiwan. Those locals, men and women alike, who had had sexual connections with Westerners, were seen as destined to contract the fatal disease. Similar patterns of the foreign connection can be found in the news media in many developing nations. For example, the link between AIDS and homosexuality has led many Africans to deny that it would become an issue for them, since homosexuality is a Western problem. China denied it was at risk because AIDS was a disease of the decadent West. Other Asian nations such as Thailand and India blamed foreign tourists for bringing the virus into their countries. In Rumania Ceaucescu dismissed AIDS as a capitalist disease. Middle Eastern Muslim leaders believed that their religion would protect them (Van der Vliet 1996). As a result, by labelling AIDS as a foreign or imported product, the locals are reassured of their immunity to the disease.

The 'foreignness' of AIDS has taken another form since AIDS epidemic became more widespread in Asia in the early 1990s. This period was the beginning of the era in which Taiwanese industries started to employ foreign labour from South and Southeast Asia. At this point the foreign connection to AIDS blaming was switched from the Westerners to South and Southeast Asians, sometimes Mainland Chinese included. Asian countries, particularly Thailand, were seen as the origin of the modern plague. Scientific reports issued by health institutions or news stories run by mainstream media made all sorts of efforts to warn the public of the dangers to the region and thus to the people. Unlike the kind of 'Otherness' assigned to Westerners, South and Southeast Asians, either blue-collar workers, sex workers, or later foreign brides were seen not only as leading a promiscuous life-style, but were simultaneously automatically categorized as socially and economically inferior to Taiwanese locals. In other words, the Taiwanese news media have adopted a First-World perspective to represent people from what is said to be the developing world in the AIDS issues. That is, AIDS had been constructed as a crisis internal to the region, cultures, peoples, indigenous character; in short, its 'Third Worldness.'

Such a First-World perspective was also evident in the Western media's representations of less developed countries. In the early 1980s, Haitians appeared to Americans as the foreign carriers of AIDS. The US media labelled AIDS a disease resulting from the 'four Hs-homosexuality, heroin addiction, haemophiliacs and Haitians' (Gilman 1988). In the 1990s, the US media assured the public that in Asia AIDS was spread by Asian-to-Asian heterosexual contact, not by contact with foreigners. Stereotypes of Asian people crop up at regular intervals throughout the First World media's sporadic coverage of Asian AIDS: poor, underdeveloped, reserved, and hidebound by custom, complacent, superstitious, and war-stricken. Visiting brothels is represented as a cultural sign of Asian masculinity, a local custom, even as something ethnic (Erni 1997). In a study of foreign media coverage of prostitution and tourism in Thailand, Suwanmoli (1998) showed that Thailand is associated with the images of 'four S's – sun, sex, sea, and sand – as they are spelled out in various travel publications. As stated by Erni (1997), the handful of media reports from the US and other First World countries has created 'a classic orientalist heterosexual "Asian AIDS" that reinaugurates the postcolonial discourse of global economic development and precolonial fantasies about militarised and leisurized masculinity' (p. 75).

There are certainly other types of foreign connections with AIDS in the world. The former Soviet Union blamed the US for manufacturing HIV as a biological weapon in laboratories, while France came up with similar conspiracy theories. Haitians suggested that African monkeys imported as pets into homosexual brothels in Haiti had spread the virus (Chirimuuta and Chirimuuta 1987). The above pattern was not found in our analysis in the Taiwanese news discourse.

'DEVIANT' GAY MEN

Once local cases were identified in Taiwan, male homosexuality appeared to be the scapegoat to blame for contraction of AIDS. Similar results can be found in other cultures, too. For example, in analysing portrayals of AIDS in its early years in popular magazines in the US, Albert (1986) found that the media were primarily concerned with homosexual patients and the socio-cultural perspectives. Baker (1986) also found that articles on AIDS were indexed under the heading 'homosexuality' in both the *New York Times* index and in *Readers' Guide to Periodical Literature* until the end of 1982.

In our study, we found that marginalization and stigmatization of gay men were both created by a sense of distance, produced in two distinct ways. First, gay behaviour was made to occur in geographic isolation, that is, in bathhouses, in certain parks, by certain riversides, and so forth. Second, gay men were portrayed as leading an 'abnormal' sex life, for which a justified price was paid by an increasing death toll. It is here that the distancing of PWA/HIVs as the 'problem group' can be seen. Because of its lack of effect on 'us,' that is, the general population or the unaffected group, AIDS is like a war merely involving gay men.

We also observed an interesting pattern of representing gay men throughout the early years of the AIDS discourse: homosexuality can be corrected. Therefore, warnings from the health and other expert sources about the danger of man-to-man sex, accompanied by confessions by regretful gay patients and explanations from gay activists (e.g., Chi Jia-Wei) who identified themselves with the heterosexual population, were typical ideological apparatuses deployed in the news discourse. In fact, the processes of marginalizing gay men in the AIDS discourse were also the most complicated when compared to other types used to isolate stigmatized groups. Safer sex practices such as condom use were not promoted among gay men. The term 'condom' actually started to appear in the AIDS discourse when the disease was found to intrude into the heterosexual families.

With the efforts being made by the AIDS advocacy groups in recent years, particularly since 1993 when gay right activists became more involved in the AIDS NGOs (Wang 1999), representations of gay men have undergone certain changes in which more diversified perspectives, though not necessarily all of them positive, can be seen. In a two-way panel survey conducted in the Greater Taipei area in Taiwan, Hsu (1998) also found that the general public's attitudes toward homosexuality became less negative from 1996 to 1997. Does it mean that gay men will be eventually accepted as members of the 'Us' group in the popular discourse, such as the news? In fact, as revealed in our analysis, gay men were not exonerated even after greater attention had been paid to the heterosexual Others. Cogently, more follow-up studies are needed to track the changes in the AIDS discourse. A caution also needs to be heeded here advising a distinction to be made between representations reflecting genuine reactions from the social relationships and those simply reflecting political correctness in the society.

SEX WORKERS AS SIGNIFIERS OF THE DISEASE

Sex, women, and disease were found to be associated to a very high degree in the study, particularly for sex workers and those who were devalued as 'loose.' In Western countries, sex workers and 'loose' women had been blamed for endangering national security, the fall of principles and mighty men (Treichler 1988; Wilton 1997). In countries struggling in the geopolitical aftermath of colonialism, purity and motherhood continue to be associated with nationalism (McClintock 1995). Within the early years of AIDS discourse in the West and in many parts of the developing world, gay men seemed to have taken the place of women in the epidemic of signification (Treichler 1988). When it became apparent that AIDS would affect the heterosexual population, AIDS discourse recycled the centuries-old stigmatization of women. While relatively privileged women were assigned the position of innocent victim or heroic conscript, powerless women such as sex workers or women in the developing world were seen as the source of infection (Treichler 1988).

The above pattern was also evident in Taiwan. Ever since AIDS began to pose a threat to heterosexual family units, female sex workers, rather than their clients, have been seen as the blackguards in the spread of the disease. This led to various ideological and institutional processes of marginalization in the news discourse. Sex workers' health was perceived as something to be controlled, rather than to be protected. The right to ultimate welfare was the undisputed privilege of heterosexual families. Stigmatization of sex workers was complicated even more by a threat related to 'foreignness,' especially posed by people from South and Southeast Asia. Foreign workers caught selling sex illegally in Taiwan or brothel sex workers in South and Southeast Asia were stigmatized tribally and denigrated as possessing devalued personality and behaviour. It has only been recently, since issues of PWA/HIVs' rights have been given an airing in the news agenda that we have been able to observe a tendency to treat the clients of the sex workers as groups to be controlled in the news discourse.

MOTHERS TO BE BLAMED

Women were represented as threats not only to their innocent clients, if they were believed to be sex workers, but also to their innocent babies if they were known to be pregnant. The possibility that a woman who is HIV positive may transmit HIV to her unborn child has given rise to another good woman/bad woman dichotomy. The pattern found in our study echoes what has been documented in literature on women and AIDS in the Western world. That is, a woman can only be accepted as part of 'Us' if she assumes the much more sympathetic, virgin role: helpmate, caretaker, mother, deceived wife or lover, puzzled daughter, compassionate physician (Treichler and Warren 1998).

INVISIBILITY OF LESBIANS

Another type of stigma concerning women in the AIDS crisis occurs among lesbians, to whom little attention has been paid. Within the mainstream AIDS discourse, 'women' are viewed by default as heterosexual. This can been seen from the statistics of AIDS risk factors regularly published by the DOH. Whereas men are categorized into heterosexual, bisexual, and homosexual according to their sexual orientation, women have to make do with just the heterosexual category for the same purpose. The media coverage has both illustrated and reinforced prevailing heterosexual assumptions about women. As pointed out by Kitzinger (1994), such representations within mainstream AIDS discourse tend to exclude large proportions of the female population. The 'innocence' label and the figure of good-woman image are used as a foil against which to judge the deviants, including lesbians.

Similarly in the US, among the lesbians with AIDS reported by the Centres for Disease Control, most are assumed to have acquired HIV through high risk practices associated with IV-drug use. Richardson (1994) pointed out that unlike reports of male cases, government statistics rarely classify cases of AIDS or HIV infection in women according to whether they are heterosexual, bisexual, or lesbian. What this means in practice is that women with multiple risks are assigned to one exposure category only, whereas men now may be placed in multiple risk categories. The construction of lesbians as essentially asexual may lead many to conclude that lesbians are neither at risk nor in need of information about risk.

MEMBERS OF 'US' TO BE PROTECTED

The foregoing discussions highlighted those groups that have been stigmatized as 'Others' in the AIDS discourse. The formation of the opposite category, the 'Us' groups depends on how 'Others' are constructed. When Westerners or South/Southeast Asians were perceived as 'Others,' the general public of the Taiwanese locals were the 'Us' group members. When gay men became the 'Others' on whose shoulders the blame could be placed, the heterosexual population was naturally entitled to be protected. In fact, members of heterosexual families, including husbands, wives, and children, have been in the forefront as 'Us' members framed in the AIDS discourse. The maverick element of this group was composed of HIV-positive women, who were treated differently, depending on how they became infected. They could only be identified as 'Us' if they did not contract AIDS sexually outside their lawful marriage, or if they did not transmit the virus to the next generation. Heterosexual men had been generally perceived as members of the 'Us' group in the AIDS discourse, but there was a growing tendency to treat them as 'Others' when more institutional control was enforced on clients of the sex workers after 1997.

In the AIDS discourse, haemophiliacs have always been people to be protected. So have been schoolchildren and health-care workers. College students were seen as the 'Us' group members after 1998, but in the earlier years of the AIDS epidemic, gay students had been excluded from the 'Us' category.

THE 'HONOURED' US

Whereas the afore-mentioned members of the 'Us' and 'Others' still fitted the victim/guilty dichotomy, we found that there was a special group of individuals, i.e., the Taiwan-born AIDS scientists, who have also been seen as 'Us' members. Dr David Ho and many others are typical examples of this type. To distinguish this group of individuals from AIDS-related victims classified as members of 'Us,' we would label them 'honoured' Us in which the general 'Us' groups are glorified by what these individuals have accomplished in their professions. Formation of 'honoured' Us is indeed culturally specific, and it is virtually a reflection of Taiwanese nationalism, springing mostly from the country's relative invisibility in the international political arena. Similar patterns of media representations can be found in international sports, awards, and occasions on which scientific achievements are acknowledged, at which Taiwan-born participants or nominees are honoured.

AGENTS AND PROCESSES OF MARGINALIZATION

Patterns of marginalization

Although Cohen (1999) identified three kinds of marginalization processes: ideologies, institutions, and social relationships, only the first two can be found in the AIDS news discourse we analysed. Marginalization through social relationships, the one we did not come across in our analysis, could be more readily identified in interpersonal communications, verbal and nonverbal, than in mass communications. Specifically, policies, laws and organizational rules about AIDS, as reported in the news, served as institutional practices of marginalization. Pertinently the agents facilitating ideological marginalization were not the news media themselves, but the sources they cited in legitimising the credibility of the reports. As can be identified in our analysis, health authorities, health-care workers, and, occasionally, experts had been widely used to inform the public of what constituted accurate knowledge, correct thinking, and appropriate behaviour. Agents of both institutional and ideological marginalization further facilitated categorizations of people into various groups according to their conformity to and consistency with the created group norms. Stigma and deviance were thus assigned to those categorized as 'Others,' whose access to the social resources may be hindered to some extent. A summary of the major groups of 'Us' and 'Others,' plus the institutional and ideological processes of marginalization found in our analysis is presented in Table 8.1.

Journalistic routines and marginalization

The fact that the news depended on the authoritative sources to impose ideological marginalization in the AIDS discourse seems to echo what research evidence says about health news coverage. That is, journalists tend to rely on medical expertise as their major source of information (Milio 1985). The imbalance found in the medical reporting is partly a result of the perspective from which many reporters view science and medicine. Although in reality, the acquisition of a knowledge of science is messy and cluttered with uncertainties, journalists usually look for simple and neat solutions, which forces them to be dependent on a handful of authoritative sources (Moore 1989). Such a practice is also evident in the reporting of AIDS-related issues. Studies in many countries such as the US, Britain (Williams and Miller 1995), and Portugal (Traquina 1996) reveal that government health officials and medical experts are still the major news sources on whom journalists rely most for the AIDS coverage. Similarly, in a content analysis of Taiwanese news coverage of AIDS from 1996 to 1997, Hsu (1998) found that authoritative sources such as health-care workers, experts or scholars, and government health officials accounted for more than half of all the sources cited in the AIDS stories.

Given the above, it appears that the patterns of stigmatization are not easily going to be changed in the news. Fortunately, since 1996, the year when the period of AIDS as a public forum for human rights began, there has been more active involvement of NGOs in the AIDS campaigns and related public relations activities. Journalists' awareness of the grassroots' influences on the public regarding AIDS prevention has increased. This was revealed in the AIDS news coverage, which gradually resorted to non-traditional sources such as the NGOs and voluntary workers (Hsu 1998), a result similar to that found in the British broadcasting media (Williams and Miller 1995). What does this tell us about AIDS stigmatization and the change it has undergone in the news discourse? Although future systematic studies are needed to document the patterns, the forces newsmakers and gatekeepers exert in the construction of social reality cannot be overlooked. It should be noted here that the ways news represents AIDS do not necessarily equate to public perceptions of the disease and those affected by it.

To conclude, the use of characterisations in AIDS discourse may help produce the very differences which exist between people in relation to the disease. Those who ran a higher risk of AIDS are characterized either as belonging to 'at-risk groups' or as 'victims.' These differences have actually highlighted already firmly established social categories. As the present research was the first extensive AIDS study in Taiwan aimed at examining representations in the news discourse, findings reported in the study could serve as an exploratory investigation into the nature and determinants of a broader context of the social constructions of AIDS. It is expected that with the results presented and discussed in the study, our understandings of how and why mass media communicate about AIDS as they do in culturally specific contexts will be significantly increased.

NOTES

1 Data presented in the study are the partial investigation results from the first author's research project, 'Scientific Reality Vs. Political Reality: Representations of AIDS in the News Discourse,' sponsored by the National Science Council in Taiwan. The authors would like to thank Dr Ting-Yu Chen, Shao-Jia Hu, Hai-Lan Yang, and Chun-Lan Shih for their participation in the project. Gratitude must also be expressed to *United Daily*, *China Times*, *Min Seng Bao*, and *Time* magazine as well as to the Department of Health in Taiwan for the use of their media materials in this chapter.

2 *Bo li chuan*: literally translated from Mandarin Chinese, glass circle, is a derogatory term referring to the gay men community. The phrase *bo li* (glass) in Mandarin Chinese implies men's butts and therefore by extension anal sex between gay men.

3 In Taiwan, it was mandatory for male college students to attend the military training camp. This policy was abolished in 1999. But young male adults are still required to serve in the army for at least two years.

4 The term 'prostitute' will only be used here when the news discourse refers to it literally. Otherwise, the term 'sex worker' preferred in the present study to avoid further stigmatisation.

5 Also marking this period was the first-ever direct election of the president held in March 1996, which was said to complete a critical step in Taiwan's journey towards full democracy.

Table 8.1 'Us' Vs. 'Others' and the Processes of Marginalization in the AIDS News Discourse in Taiwan (1984-1999)

Period	Major 'Us'	Major 'Others'	Ideological marginalization	Institutional marginalization
1. Western import (late-1984–mid-1985)	Taiwanese locals	Westerners; gay men	Intrusion of patients' privacy Detailed descriptions of patients' sex life	Ignorance of local AIDS policy
2. Gay men's disease (mid-1985–late-1988)	Heterosexuals; HIV negative college students; haemophiliacs	Gay men; people with occasional homosexuality: gay activists; HIV positive college students; foreigners	Criticisms of homosexuality Regretful confessions from HIV-positive gay men. Urges for one-to-one sex among gay men Detailed descriptions of sex life Rejection of gay teachers Prevention of teenagers from homosexuality Claims of patients' right to education Claims that haemophiliacs are innocent	Blood tests urged AIDS not seen as a legalized infectious disease "Innocent" ID cards for HIV-negative gay men Dismissal of gay men from military training camp Dismissal of gay men from school Mandatory testing in the military AIDS students not allowed to have close contacts with others Mandatory testing in some colleges
3. Intruder to family (late-1988–mid-1991)	'Good-woman'; mothers; babies; heterosexual men	'Loose' women; foreigners; gay men; sex workers	Warning: Be careful when making friends with foreigners Warning: Don't hurt the family and the next generation Use of 'time bomb' metaphor on gay men HIV-positive men's denial of homosexual connection Advice: Restraints from promiscuity	Suggestion: Blood tests for pregnant women Suggestion: Caesarean birth for HIV positive women Foreign visitors required to be tested
4. South/Southeast Asian import (mid-1991–early-1993)	Taiwanese locals; heterosexual men; mothers; wives; health-care workers;	South and Southeast Asians; sex workers; gay men	Warning: AIDS widespread in South and Southeast Asia; men should not visit brothels in those regions Warning: Foreign workers should be sexually discreet Warning: Hiring foreign workers is	Repatriation of HIV-positive foreign workers Foreign workers required to be tested Suggestion: Condom use; blood tests

	students; AIDS scientists with Taiwanese ethnicity	dangerous Emphasis on family values and personal responsibility		
5. Site of identity change (early-1993– late-1996)	HIV-positive women infected by contaminated blood products or lawful husbands; babies =>Women in general; schoolboys	Gay men and bisexuals; sex workers; foreign labourers; mothers transmitting virus to babies =>Rejected AIDS activist; HIV-positive foreign celebrity	Warning: Underage sex workers are not safe Warning: AIDS babies are a social burden Advice: Don't hurt HIV-positive schoolboy again Warning: HIV positive foreigner may pass the virus to Taiwanese locals	Warning: Promiscuous pregnant women should be tested Protest from women's groups that women are stigmatized HIV-positive wives infected from husbands can file for divorces Sanctions on AIDS voluntary workers intruding patients' privacy Accurate AIDS knowledge of school teachers demanded Protection of patients' privacy in hospitals Penalties for violating patients' rights to school, medical care and work Denial of Magic Johnson's entry to Taiwan Repatriation of HIV positive foreigners
6. Public forum for human rights (late-1996– late-1999)	PWA/HIVs infected by contaminated blood products; Haemophiliacs; AIDS scientists with Taiwanese ethnicity; young people	People with 'abnormal life-style'; ethnic minority (e.g., natives); foreign or mainland Chinese brides; clients of sex workers	Warning: Sympathy for 'innocent' victims'; people with "abnormal" life-style deserve the disease Emphasis on AIDS scientists' achievements Warning: Be careful when marrying foreign or mainland Chinese brides	Guarantees of PWA/HIVs' right to school, work, but only 'innocent' victims deserve free medical care Revision of anti-discrimination law National indemnity for people infected by contaminated blood products Introduction of the combination therapy Establishment of more half-way houses for PWA/HIVs Foreign brides need to be tested

REFERENCES

Albert, E. (1986) 'Illness and Deviance: The Response of the Press to AIDS,' in: D.A. Feldman and T.M. Johnson (eds) *The Social Dimensions of AIDS: Method and Theory.* New York: Praeger, pp. 163–78.

Archer, D. (1985) 'Social Deviance,' in: G. Lindzey and E. Aronson (eds) *Handbook of Social Psychology* (3rd ed., Vol. 2). New York: Random House, pp. 743–804.

Baker, A.J. (1986) 'The Portrayal of AIDS in the Media: An Analysis of Articles in the New York Times,' in: D.A. Feldman and T.M. Thomas (eds) *The Social Dimensions of AIDS: Method and Theory.* New York: Praeger, pp. 179–94.

Bardhan, N. (1996, August) *Frame of Blame: Semiosis of Newstrack's Representation of AIDS in India.* A paper Presented to the Annual Meeting of the Qualitative Studies Division, Association for Education in Journalism and Mass Communication, Anaheim, California, USA.

Best, J. (1990) *Threatened Children: Rhetoric and Concern about Child-Victim.* Chicago: University of Chicago Press.

Blendon, R.J. and K. Donelan (1988) 'Discrimination Against People with AIDS: The Public's Perspective,' *New England Journal of Medicine* 319: pp. 1022–6.

Bloor, M. (1995) *The Sociology of HIV Transmission.* Thousand Oaks, CA: Sage.

Bradley, R.J. (1998) *Latent Virus: Early Coverage of the AIDS Epidemic by the Canadian Press.* A Doctoral Dissertation Submitted in Partial Fulfilment of the Requirements for the Degree of Doctor of Philosophy at The University of Western Ontario London, Ontario, Canada.

Cantor, N. and W. Michel (1979) 'Prototypes in Person Perception,' in: L. Berkowitz (ed.) *Advances in Experimental Social Psychology* (Vol. 12). New York: Academic Press, pp. 3–52.

Chirimuuta, R.C. and R.J. Chirimuuta (1987) *AIDS, Africa and Racism.* Derbyshire: R. Chirimuuta, Bretby House.

Cohen, C.J. (1999) *The Boundaries of Blackness: AIDS and the Breakdown of Black Politics.* Chicago: University of Chicago Press.

Crocker, J.B. Major and C. Steele (1998) 'Social Stigma,' in: D.T. Gilbert, S.T. Fiske and G. Lindzey (eds) *The Handbook of Social Psychology* (4th ed.). New York: McGraw-Hill, pp. 504–53.

Department of Health (2000) *Control of Communicable Diseases* [On-line]. Available: http://www.doh.gov.tw/english/1996stat/appendix.html.

Department of Health (2001) *News Release* [On-line]. Available: http://www.cdc.gov.tw/g/control.

Erni, J.N. (1997) 'Of Desire, the Farang, and Textual Excursions:

Assembling "Asian AIDS" ' *Cultural Studies* 11(1), pp. 64–77.

Foucault, M. (1979) *Discipline and Punish: The Birth of the Prison*. New York: Vintage Books.

Frankenberg, R. (1994) 'The Impact of HIV/AIDS on Concepts Relating to Risk and Culture within British Community Epidemiology: Candidates or Targets for Prevention?' *Social Science and Medicine* 38(10), pp. 1325-35.

Freimuth, V.S., R.H. Greenberg, J. DeWitt and R.M. Romano (1984) 'Covering Cancer: Newspapers and the Public Interest,' *Journal of Communication* 34(1): pp. 62–73.

Freire, P. (1972) *The Pedagogy of the Oppressed*. New York: Continuum.

Gilman, S.L. (1988) *Disease and Representation*. Ithaca, NY: Cornell University Press.

Goffman, E. (1963) *Stigma: Notes on the Management of Spoiled Identity*. Englewood Cliffs, NJ: Prentice-Hall.

Goldin, C.S. (1994) 'Stigmatisation and AIDS: Critical Issues in Public Health,' *Social Science Medicine*, 39: pp. 1359–66.

Government Information Office (2000) *The Republic of China Yearbook*. [On-line]. Available: http://www.gio.gov.tw.

Hsu, M. (1998) *Issue Importance and Source Reliability of AIDS in Taiwan: A Comparison of the News and Campaign Agenda-Setting*. A Paper Presented to the Annual Meeting of the Health Communication Division, International Communication Association, Jerusalem, Israel.

Kitzinger, J. (1994) 'Visible and Invisible Women in AIDS Discourses,' in: L. Doyal, J. Naidoo and T. Wilton (eds) *AIDS: Setting a Feminist Agenda*. London: Taylor and Francis, pp. 95–109.

McClintock, A. (1995) *Imperial Leather: Race, Gender and Sexuality in the Colonial Context*. London: Routledge.

Milio, N. (1985) ' "Political" Information Is Essential,' *World Health Forum* 9, pp. 501–4.

Moore, M. (1989)'Beware the Bracken Fern,' in: M. Moore (ed.) *Health Risks and the Press: Perspectives of Media Coverage on Risk Assessment*. Washington, DC: The Media Institute, pp. 1–18.

Plummer, K. (1979) 'Misunderstanding Labelling Perspectives,' in: D. David and R. Paul (eds) *Deviant Interpretations*. London: Marin Robertson, pp. 85–121.

Richardson, D. (1994) 'Inclusions and Exclusions: Lesbians, HIV and AIDS,' in: L. Doyal, J. Naidoo and T. Wilton (eds) *AIDS: Setting a Feminist Agenda*. London: Taylor & Francis, pp. 159–70.

Riggins, S. H. (1997) 'The Rhetoric of Othering,' in: S.H. Riggins (ed.) *The Language and Politics of Exclusion: Others in Discourse*. Thousand Oaks, CA: Sage, pp. 1–31.

Rosch, E.H. (1978) 'Principles of categorization,' in: E. Rosch and B.B. Lloyd (eds) *Cognition and Categorization*. Hillsdale, NJ: Erlbaum, pp. 27–48.

Sarbin, T.R. (1967) 'The Dangerous Individuals: An Outcome of Social Identity Transformation,' *British Journal of Criminology* 7, pp. 285–95.

Simpkins, J.D. and D.J. Brenner (1984) 'Mass Media Communication and Health,' in: B. Dervin and M.J. Voigt (eds) *Progress in Communication Sciences*. Norwood, NJ: Ablex, pp. 275–97.

Suwanmoli, M. (1998) *Foreign Correspondents in Bangkok and Foreign Media Coverage of Prostitution and Tourism in Thailand*. A Doctoral Dissertation Submitted in Partial Fulfilment of the Requirements for the Degree of Doctor of Philosophy at the University of Wisconsin, Madison, USA.

Todorov, T. (1982) *The Conquest of America*. New York: Harper.

Traquina, N. (1996) *Portuguese Journalism and HIV/AIDS: A Case Study in News*. A Paper Presented to the Annual Conference of Association for Education in Journalism and Mass Communication in Anaheim, CA, USA.

Treichler, P. (1988) 'AIDS, Gender and Biomedical Discourse,' in: E. Fee and D.M. Fox (eds) *AIDS: The Burden of History*. Berkeley, CA: University of California Press, pp. 136–51.

Treichler, P. and C. Warren (1998) 'Maybe Next Year: Feminist Silence and the AIDS Epidemic,' in: N.L. Roth and K. Hogan (eds) *Gendered Epidemic: Representations of Women in the age of AIDS*. London: Routledge, pp. 109–52.

Van der Vliet, V. (1996) *The Politics of AIDS*. London: Bowerdean Publishing Company.

Wallack, L. (1990) 'Mass Media and Health Promotion: Promise, Problem, and Challenge,' in: C. Atkin and L. Wallack (eds) *Mass Communication and Public Health*. Newbury Park, CA: Sage, pp. 41–50.

Wang, Y. (1999) *A History of Gay Rights Movements in Taiwan*. Taipei, Taiwan: Cheerful Sunshine Publishers (in Chinese).

Watney, S. (1987) *Policing Desire: Pornography, AIDS and the Media*. London: Methuen.

Weiss, C.H. (1974) What America's Leaders Read. *Public Opinion Quarterly* 38, pp. 1–21.

Williams, K. and D. Miller (1995) 'AIDS News and News Cultures,' in: J. Downing, A. Mohammadi and A. Sreberny-Mohammadi (eds) *Questioning the Media: A Critical Introduction* (2nd ed). Thousand Oaks, CA: Sage, pp. 413–506.

Wilton, T. (1997) *Engendering AIDS: Deconstructing Sex, Text and Epidemic*. Thousand Oaks, CA: Sage.

CHAPTER 9

AIDS AND CIVIL SOCIETY IN TAIWAN[1]

EVELYNE MICOLLIER

In relation to economic growth and political liberalization, the emergence of a civil society is one of the most significant social transformations which has taken place in Taiwan since the 1980s. The development of the non-profit sector has embarked on a new and unprecedented phase. This process is a dynamic component of social change and offers an interesting perspective on the emergence of a 'civil society', a concept sure to trigger off debate among scholars when applied to Chinese and/or Taiwanese contexts (Huang 1993; Ma 1994). While the legal framework and historical background of civic bodies are both highly relevant to law and political science, studying the working methods of these organizations in daily life, human relationships, team building and networking at a micro-social scale is highly consistent with an anthropological approach. Social organizations have the capacity to access those margins of society government bodies cannot easily reach. This process allows the state to delegate the management of politically sensitive social issues. Although the government has been slow to act in launching a national offensive, a modern AIDS campaign has gradually taken shape with the help of the non-profit sector – secular and religious organizations[2] – working in conjunction with official bodies.

I have done ethnographic fieldwork in Taipei. For that purpose, official bodies as well as social organizations involved in AIDS prevention and care, were approached.[3] I visited regularly the service in charge of PWA/HIVs (People living with AIDS/HIV) in the Taipei hospitals appointed by the government, and worked with two secular social organizations involved in the fight against AIDS. This approach enables me to be a participant-observer, to know and interview activists from diverse social categories, social workers, journalists showing an interest in AIDS-related issues, people suffering from HIV/AIDS, health personnel in medical institutions and in officials working in health bureaus or in the headquarters of the DoH. The following topics will be discussed in this paper: The emergence of a civil society is investigated through an analysis of the development of the non-profit sector and the working methods of local NGOs. Specific questions related to the HIV/AIDS epidemic, a sensitive health issue, have shed an original light on the debate about civil society: official responses echo non-official organized responses to the epidemic threat. Finally, AIDS memorial rituals are described as voices of society, and the controversial issue of sex education is introduced.

THE EMERGENCE OF A CIVIL SOCIETY

In contrast to the kinship group, civil society is part of the political community. Representative of progressive forces which cannot deploy themselves within the framework of a backward state which has a monopoly on social change and political power, it organizes itself as the opposition to the State.[4] Considering the Chinese context, Hsu (1994) has selected the word 'society' rather than 'civil society', arguing that a city-state organization has never existed in China, and that the notion of civil society is primarily related to the social reality of Greek and Roman antiquity. Indeed, the concept of the 'public sphere' borrowed from Habermas (1989) is to be preferred when applied to Chinese culture (Huang 1993, cited by Kwok 1994). The growing role of the non-profit sector and the development of a civic culture are among the preliminary conditions for the emergence of a democracy (Wachman 1994:35).

In the early 1980s, progressive forces found themselves gathered together in a political organization 'Outside the Party' (*Dangwai*): Taiwan was ruled under a regime of martial law by the 'Nationalist Party' (*Guomin dang*). Political pluralism only came into effect in 1986 with the foundation of the 'Progressive Democratic Party' (*Minjin dang*) and was consolidated in 1987 with the lifting of martial law. This process of political trans-formation allowed progressive forces to diversify, reshaping themselves into non-political social organizations. For a decade now, civic associations have been taking various forms, diverging in both methods of working and the social purposes which they espouse. During the 1980s, civic freedom was gradually insinuated. In this process, religious freedom was even encouraged by the nationalist government, which saw it as a remedy against the on-going erosion of traditional values and morality (Vermander 1995:11). Debate about long-tabooed matters is nowadays allowed and self-censorious behaviour is steadily being abandoned. Cultural, ethnic and linguistic plurality in Taiwan is now clearly taken for granted by people from every ring of the whole social spectrum.

The role of tensions arising from identity in the process of democratization is well documented (Wachman 1994; Geoffroy 1997). Lay associations show non-traditional forms: they are centred neither on the kinship group, on corporate networks, on locality, on proximity. Collaboration involving Taiwanese and foreign NGOs, religious groups which do not share religious affiliation – Christian and Buddhist groups – in the field of public health and education is now the order of the day. This seems very upbeat but there is a downside. Many local NGOs rely on one person, or at best a few persons and never on the whole team. Without these charismatic people at the helm, the NGO is drained of efficiency either by lack of funds or a shortage of human resources. Motives for joining are generally linked to the personality or status of a president rather than to a genuine involvement in a cause. Civil society may remain weak if some actors are not intimately drawn to cause by either beliefs or practices. As Cabestan (1999:120) put it, many people are unable to accept the restrictions imposed by an organized action, which is not linked to their own immediate interests. This tendency may contribute to the slowing down of the maturing process of Taiwanese civil society. However, this feature may not be culturally bound as Cabestan suggests. Numerous changes have taken place in Taiwan during the 1990s, and they clearly show a diversification of society and social dynamics, which may be interpreted as phenomena part of a broader 'globalizing' process: this trend suggests that Taiwanese society is entering in the 'post-modernist' era described in capitalist societies of the Western world. It is thus difficult to recognize a general conservative or progressive trend.

The non-profit sector can be divided into two categories: non-governmental organizations (NGOs) (*minjian tuanti*) and endowment-centred foundations (*jijinghui*). By 1997, the number of Taiwanese NGOs including all types of political organizations had reached 12000, a 50 per cent rise compared to the early 1990s. Membership figures are high: one Taiwanese out of five is an NGO member. More than 60 per cent of the current total number of registered NGOs have been created either in the 1980s or in the 1990s. Social service oriented, public interest, and charitable organizations account for 30 per cent, while academically, culturally and internationally aligned bodies make up more than 40 per cent. According to Hsiao (1995:239), although related, two social changes regarding NGOs in Taiwan are yet distinguishable: 'One is the rise of a social movement sector within the NGOs, the other the self-transformation of many already well-established NGOs.' Emerging social movements urging social reforms and changes in state policies can be classified into four categories in terms of their objects of concern:

- Consumer protection, pollution, rising housing costs, and conservation
- The rights of disadvantaged or stigmatized social groups such as ethnic minorities (language rights, land control, and cultural identity), the elderly, the handicapped, veterans, and certain religious groups.

- The state's corporatist mode of control over key social groups, such as workers, farmers, students, women, teachers, and intellectuals.
- Politically sensitive issues such as the relations between Taiwanese and Mainland Chinese people, and human rights.

More than one hundred specific individual social movement organizations can be identified in terms of their objectives, social bases, and mobilization strategies. Most of them are grassroots and locally based, thus constituting the 'new sector' of Taiwan's NGOs (Hsiao 1995:240).

In 1997, there were 1600 foundations, which could be defined into three categories: most of them (70 per cent) are private and independent, 25 per cent are corporate, and 5 per cent are semi-governmental or governmental.[5] Recently created non-governmental foundations dominate the sector. The increasing number of corporate foundations shows the growing interest of the private business sector in social issues. Following the same patterns as NGOs, welfare and charitable foundations constitute top-ranking categories in terms of numbers. Research, education, culture, foreign exchanges, and social involvement comprise the other high-ranking categories. Most of the foundations are operative rather than grant-giving organizations. This original feature suggests that foundations are not clearly differentiated from NGOs except in legal terms. The famous Buddhist foundation *Ciji*, is the most significant private foundation in terms of endowment and lay support. On the strength of its four million members, the organization is involved in social services related to education, health, and culture, not only in Taiwan but also in countries afflicted by human or natural disasters. The success of *Ciji* may be traced to the rise of a new conservatism (Laliberté 1998). The organization refers to some basic values of Taiwan's cultural matrix: 'It has succeeded because it appeals both to "timeless" Chinese/Taiwanese values yet also quick to adopt new forms of group organization and models of "love" familiar to lay membership as it has changed over time.' (De Vido 2001:94) For instance, *Ciji* 'promotes and reproduces an essentialist notion of feminine nature, of female as synonymous with Mother, as a self-sacrificing, infinitely forbearing, compassionate nurturer of others: the uncontested norm in Taiwan society' (De Vido 2001:95).

Indeed, religious organizations benefit the most from people's donations. Taiwanese attitudes towards philanthropy tend to favour traditional forms to more progressive secular forms of social solidarity. Such support of the Taiwanese public opinion for selected social organizations is one of the conservative elements remaining in a definitely emerging pluralistic society. Critical analysis of society by academics and heated debates in academic circles, the vitality of the literary scene, and the activism of the queer and

226

homosexual movements (*kuer yundong, tongzhi yundong*) demonstrate simultaneously the strength of progressive elements.

RESPONSES TO THE HIV/AIDS EPIDEMIC

The first case of HIV infection was reported in 1984 by the DoH 'Department of Health' *weisheng shu,* the highest governmental health body. From December 1984 to March 2000, almost 22 million blood samples were tested. The epidemiological data released in December 2000 by the DoH were as follows: the official figure shows one of the lowest infection rates in the region with 2773 'People infected with HIV' (PWH) including 905 full blown AIDS people 'People with AIDS' (PWA). More than 90 per cent of them are Taiwanese male nationals.[6] The main channel of transmission is sexual (85 per cent of PWH), more precisely heterosexual (41 per cent), bisexual (16 per cent), gay male (28 per cent). Bisexuality is not clearly defined. According to my ethnographic data, people included in the category are often married men, fathers, and homosexuals in their behaviour and attitudes. Looking at the problem from the perspective of age, people ranging from twenty to thirty-nine constitute 70 per cent of officially declared PWH. Turning to social indicators, it is worth noticing that 22 per cent of HIV infected people pertain to the social category 'unemployed' even though the unemployment rate (3 per cent in 2000) is fairly low in Taiwan. One very specific epidemic trend is the ratio male/female among reported HIV infected people, which is twelve men to one woman (women accounting for only 7.7 per cent of reported HIV infections). This figure is indeed surprising, knowing that the main epidemic channel is heterosexual transmission and that women are more vulnerable to HIV infection than men. Data show that sexual transmission is the most common infection route suggesting that AIDS control policies should focus on prevention. For that purpose, sex education programmes are gradually being introduced in schools.

The sex industry is expanding and commercial sex work is facilitating the spread of HIV infection: estimates give a figure of more than 50,000 prostitutes working in Taipei alone (*The Echoes of the ROC,* Sept. 21, 1997). Another risk factor is an increasing mobility of the population. The Taiwanese are quite well off on a regional scale; they have plenty of opportunities to travel both inside and outside the country either for business or tourism. Since 1989, an increasing number of migrant workers have been arriving each year from Southeast Asia (Philippines, Thailand, Indonesia) to work legally in Taiwan for a maximum of three years (Chang 1999: 14). In 2000, 310 000 were officially registered.[7]

AIDS care is not neglected. Treatments for PWH are available, commonly accessible, and established from therapeutic trials. Testing and treatment sites are of good quality. Compared to Thailand for instance, the infrastructure for AIDS prevention and care, is better set up. As far as access to recent poly-therapies is concerned, the Taiwan case is unique in Asia, being one of the few countries in the world where treatment is free of charge for the patients as long as they are covered by the National Health Insurance (covering 96 per cent of the population in 1997).[8]

Since 1992, NGOs and volunteer groups supported by the DoH have launched an AIDS campaign, and have developed help and care networks. Their activities include organizing cultural events, conferences, sex education training, running hotlines, websites, developing sex education programmes and insinuating educational messages through the media in the press and on TV, in leaflets, brochures, and the like. Starting from 1997 and following a ten-year plan, the DoH is modernizing the system for controlling communicable diseases including AIDS.[9] In AIDS control, the main focus is the introduction of new therapies and the launching of more efficient educational programmes for prevention.

Although epidemiological data are less alarming than in other Asian countries, by 1998, the spread of the virus had accelerated up to one new reported HIV-infection per day.[10] Because of its exceptional political situation (Taiwan is not a member of the UN), the island manages to control the epidemic risk with more independence than other states which are curbed by their rights and obligations to the UN. Despite its position as an outsider, Taiwan tends to act along the lines of UN recommendations for obvious health reasons and also for diplomatic motives. National responses are part of the state planning structure, which has addressed private and public sectors, civic collaboration, and schools. Official and non-official organized responses have to be matched. People at risk cannot be educated, informed, tested, and receive care in a context in which a mixture of silence, fear and stigmatization is the most common attitude towards the illness and towards people infected by the virus. From this perspective, sexual risk has to be clearly contextualized in order to make 'culturally appropriate interventions' (Brummelhuis and Herdt 1995:15). In Taiwan, three categories of the population are primarily involved in AIDS prevention: HIV-infected people, politicians, and health workers. HIV-infected people could organize themselves and claim their rights. Conscious of voters, politicians do not dare to lead the campaign. The awareness of health workers still has to be raised as recent studies have shown, assessing the attitude of fear and ignorance prevailing among health personnel (Yuan *et al.* 1994; Ting and Twu 1997).

The DoH has designed a number of policies designed to control the epidemic. The Department co-operates with other official bodies as the Ministry of Education (*Jiaoyu bu*) and the Ministry of Defence (*Guofang bu)*, and with local NGOs. In principle, involvement in the official AIDS campaign is required from all administrative levels. Non-official organized responses to the epidemic are complementary and are indispensable to improving efficiency of institutional responses. It is important to note that only three associations are exclusively involved in the fight against AIDS: the 'Light of Friendship for AIDS Prevention and Control' *(Yiguang aizi fangzhi xiehui)*; the 'National Association for AIDS Control' *(Zhonghua minguo aizibing fangzhi xiehui)*; and the 'Hope workshop' *(Xiwang gongzuofang)*. Membership, the goals and the working methods of these organizations will be examined in more detail below.

The 'Light of Friendship for AIDS Prevention and Control' (*Yiguang xiehui)* is an NGO funded mainly by the DoH. Numbering about 200 members, the association was created in 1992. In 1995, it split up into two on the basis of divergent standpoints on priority actions. The services provided by the *Yiguang* are focused more on providing information and education for AIDS prevention. The association has no links with other Taiwanese or foreign organizations. It is interesting to note that the president is head of the Taipei Health Bureau (*Taipeishi weishengju)*. Based in Taipei, the *Yiguang* has also a small branch in Taizhong, the third Taiwanese city. The staff includes two social workers and three volunteers in Taipei and only one social worker in Taizhong. Documents including books, periodicals, audio- or videotapes, and the association's own publication (a monthly periodical) are freely available to the public during the regular working hours every week. A website (www.lofaa.org.tw) and a hotline are also run by the *Yiguang*. Educational training, informing through media and publications, free condom distribution in public places (such as main railways station, bars, and night clubs) are its main activities. Information and education may specifically target vulnerable groups such as homosexuals and commercial sex workers (CSWs). Other services such as free anonymous HIV tests, island-wide HIV/AIDS prevention and education activities, the internet as a channel for prevention and education, various training, and global interaction involving GOs and NGOs are newly available. Further information on the *Yiguang* can be found on its website.

The 'National Association for AIDS Control' (*Zhonghua minguo aizibing fangzhi xiehui)*, is more medically oriented as most members are health workers and providing care for and help to the patients, are its main activities. However, prevention, including some educational training in schools is also one of its undertakings. The monthly periodical published by the association is designed mainly for medical personnel. The staff includes physicians, nurses, and volunteers. The main office is in Taipei with a branch in Gaoxiong, the second city of Taiwan and the biggest harbour of the island. A monthly periodical 'AIDS Prevention and Care' (*Aizibing fangzhi jikan*) published by the association is distributed to members, and to individual subscribers and institutions such as libraries, medical schools, institutes of public health, and healthcare services. The president, a physician and professor who is also involved in the social sciences, is chief of the 'Clinical Virology Division' of Taipei Veterans General Hospital. He gives educational training to military trainees, students, and Southeast Asian migrant workers at worksites. A hotline is available for advice and information.

The 'Hope Workshop' (*Xiwang gongzuofang*) operates within the framework of the 'National Academic Society for Preventive Medicine' (*Zhonghua minguo yufang yixue xuehui*), an academic association which covers a whole range of health workers, researchers, and professors specialized in public health or other medical disciplines. The Society is involved in all priority health issues such as early testing for cancer, anti-tobacco campaigns, and prevention of communicable diseases including STDs and HIV/AIDS. The 'Hope Workshop' is the main organizer of the December 1st World AIDS Day annual campaign in Taipei. In its efforts to coordinate World AIDS Day activities, the association is supported financially by the DoH and the 'National Academic Society for Preventive Medicine'. Since December 1995, World AIDS Day has been celebrated in Taiwan by stressing AIDS prevention through information and education, and by condom promotion.

Another association, the 'ROC Association for HIV/AIDS patients Rights Advocacy', is striving for legal changes in the status and rights of HIV-infected people. The aim is to obtain appropriate medical services for HIV positive patients and the right for them to continue working. The association is fighting for the right of HIV positive patients to be awarded an allowance as disabled people such as the right recognized in France. Patients in Taiwan do not yet benefit from such an allowance. Cogently, its secretary is a former staff member of the 'Hope Workshop' and that the two associations organize joint activities.

The 'Hope Workshop' did try to create a 'mid-way house', which did not work out in the wake of strong local opposition against the project. Enjoying the advantage of owning a house and for that reason, having more chance to succeed, a Roman Catholic group attempts to launch the project again. When I interviewed the head of the 'Communicable Disease Control Division', she explained the current problems related to the 'mid-way house project': 'The DoH was supporting the project in spite of obstacles: but firstly, difficulties were raised by neighbours angry about a fall in local housing prices; secondly, this housing system is not very appropriate to the Chinese and/or Taiwanese cultural contexts. Only a few HIV-infected people need this type of housing. The DoH encourages patients to be helped in the traditional family context as for any other illness'.

Indeed, the family plays a major role in patient care: traditional conceptions of illness assume that, if a family member is ill, all the family is in fact affected. The family supports and provides care to the patient as the principal aim is to restore family harmony as soon as possible. In Taiwan, health policies are still partly drawn from traditional practices and ideas. Health care is still currently provided by the female members of the family – mothers, spouses, sisters, daughters-in-law – instead of nurses as it is the case in all modern Westernized health care systems. Nursing training was introduced quite recently into the educational system (1935) (Lu 1990:31). The first missionary nurse had arrived in China in 1884. Although China has an old medical history, professional nursing dates back only to the nineteenth century when modern Western medicine was introduced by Christian missionaries.

According to Su Yi-Hung, chief nurse at the Taipei Veterans General Hospital, most AIDS patients are helped and supported by their family. Informed by her thirteen-year experience of working with AIDS patients (about one hundred), she claims that 90 per cent of the families are ready to support HIV infected relatives, men tending to keep their distance and be less involved than women (*The Echoes of the ROC* March 1999). Published in an official news periodical, this figure may be greatly overestimated, a fact found our ethnographic data tends to support: most HIV-infected people do not inform their relatives about their HIV status when the infection is a-symptomatic. On the basis of regular visits to a Taipei hospital in services designed for AIDS patients, I have noticed that even in the case of hospitalization, only a limited number of family members visit AIDS patients.

AIDS MEMORIALS AS VOICES OF SOCIETY[11]

International AIDS memorial ceremonies, such as the 'Quilt Ceremony' and the 'Candlelight AIDS Memorial', have been born in the wake of the abrupt disappearance of so many young people and the distress following the disastrous consequences of the epidemic. They are part of the so-called 'new rituals' aimed at mourning and commemorating people who have died of AIDS; they are definitely performed on an international scale on World AIDS Day (1 December) but take specific cultural forms. These rituals show an aspect of social change related to AIDS (*Ethnologie française* 1998).

They are now currently celebrated in Taiwan, and the specificities of these rituals in the Taiwanese cultural context give clues to hear some voices in society, which usually remain silent.

Since 1995, a Taiwanese Quilt has been conceived in co-operation with the international NGO 'Names Project' created in California in 1987 and is shown in various Taiwanese cities for World AIDS Day (Chang *et al.* 1997). The Quilt ceremony has two levels of significance – individual and activist: each patch, each name pronounced while the patchwork is shown, underline the uniqueness of each deceased person; the patchwork configuration, the fact that the association will collect the individual patches, put them together and show them to the world to stress the disastrous consequences of the epidemic, bring about the social significance of death due to AIDS (Fellous 1998:80). The Quilt's unique feature is that the personal mourning healing process and the collective activist campaign are closely interwoven. Interestingly, the text in Taiwanese patchworks is often written in English. Moreover, angels and crosses, both Christian symbols, are used to talk about death and to commemorate the dead. Is it a way of 'Othering' the disease, stressing its foreign nature by using an imagery obviously related to Western culture? The imputation of the AIDS disease on the Other is now well documented in a number of cultures.[12] For instance, in Japan, an infected and infecting mother is no longer addressed in Japanese but in English. Her body has become foreign (Buckley 1997:290). However, we need to be careful in our interpretation: local culture changes the meaning of foreign symbols, which lose their exogenous nature in the process. Moreover, the fact that Christian groups are involved in the AIDS campaign and could insinuate such meaningful images for their own purposes has to be acknowledged.

Love and sexuality from the West are referred to with the juxtaposed evocation of sexual liberation and Christian universal love. The English language and Christian symbols are commonly used in the educational messages of the AIDS campaign. The repetitive figuring of the cross in the Quilt to symbolize death, of angels and children in 'The Book of Silent Love' (Zhi *et al.* 1997), an educational book about safe sex published by the 'Chinese Society of Preventive Medicine', show the current need to refer to a foreign culture in order to talk about love and sex, the need for a 'screen discourse' imbued with a mediator role.

The Taiwanese 'Candlelight AIDS Memorial' called, *fangshui deng,* literally 'throw the lanterns in the water', commemorates the death of PWA and addresses a prayer of hope for PWH.[13] Organized in Taiwan since 1994, this ritual gathers patients, relatives, and activists. Some people hide their HIV status and only a few family members attend the ceremony. The public and journalists were not admitted in 1997 as HIV-infected people were worried about being identified and discriminated against. In 1999, this censoriousness of social stigmatization seemed to have improved. Indeed, journalists have been allowed to report and take photographs.[14] A short article about the event with a picture, has been published in the official *Echoes of the R.O.C.* (Dec. 11, 1999: 4).

The lotus flower shaped lanterns, a traditional appurtenance in Buddhist death rituals, were thrown one by one into the river at dusk by each participant. Participants watched over them as they floated in the water from the starting point of their journey, and were busy putting them into the flow again if the journey was impeded by any obstacle. These ritual sequences may be an efficacious measure as they assume a structural role. White is the traditional colour of death in China: lanterns are therefore white for the dead and pink for the PWH, symbolizing hope.

PWH or volunteers involved in the fight against AIDS may interpret death from AIDS as an unnatural premature death. Moving this death away from the living people is therefore necessary. The function of the ritual is then to prevent the dead, who might come back as 'wandering souls', from harming the living. These ideas are rooted in popular religion or more precisely in popular Buddhism, which is fully integrated into popular religion. It is important to distinguish two *a priori* contradictory sets of ideas for a better understanding of the distinctive meaning of these ritual practices:

- On one hand, the ritual commemorates the deaths of PWA. As an international and activist memorial, one of its goals is to raise public awareness about AIDS and to show the reality of the human distress of people suffering from AIDS. Indeed, PWH live under the threat of biological death as well as of social and symbolic death, stemming from the stigmatizing attitude and behaviour of the people around them.

- On the other hand, if the ritual is related to a death traditionally perceived as unnatural and premature, PWH and activists are taking upon themselves the shame spread on family members and relatives. This death is perceived as harmful and inauspicious to the group. The ritual is then a means to escape from this 'non-ominous death', to restore family and social harmony.

If this interpretation of the ritual is valid, participants and initiators of the memorial ceremony may be embedded in traditional cultural representations. This ritual may then reveal a world view in transition (moving through a continuum with polarities—a traditional worldview and a globalizing one) in these groups of activists fighting against AIDS who simultaneously question important taboos regarding sexuality, claimed as non-standardized, and regarding death. The voice of the people is brought out through this case study, and deserves to be heard as a voice from a kind of 'underground', 'alternative', or 'non-politically correct' civil society. Needless to say that further research is needed on this topic.

THE NEED FOR SEX EDUCATION

The purpose of a section of the 'Mercy Memorial Foundation' (*Xingying jijinghui*), the 'Center for Family Life and Sex Education' (*Jiating shenghuo yu xingjiaoyu zhongxin)*, is to elaborate and develop sex education programmes in co-operation with two state bodies—the DoH operating as a funding agency, and the 'Bureau of Social Affairs' institutionally affiliated within the Ministry of Education (*Jiaoyu bu shehui ju)*. The foundation favours international exchanges, particularly trans-Asian cooperation and is currently working on projects with the Hong Kong-based 'Sex Education Associates', with the international 'Asia Sex Education Committee', and with the Shanghai 'Chinese Association of Sexology' (*Zhongguo xing xuehui)*, which now have representatives in every province of mainland China. Some associations provide information services since 1989.

Since the late 1980s, Prof. Yen (1989), professor of health education at National Taiwan Normal University, president of the 'Asian Federation for Sexology' (*Yazhou xingxue huiyi)*, and executive director of the 'Mercy Memorial Foundation', has vigorously supported the introduction of sex education in schools on a national scale. His long-term, pioneering work has ineluctably shown the need for sex education to solve a number of social and health issues in a society facing rapid and drastic social changes, and the need for a better understanding of human sexual life at an individual level as well as at a societal level. To illustrate this, I will quote the summary of a paper, which he delivered at a 1988 conference. In this, he discussed the relevance, definition, objectives, and contents of sex education, and reviewed a number of essays related to sex education collected between 1977 and 1989. Based on the ideas about sex knowledge, attitudes, sexual behaviour, and sex education expressed in the materials, he had drawn a few concluding lines:

- The lack of sexual knowledge was a common phenomenon
- The source of what knowledge there was came mainly from peers.
- There was a general support for sex education and a gradual acceptance of premarital sex, although the society still showed signs of conservatism towards sex.

- Data on premarital sex were analysed and compared in several essays.
- The emphasis on sex education designed for local students should be focused on knowledge about gendered relations, as well as the biological and psychological aspects of sexuality.

Nowadays, research fellows affiliated with the 'Mercy Memorial Foundation' draw their results from both field studies and documentary research. On the basis of these manuals are compiled which are more in keeping with the times and educational videotapes. Personnel from the educational sector (professors, teachers, directors) are welcome to ask for information, training, and educational materials. Recent surveys were conducted among four groups of the population (parents, teachers, experts, students) using the KABP 'Knowledge, Attitude, Belief, and Practice' method. The results of these surveys are being used to realign the contents of sex education programmes. In September 1998, the foundation released the results of a recent survey on the sexual behaviours of young people. This survey reports on information channels about sex: for 34 per cent, sex knowledge comes primarily from books; for 17 per cent from school; for 13.3 per cent, from sexual partners; for 12.8 per cent, from friends or classmates; the last informative channel, the family context (parents), account for 7 per cent of young people. The results were widely available on a number of Internet websites.

In 1998, sex education was still a new discipline in schools, and was being introduced into fields such as education, biology, psychology, and social work. A large-scale national programme is difficult to implement in the face of the opposition from a certain number of teachers and parents. Sex education is designed to be taught at all educational levels from kindergarten to university. Since 1995, sex education has been included in the following university departments: social work, public health, psychology, and health education. It was already compulsory in health education programmes (*guozhong*: high school level) and exclusively female nursing training (*gaozhong*: senior high school level) of public schools. In universities, it was part of the compulsory self-defence classes (*ziqiuke*).

CONCLUDING REMARKS

Civil society in the Taiwanese pluralistic society as observed through the lens of social organizations is still in the process of maturing. Its emergence does not automatically generate structural changes allowing progressive voices to be heard. Moreover, social order could be strengthened and conservatism may be on the rise, seized on as a way for the people to face the drastic and rapid transformations challenging Taiwanese society. For instance, a rather conservative religious organization as the Buddhist Foundation (*Ciji hui*) is the most favoured social organization as both the amount of funds raised and high membership figures show.

These cautionary remarks are not intended to dispel a more encouraging view on the on-going development of a civil society. A few progressive Chinese language publications are concerned with AIDS and gender-related topics.[15] The publications and research of the 'Sex Center' at the Central University offer progressive views, as well as movies such as 'Meili Shaonian' and 'Bu zhi shi xiyan' directed by Mickey Chen. However, the readership of all these publications is still limited, and the existence of these works does not demonstrate that progressive voices are heard in society and have an impact on most social actors. Moreover, in her content analysis of AIDS campaign messages and news coverage, Hsu (1998) has shown that themes dealing with attitudes toward PWA/HIVs and their civil rights are almost inexistent constituting less than 2 per cent of the total.

I will recall also here the results of a 1997 poll showing high interest in volunteerism among young people (Wu 1997): 'Young people most commonly volunteer their time in social welfare services, community development programs, counselling for youngsters or adolescents, health care services and environmental protection programs, in that order. Up to 90% of the respondents hold a positive view of voluntary services, saying volunteerism can not only promote social harmony but also contribute to one's own growth or self satisfaction. Most local young people want the government and private enterprises to play a more active role in promoting voluntary services. Encouraged by the survey findings, the National Youth Commission will launch programs aimed at pooling the resources of the government and the private sector to create a clean living environment.'

Traditional values such as promoting social harmony, confronted by 'globalizing' values such as the rise of individualism account for the motivation of young people involved in volunteerism. Following widespread protests denouncing governmental inertia about environmental issues, these currently stand high on the political agenda, becoming a political stake in both local and national elections. Ecological and Buddhist groups, or one or the other, have increased the awareness of the population about environmental protection through campaigns, thus urging the government to take concrete measures.

The activist movement against AIDS is embedded in a global context but its practices and claims are 'contextualized' and reinterpreted through local meanings as some aspects of the AIDS memorials and the AIDS campaign have shown. Finally, our case-study of the AIDS campaign has shown through the working methods of social organizations involved in the fight against the disease, state policies, and the difficulties encountered in implementing sex education programmes that an epidemic threat such as the AIDS disease is a challenging social issue in a democratizing society.

NOTES

1 The draft of this paper was presented at *The 2000 North American Taiwan Studies Conference, June 16–19, Harvard University, Mass.* Some parts of it have been revised from Micollier, E. 2000a.
2 Unfortunately I did not have the opportunity to work as a participant-observer with religious organizations as I had to select a few organizations to work with and I chose to focus on secular social organizations. It seems to me that these latter organizations were more significant in the analysis of the development of a civil society and of a pluralistic society in Taiwan. Indeed, as mentioned elsewhere in the paper, religious organisations were encouraged to blossom by the Nationalist government in contrast to secular social organizations, which develop during the 1980s accompanying the process of democratization.
3 Field research was carried out in 1997 (4 months) thanks to the support of the 'Centre for Chinese Studies', National Central Library, Taipei, and of the CNRS-SHS Dept, 'National Programme on AIDS', Paris.
4 Aristotle and most political theoreticians until the eighteenth century, include the State in the political community. In the nineteenth century, civil society is opposed to the State, an idea conceived by Hegel and systematized by the Marxists (Gramsci, 1930s), see Gresle F., Panoff M., Perrin, M., et P. Tripier (1990: 306).
5 Data from 'Taiwan Report: The Non-profit Sector in Taiwan: Current state, New Trends and Future Prospects' (1998).
6 As in Japanese official figures, the categories 'foreigner/local' are the first reported distinction, cf. Buckley, S. (1997: 265).
7 The trend has been reversed this year following an official policy aimed to restrain foreign labour in sectors in which they are competing with local workers., cf. *The Echoes of the ROC*, Sept. 21, 2000: 2.
8 Patients are not reimbursed only when they ask for a very recently commercialized medication, which is not yet on the list approved by the DoH. On the National Health Insurance Scheme introduced in 1995, cf. 'National Health Insurance' *Public Health in Taiwan* (1997); Ku Yeun-Wen (1998).
9 See 'Control of Communicable Diseases' *Public Health in Taiwan*, 1997: 52–72.
10 *The Echoes of the ROC*, March 11, 1999.

11 This part is revised from Micollier, E. 2000b.
12 See Sontag, S. 1993; Farmer, P. 1992; in Japan, cf. Buckley, S. 1997; in Taiwan, Hsu *et al.*'s paper in this volume, in Taiwan and China, Micollier 1999.
13 I attended this ceremony (part of World AIDS Day activities) late afternoon on Dec. 29 of 1997 taking place in Taipei along the Yun-non River; the 'Hope workshop' was granted the authorization to organize it since 1994.
14 Although HIV/AIDS-related news reports may reinforce the process of stigmatization. For an overall analysis of these reports, and in particular in relation to the stigmatization of PWA/HIVs, see Hsu *et al.*'s paper in this volume.
15 Among them, see the daily paper 'Li-Bao', the weekly magazines 'POTS' and 'Stir', the journals 'The Isle Margin' and 'Awakening'.

REFERENCES

Brummelhuis H.T. and G. Herdt (eds) (1995) *Culture and Sexual Risk. Anthropological Perspectives on AIDS.* Amsterdam and Philadelphia: Gordon/Breach Ed.

Buckley, S. (1997) 'The Foreign Devil Returns: Packaging Sexual Practice and Risk in Contemporary Japan,' in: L. Manderson and M. Jolly (eds) *Sites of Desire, Economies of Pleasure. Sexualities in Asia and the Pacific.* Chicago and London: University of Chicago Press, pp. 262–91.

Cabestan, J.P. (1999) *Le système politique de Taiwan.* Paris: PUF, coll. 'Que sais-je?' N. 1809.

Chang H, Ho C., Shih An-Ti, Chien Ching-Shu and Tang Shao (eds) (1997) *Taiwan aizibing beidan gushi.* (Stories from Taiwan's AIDS Quilt). Taipei: Chinese Society of Preventive Medicine, bilingual Chinese-English, 24 pp.

De Vido, E.A. (2001) 'An Audience with Venerable Master Zheng Yan', *The Taipei Ricci Bulletin*, Taipei Ricci Institute, pp. 77–102.

Ethnologie française (1998) N. spécial 'SIDA: deuil, mémoire, nouveaux rituels,' Vol. XXVIII N. 1.

Farmer, P. (1992) *AIDS and Accusation.* Berkeley: University of California Press.

Fellous, M. (1998) 'Le Quilt: un mémorial vivant pour les morts du SIDA' *Ethnologie française* N. spécial 'SIDA: deuil, mémoire, nouveaux rituels' XXVIII(1), pp. 80–6.

Geoffroy, C. (1997) *Le mouvement indépendantiste taiwanais.* Paris: L'Harmattan.

Gresle F., M. Panoff M., M. Perrin M. and P. Tripier (1990) *Dictionnaire des sciences humaines*. Paris: Nathan.

Habermas, J. (1989) *The Structural Transformation of the Public Sphere: An Inquiry into a Category of Bourgeois Society.* Cambridge: MIT Press.

Hsiao, Hsin Huang M. (1995) 'The Growing Asia Pacific Concern among Taiwan NGOs' in T. Yamamoto (ed.) *Emerging Civil Society in the Asia Pacific Community.* Tokyo, Japan Center for International Exchange, pp. 239–44.

Hsu, Cho-Yun (1994) 'Development of the State-Society Relationship in Early China' in: L. Vandermeersch (ed.) *La société civile face à l'Etat dans les traditions chinoise, japonaise, coréenne et vietnamienne.* Paris: EFEO, Etudes thématiques 3, pp. 1–16.

Hsu, Mei-Ling (1998) 'Issue Importance and Source Reliability of AIDS in Taiwan : A Comparison of the News and Campaign Agenda-Setting,' Paper presented at the annual meeting of the Health Communication Division, International Communication Association, Jerusalem, July.

Huang, P. (ed.) (1993) 'Symposium 'Public sphere/Civil society' in China? Paradigmatic issues in Chinese studies,' *Modern China* 19(2), pp. 107–216.

Ku, Yeun-Wen (1998) 'Can we afford it? The development of National Health Insurance in Taiwan,' in R. Goodman, G. White, H.J. Kwon (eds) *The East Asian Welfare Model – Welfare Orientalism and the State.* London: Routledge, pp. 119–38.

Kwok, D.W.Y. (1994) 'Moral Community and Civil Society in China: Enigmas viewed from the Traditions of Protest and Political Advice,' in: L. Vandermeersch (ed.) *La société civile face à l'Etat dans les traditions chinoise, japonaise, coréenne et vietnamienne.* Paris: EFEO, Etudes thématiques 3, pp. 17–28.

Laliberté, A. (1998) 'Tzu Chi and Buddhist Revival in Taiwan. Rise of a new conservatism?' *China Perspectives* 19, pp. 44–50.

Lu, Zxy-Yann Jane (1990) *Ill fate: Women's illnesses experiences in the pluralistic health care system of Taiwan.* Ph. D. dissertation, University of Michigan.

Ma, Shu-Yun (1994) 'The Chinese discourse on civil society,' *The China Quarterly* 137, pp.180–93.

Micollier, E. (1999) 'L'Autre : porteur originel et/ou vecteur privilégié du VIH/SIDA (Chine populaire-Taiwan),' in: C. Fay (ed.) 'Le sida des autres : constructions locales et internationales de la maladie,' *Autrepart* (Cahiers des sciences humaines), IRD-L'Aube 12, pp. 73–86.

Micollier, E. (2000a) 'Emergence de la société civile à Taiwan: vers une gestion collective des problèmes de santé,' in: C. Chaîgne, C. Paix and

C. Zheng (eds) *Taiwan. Enquête sur une identité*. Paris, Karthala, pp. 309–31.

– (2000b) 'Analyse de la campagne de prévention à Taiwan,' dans M.E. Blanc, L. Husson and E. Micollier (eds) *Sociétés asiatiques face au SIDA*. Paris, L'Harmattan, coll. «recherches asiatiques», pp. 229–52.

Public Health in Taiwan. Taipei: DoH, Executive Yuan 1997.

Sontag, S. (1993) *La maladie comme métaphore. Le sida et ses métaphores*. Paris: C. Bourgois.

'Taiwan Report: The Non-profit Sector in Taiwan. Current state, New Trends and Future Prospects' (1998) Background Paper delivered at the International Conference on Philanthropy, Asia Pacific Philanthropy Consortium, Bangkok, January.

Ting Chih-Yin and Shing-Jer Twu (1997) 'Aizibing fengxian yishi de linchuang fanghu ji zhaohu yiyuan,' (AIDS Risk, Physicians Clinical Precautions and Willingness to Treat AIDS Patients) *Zhonghua weizhi* (China Journal of Public Health, Taipei) 16(3), pp. 231–43.

Vermander, B. (1995) 'Religions in Taiwan today,' *China News Analysis* July 1, N. 1538-9, pp. 1–15.

Wachman, A.M. (1994) *Taiwan: National Identity and Democratization*. New York: M.E. Sharpe.

Wu, S. (1997) 'Poll: Interest in volunteerism high', *The China Post* 12 Sept., p. 18.

Yuan H.S., Pan J.Y. and J.W. Chen (1994) 'Wu zhuanji zhixiao gaonianji husheng dui aizibing zhishi taitu ji huli yiyuan zhi tantao,' (AIDS Related Knowledge, Attitudes and Willingness in Caring for Patients Among Senior Nursing Students from a 5-Year Junior College and Vocational Schools), *Huli zazhi* (Nursing Journal, Taipei) 41(3), pp. 41–51.

Zhi Xiao, Zhang Wei, and Ai Mo (1997) *Tongzhi zhi zhenbian shu* (The Book of Silent Love). Taipei: Chinese Society of Preventive Medicine, 45 pp.

CHAPTER 10

SEX EDUCATION FOR VIETNAMESE ADOLESCENTS IN THE CONTEXT OF THE HIV/AIDS EPIDEMIC: THE NGOS, THE SCHOOL, THE FAMILY AND THE CIVIL SOCIETY

MARIE-EVE BLANC

In Vietnam, since the beginning of the 1990s the HIV/AIDS epidemic has inspired a plethora of debates on sexuality and produced changes in education and in sex education, preventive education in particular. Indeed education is the only response available and indeed the cheapest one in poor and developing countries to prevent the spread of the HIV virus, in spite of the many efforts made to give wider access to anti-retroviral medicines. Straightforward as they may seem, these changes in education came up against a host of cultural, moral and social obstacles.

Sexual taboos are linked to the Confucian culture of sexual division, which means a division of female and male bodies. The sexual division there is complicated by a hierarchy of age, which is a second obstacle to easy communication between the young and the old. At school and out of school, sex education is a sensitive matter. The subject raises awkwardness inconvenient between teacher and pupils and the situation in a coeducational school represents a site for social discomfiture because it presents a difficult situation for people to manage and still preserve their social 'face'.

Many people think that the opening up of the country to the world, the transformation of the content disseminated by mass media and access to the Internet has automatically produced a wide wave of social change and sexual emancipation. Nowadays, it is assumed that early sexual relations are tending to increase, as a higher abortion rate can be observed in young girls younger than eighteen.

We will try to show how sex education is carried out at school and also out of school, taking due note of the taboos families and teachers have to deal with. We will analyse the role of the foreign NGOs in the production of a new sex education and HIV/AIDS prevention materials as well as examining their innovations and the limitations placed on them by extant conceptions of the body and of educational methods. And finally we will analyse the reactions of the civil society (mass organizations and

Vietnamese NGOs) which is trying to find 'its way,' in spite of a traditional education coupled with a strong social control over the youth.

This paper is based on fieldwork data collected in 1999 and 2002 in Hanoi and in 2000 in Ho Chi Minh City among young people in urban areas.[1] We choose to illustrate our discussion with this population because big cities are located at the crossroads of influences and are places with intensified development and therefore in the forefront of social changes.

THE AIDS EPIDEMIC IN VIETNAM: THE BIRTH OF EDUCATIONAL NEEDS AMONG THE 'YOUTH'

Needs in education are often linked to various changes both social shifts and fundamental technological innovations. Sex education seems to follow the same rule, but is more emotionally charged as it leads to moral and societal discussions because 'Youth' management, differs profoundly both institutionally and culturally in many countries as shown by Olivier Galland (2001:628). What is seen as 'normal' in one society, one family or even one person may be thought of as deviant in another. Should sex education take place in the classroom or is it a private issue, better addressed by parents individually?

In our survey of literature, we observed that in every country, initially sex education is implemented in school which it is linked to a primary scientific instruction. In a second phase, sex education becomes increasingly widespread, reaching all the population with more attention paid to individual and psychological aspects of sexuality.

For instance, in France, the first law implementing sex education at school, designated Fontanet's Circular dates back to 23 July, 1973. It was introduced after a period of emancipation and liberalization in French society between 1967 and 1973. During this period, an institutional discussion about contraception and abortion was held. This text produced under the auspices of Minister Joseph Fontanet allowed many questions about biological aspects on sexuality to come out of the shadows where they had been lurking and emerge into the full light of day in the school curriculum. At this time, admittedly in a relative conservative social context, it was thought best for sex education to hover somewhere in between total sex education and a limited amount of scientific information which would leave families as the main institution shouldering the task of educating children about the moral and emotional aspects of sexual behaviour. France is certainly not the only country to follow this path. 'For over a century, American sexuality education in schools has primarily focused on bio-medical aspects of human sexuality and instilling traditional sexual morals in Youth' (Elia 2000:122–9). In early twentieth century, sex education was inspired by principles of eugenics and neo-Malthusian philosophy which developed the idea of 'free pregnancy' and new contraceptive methods (Jaspard 1997:34–8). Durkheim participated in this discussion where religion was confronted by science. But he thought that 'anxiety over sex existed in every culture and therefore, must be a real and not an imaginary issue' (Pedersen 1998:135). Positivism and scientism could not be the panacea to prevail against the Judaeo-Christian morality governing sex and the latent fear of female emancipation.

In France, the AIDS epidemic offered the opportunity for a second discussion on reproductive health and, from 1988 to 1998, led to the conclusion that a good sex education and health information were not enough to inculcate responsible behaviour in their sexuality among young people. However, some studies have shown that sex education at school delayed the average age to the first intercourse (Dawson 1986; UNAIDS 1997). A new circular on sex education and AIDS prevention to replace Fontanet's Circular was issued on 19 November, 1998. The main objectives of this new law are to be more efficient and extend sex information and education to every school at secondary level. The overriding idea is to provide the young with self-awareness of their own bodies and respect for others, a right to intimacy, and to encourage positive self-esteem. It would seem fair to say that this response is designed to prevent side effects of sex emancipation.

The Vietnamese case is slightly different. Firstly, Vietnam is a developing country and consequently social change has been faster and more profound these last few years compared to the pace in France. Sex emancipation in young people and the AIDS epidemic happened at the same time scarcely ten years ago with the implementation of the *Doi Moi* renovation policy. The atmosphere prevailing in a Sino-Vietnamese culture implies strong control over the young. Therefore, taking account of the social needs in sex 'culture' and unequivocal information are crucial. Where do the young Vietnamese go to ask about and search for information about sexuality?

In our survey about sexuality and AIDS in a questionnaire, we asked 407 young men and women aged between fifteen and twenty-nine living in Ho Chi Minh City about their sources of information about sexuality. They told us that neither school nor their parents were their main sources. Books and newspapers seem to be the information sources most consulted (20.2 per cent). Books and printed matter are more convenient for an individual use and appealed to a perceived need for privacy and intimacy. There is no real difference between boys and girls. This can probably be attributed to the coeducational system. The young people told us that they received enough information on AIDS (84 per cent), but the quality does not match the quantity in their opinion. Fifty-six per cent of the young people said that they never talk about AIDS with their parents.

Table 10.1 Main sources of preventive HIV/AIDS information of the young (Ho Chi Minh City – 2000) according to gender

	Boys	Girls	Together
School	16.4	17.5	16.9
Books, newspapers	20.0	20.4	20.2
Radio	13.9	12.1	13.1
TV	17.7	19.4	18.4
Family	8.1	8.6	8.3
Friends	10.7	9.6	10.2
Community (mass organizations, youth clubs …)	12.9	12.2	12.6
Other	0.1	0.0	0.1
No answer	0.2	0.3	0.2
Total	100	100	100

If we look at the age brackets, the older the people were the more they continue to seek information in books. Subsequently, considering these results, school was replaced by the community. In the workplace, most Vietnamese individuals are involved in mass organizations (trade unions, and the like) linked to their professional work or branch, like the farmers' association, for instance.

Table 10.2 Main sources of preventive HIV/AIDS information of the young according to age

	15–18 years old	19–24 years old	25–29 years old
School	19.6	15.8	7.6
Books, newspapers	19.6	20.7	20.9
Radio	12.1	13.9	14.6
TV	18.7	18.0	19.0
Family	9.0	7.5	8.2
Friends	9.5	11.3	8.9
Community (mass organizations, youth clubs …)	11.2	12.4	20.9

Other	0.0	0.1	0.0
No answer	0.2	0.3	0.0
Total	100	100	100

School and books are the favourite means resorted to by the sons and daughters of craftsmen, merchants, shop-keepers and intellectuals. But school is relegated to the third position for the sons and daughters of farmers and workers, who find a better access to information in TV. Probably, this is because of their early dropout rate from school compared to the others. Young people in rural and former rural families tend to ask their friends and peers in the community a little more frequently than the others do.

Table 10.3 Main sources of preventive HIV/AIDS information of the young according to father's profession

	Farmers, rice farmers, farm labourers	Craftsmen, merchants, shop keepers	Intellectuals, profession, civil executive managers	Skilled and unskilled workers
School	15.3	19.0	18.4	13.6
Books, newspapers	19.4	22.3	19.5	20.8
Radio	15.3	12.3	12.9	14.3
Television	19.7	18.7	17.6	17.5
Family	5.8	7.7	9.6	7.8
Friends	11.9	8.0	9.2	12.3
Community (mass organizations, youth clubs...)	12.6	11.0	12.1	13.6
Other	0.0	0.3	0.0	0.0
No answer	0.0	0.7	0.7	0.0
Total	100	100	100	100

In *The Sexual Revolution* (1936), Wilhem Reich showed that the combination of patriarchal culture and the monogamous marriage produces a strong control over the sexuality of the young (adolescents and non-married young adults) and markedly repressed the pleasure and desires of the young. The Confucian culture is an important element, indeed a pivotal point in understanding the Vietnamese response to preventive education in the context of the HIV/AIDS epidemic. This country was under the domination of the Chinese for more than ten centuries. The domination of the Chinese culture in the Vietnamese society can be observed in the ancient laws, for example, the Code of the Lê dynasty (fifteenth century) and the Code of Gia Long (belonging to the Nguyên dynasty, nineteenth century) are very similar to contemporaneous Chinese Codes (Blanc 2001:408–11). The central unit and the smallest social entity in such a society is the family. As in China, the family is the basis of Vietnamese society. Under such circumstances, the young and the next generation constitute an important stake for the families. The next generation will ensure the worship of the ancestors is continued. The Kinh, another name for the Viêt, the dominant ethnic group in Vietnam, is a patrilineal and patrilocal society. A son has a great value in the family, but according to the Code of the Lê dynasty (sixteenth century), girls could be equal to boys in worship and inheritance (Blanc 2001:421). In Vietnam it seems to have been a recurrent aspect throughout history that the inequality between men and women has persisted in spite of a Southeast Asian influence which tends towards according equality between males and females.

During my fieldwork, as I was surveying on HIV/AIDS prevention among young people, I was confronted by a fear and a reluctance on the part of adults to talk about this topic. This attitude prevailed mostly in the Hanoian puritan context. Even the teachers and the preventive health workers seemed to be opposed to the survey at school and also to the idea that I should not interview the young by myself because I might introduce uncontrollable conceptions of sexuality into the impressionable young minds. AIDS was considered to be the disease of drug users and prostitutes. They were not completely wrong because the beginning of a sexually active life is less dangerous in terms of susceptibility to disease and multi-partnerships are less common too. Obviously, young people in Vietnam form a category of the population they want to protect from an abundance of sexual knowledge and from early sexual intercourse, although sex education may delay sexual intercourse as noted earlier in this chapter. This may be especially the case of those who are at school and probably the members of the elite of the nation are overprotected. Virginity before marriage has a great value in Vietnam and theoretically sex before marriage is not allowed to the young (Khuat Thu Hong 1998:56). We asked boys and girls about sex intercourse before marriage, and the girls seemed to be more conservative than the boys.

In a survey carried out in February 2002 in Hanoi among 493 men aged from eighteen to fifty-five years old, 74.4 per cent of the participants said that virginity in women is important. But 18.8 per cent of the students in the sample said that they had experienced their first sexual intercourse with a woman before the age of twenty. And 47.8 per cent of the single men said they already had sex with women. These figures show that premarital sex is widespread in urban areas in Vietnam today.

Table 10.4 Do you think you will have sex before marriage?

	Boys	Girls	Together
Yes	16.8	2.1	9.5
No	43.6	73.8	58.7
I don't know	31.4	15.5	23.4
Married	5.5	4.8	5.1
No answer	2.7	3.7	3.2
Total	100	100	100

A recent survey under the auspices of the United Nations (UN) has shown that adolescents in Vietnam 'are at high risk of unwanted pregnancy, maternal morbidity and mortality, sexually transmitted infections (STIs) including HIV/AIDS....' (UN 1999:53). The report of the UN related that: 'Young people have very limited access to information and services on sexual and reproductive health, including family planning. Nationally, about 15 per cent of all births are by women aged less than nineteen years old (Ministry of Health, 1998) and it is estimated that unmarried women (most of whom are adolescents) account for 39 per cent of total abortions (NCPFP, 1997). By August 1999, around 50 per cent of all new HIV infections were occurring among those under 30 years old (up from 45 per cent at end 1998), and almost 8 per cent of reported cases involved those under 20 years old (Ministry of Health)'. For a good understanding of this situation, it is important to know that the legal age for marriage is eighteen for a girl and twenty for a boy. Cogently, the family planning programme requires no more than two children per couple and advises the young family to wait a few years before having babies. Generally, the family planning centres are designed to give counselling or provide contraception for married people and not to adolescents or singles. Social policy, family planning, taboos, morality, protection and silences from the adults do not prevent the young trying their first sexual experiences unmarried and without contraception.

The government of Vietnam has now indubitably realized that sex education is essential and, in implementing this, it has followed more or less the same development as that in Western countries with an emphasis on sex education at school and information provided through books. This is because it is indelibly still wed to the Confucian *habitus*. Since the *Doi Moi* policy, many books giving sexual information ranging between a biological or medical popularization and a morality of marriage have appeared. What did sex education mean in Vietnam in 1989? 'Sex education is a system of medical measures and educational reforms for children, adolescents and young adults which give the right behaviour in sexuality' (Tran Dang Kieu Minh *et al.* 1989:13). Most of those books were produced at the time of the promulgation of a new law on marriage and family in 1996. Some of them are written only to young men or for young women and give a basic knowledge about sexuality, with more emphasis on the female genitals than the male. This literature respects the traditional sexual division of bodies and genders. Sex education for children and young people not yet married has been produced solely to advise abstinence and its obvious purpose is to shape good citizens with respect for family planning and the marriage law.

Nevertheless, sex education is provided in school. Theoretically, a young Vietnamese who attends school until the end of the upper-secondary level (grade 12, seventeen-eighteen years old) could have listened to ninety minutes of sex education lessons (in the curriculum of biology and through civic education lessons will learn about 'social diseases' like drug abuse, HIV/AIDS, and the like). But these lessons are sometimes forgotten by the teachers who feel uncomfortable dealing with this very sensitive matter. Teachers are victims of their own education and the morality of families too. Indubitably, coeducational school has a positive impact on general knowledge and gives equality to both boys and girls, but the coeducational system in Vietnam has side effects for sex education efficiency. Because of the traditional sexual division, uneasiness and discomfort are experienced when having to teach about sexuality to boys and girls at school. The sex taboo linked to this sexual division arouses discomfort either in female teachers or female pupils. Speaking about sex or genitals in a mixed classroom could be construed as being very impolite, amounting to an insult. Few studies in Asia have noted this difficult aspect in sex education, and when they have, have explained it on the basis of a more conservative society and an existing gender bias (Bhasin and Aggarwal 1999:531). The parents who pay mounting school fees each year also want lessons and matters focused on useful skills and knowledge which will enable their children to find a good job quickly at the end of their study. Education in Vietnam is linked to the economic and development stakes which has led to overload in the curriculum programme. The goal to be reached is the development of the country and the young are involved in the economic competition. This is why the educational system prefers computer or foreign languages lessons to sex education. We also noted that sex education is provided too late with regard to the beginning of puberty.

The second problem is that many children now leave school earlier than before, at an average of ten years old, because of the cost of school. Going to school is too expensive for some families to afford, mainly in rural areas or in the suburbs of Ho Chi Minh City where migrant people live in the slums. Paradoxically, in spite of a socialist policy, education in Vietnam is not free of charge. In poor areas, the schools are deprived and depend on the financial support of each family. Now we could observe that in the poorest places, where children are illiterate, the rate of HIV infection among adolescent people is increasing rapidly. No school and no education for them spell no possibility at all to find an honest job. They can survive only by trafficking in drugs or sex. And today in Vietnam the two main factors facilitating HIV contamination are intravenous drug use (IDU) and commercial sex work (CSW). Consequently there are two kinds of young people in Vietnam: those who are at school and those who live on the street.

Since the early 1990s, the beginning of the AIDS epidemic in Vietnam, an awareness of the problem has dawned. UNICEF, the Ministry of Education and Training, the foreign NGOs and the Vietnamese mass organizations involved into the HIV/AIDS prevention have tried to conceive new means to introduce sex education and preventive information on STDs in and out of school, using new methods like peer education, 'life skills' curriculum, distance education, prevention coffee shop and so forth. The upshot has been that each institution or organization has worked and produced a sex education programme reflecting its point of view using the means at its disposal, without any real co-ordination and without implementation at a national scale. So in Vietnam a host of pilot projects are located in several provinces and not only in Hanoi or Ho Chi Minh City. Sometimes little towns or small villages are chosen for testing new projects on sex education. The pilot projects are mainly implemented by foreign NGOs and they seem to represent 'test labs' for the government before it sets up a new social policy in the Vietnamese way. The government is very careful with this question and also seems to manage the sensitivity of the population (mainly the parents from urban areas), who may reject such educational policy because of questions of morality. The fear of raising awareness of young people still continues, but now it is linked to different reasons. The main one is linked to a cultural problem. Vietnamese institutions like the Youth Union are open to new methods, but with respect for the culture and the national identity. The books and other manuals I have been able to collect from 1995 up to now, have shown me that conceptions of who young people are, what adolescence is, and sexual maturing were not the same for the Vietnamese and the Westerners of the NGOs.

A MISCONCEPTION ABOUT THE VIETNAMESE YOUNG PEOPLE: A SLOW, LONG MATURING PROCESS

Notions of childhood, adolescence, and 'Youth' are not always present in each society. Those categories are produced by an institutional system. Philippe Ariès (1973) showed how the notion of childhood appeared in the French society in the seventeenth century. The notion of long childhood is linked to the success of educational institutions. Ariès said that the time of childhood is coterminous with the time of schooling. Who are the 'Youth' in Vietnam? What does it mean to be young there? To which age bracket does the young category correspond? In contrast to many developing countries, Vietnam has a good level of education and a high level of literacy, even though there are a few educational problems in remote, poor, rural areas. The good level of education is ineluctably linked to the ancient Confucian tradition which produced mandarins and a bureaucratic system for management of the State through a system of academic competitive examinations held every three years, until the last one held in 1919. So the presence of an educational system very early in Vietnam contributed to a long maturing of the young people.

The traditional stratification of ages in Vietnam is different from that in the West. Also, education and the management of the youth are called upon to answer to different objectives there. In Vietnam you can be considered a young person up to the age of thirty, and even above. The other institutions which play important parts in the definition of the young people are marriage and family. In Vietnam a man becomes a man when his wife has given birth to a son, to a new generation. And a woman ceases to be a young lady when she marries. The average age at marriage is about twenty-five years old that is very late in the context of a developing country. Age at marriage was continually delayed throughout the twentieth century. During the French colonial period, the law was changed and laid down the obligation to comply with a legal age at marriage (eighteen years old for the girls and twenty for the boys). Below this age it is impossible to get married. Pertinently early marriage was considered a savage or uncivilized practice and the Vietnamese wanted to differentiate themselves from the other ethnic groups like hill tribes in Northern or Central Vietnam. Now, in urban areas, marriage is delayed because of study and professional competition.

Marriage is also another step towards being part of an older generation, but does not mean that young married people are allowed more autonomy, independence, or responsibility with regard to their family. Traditionally in Vietnam, the eldest generation keep the power over all the family. Frequently, three or four generations share the same house together and resources are held in common. The grandfather and/or grandmother (*ông bà nôi*) from the father's lineage exercises authority over their children and grandchildren. They are the ones who decide how much money will be paid on such things as education, health care, and the like and even the choice of a spouse. This authority leads to irresponsibility in the younger generations. Maybe, this is why the period of 'Youth' seems to be longer than the Western case. Under such circumstances we can say, as suggested by Galland (2001: 617 & 637), that the 'Youth' is a real phase of the life in Vietnamese people and not a rite of passage which is fairly brief. Adolescence and Youth are distinct. Youth is a necessary phase between the time of adolescence and adulthood. Although it is so readily observable, many specialists in education do not pay attention to this specific point in Vietnam.

The socialization of young people does not come in a fixed passage. A great deal depends on the social origins of the parents, the urban or rural environment, the regional culture, and level and duration of schooling. Socialization is a process by which individuals learn about social norms and this process makes the transmission of culture between generations possible. Pertinently, socialization is not bound to just two alternatives by the family and the school (following traditional, patriarchal, and Confucian values), there is yet a third method. In the case of Vietnam, we have to pay inescapable attention to the very important and numerous mass organizations like the Youth Union (YU). The YU is present at each of the four levels of administration: national, provincial, district, and village (or ward in urban areas) level. This mass organization develops a socialization of another kind, based on the management of the young people's free time. This is another form of training for good citizenship according to the ideas of Uncle Ho, a blending between a scout movement and a mini-school for the Party (following socialist and community values). In actual fact the three kinds of socialization could be put one on top of the other, and then the systems of values resemble an ecumenical system. At least this was so until recently, but social changes have meant new population settlements in the suburbs of the big cities, and the growth of slum areas and such new settlements do not have schools or the infrastructure of mass organizations. The lack of social and educational structures appears to be not merely attributable to the recent urbanization but can also be put down to a fear of delinquency. This lack is leading to severe social problems and to symptoms of anomie in this society.

The Youth Union also manages to eliminate age differences. One age corresponds to particular activity in the Union and crucially gender is also important in this cutting out of age. The Vietnamese Youth Union produces important literature on adolescent development. YU disseminates a socialist representation of puberty which is based neither only on the physiological

251

development of the body or on the psychological development of the adolescent. It gives educational guidelines in order to produce good and healthy citizens. This Union plays its part as an ideological State apparatus perfectly. It goes without saying that the development of girls and boys is not the same and the conception of the maturing of the body can be found in the contents of schoolbooks. Cogently some differences between the traditional family conception of maturing and its socialist counterpart are also patently present. The socialist conception of adolescent maturation is shorter than the traditional one, and more egalitarian for the girls. The socialist conception is mid-way between the traditional Vietnamese idea and that of the Western world. The Youth Union makes constant conscientious efforts to respect the identity and culture of the people, even if the people have changed their conceptions and matched their behaviours to such alterations. The upshot is that Vietnamese identity or culture extolled by the YU seems to have now passed into the realms of mythology. Compared to the YU, it is evident that the foreign NGOs have played a great part in the change of the definition of the adolescent during the past ten years, the period in which the AIDS epidemic has spread. In such a welter of what might seem to be confused and confusing change, it is important to remember that in Vietnam, it is always possible to add things. It is a typical element of an ecumenical system, that the traditional definition of the individual maturing also remains alongside more modern conceptions.

At the beginning of the AIDS prevention campaign and with the implementation of the first information programmes by the foreign NGOs acting as consultants, the contents were not adapted to the local culture. The model did not respect the different steps of the traditional concept of maturing. The contents of the sex education programme and its methods collided with an educational system and a conception of education that was totally different. It was the time of the introduction of the chrono-biological transformations associated with puberty. Some problems occurred with the translation of some notions mainly from English into the Vietnamese language. One problem was that the Vietnamese specialists in education continued to give general preventive information, but failed to follow this up with preventive education. They appealed again and again to the responsibility of citizens (meaning adults not adolescents) in their efforts to fight against the epidemic. Their health campaign was still replete with the old revolutionary propaganda methods. Since 1997, Vietnamese specialists have begun to think about puberty 'in Vietnamese style'. Step by step they have integrated another chrono-biology of maturing. They have started to use the notion of *vi thành niên* (meaning literally 'minor' or 'not mature') for an equivalent to 'adolescent'. The Vietnamese adolescent is a human being who is not yet ripe intellectually and physiologically. He is not ready for sexual intercourse. This revealed to us that rethinking about sex education was an opportunity for asserting the Vietnamese identity. The goal of such sex education is clear: avoid early sexual intercourse among the young before marriage, without preaching that chastity is the best way to fight HIV infection.

The other foreign NGOs and UN agencies (like UNICEF and UNFPA) have continued to think about the cultural problem in the implementation of a new sex education programme at school and outside school and adapted a new notion *thanh thiêu niên* (which means becoming a young man), which resembles Western notions of 'Youth' or adolescents and post-adolescents more closely. UNICEF worked on a pilot project of 'Life Skills', which included sex education in a set of knowledge and attitudes that adolescents needed to learn in order to manage their health, respect others, and develop self-esteem by themselves. This programme was tested in only one school in Hanoi and in some other provinces at the fifth and eighth grades (respectively, ten- and thirteen-year-olds). This project was the first one to provide sex education at school in Vietnam so early. For instance, in Thailand, the newly targeted audience is composed of children in *kindergarten*, who are to be given sex education by 2002. This new curriculum aims to teach children at an early age about the changes that will occur in their bodies as they grow older. The aim is to support reproductive health and eradicate taboo (Thailand Department of Mental Health, Depart. of Health and Education Ministry, July 2000). At present the Vietnamese mentality is not really open to this. Changing the mentality will take time especially if there is no implementation of a specific public policy. Realizing this makes the linguistic aspect of sex education in Vietnam more comprehensible. At the moment it is an important obstacle and could explain the different theories about the fuzzy category of the Vietnamese Youth. What is adulthood in Vietnam? This is best described as an achieved status, being a member of the village council and a notable. I remember that a specialist in preventive medicine at the Ministry of Health told me that 'to be young in Vietnam is to be sexually active and attractive. This could last until the age of fifty.'

This leaves no doubt that sex education should be reconceptualized. Without any theory, education is not education. Importantly, education is not the panacea to prevent the HIV infection. 'Education is a cognitive process, AIDS is behavioural' (Hochhauser and Rothenberger 1992:103). Sex education could be an effective prevention strategy. It is most likely to be useful in changing knowledge and attitudes, but less effective in changing behaviour. Indeed it is very difficult to measure the impact of sex education on adolescent behaviour. The correlation between knowledge and behaviour is hard to show. Indubitably the state of play in Vietnam is that there is education and there is sex information. Many Vietnamese teachers think they give sex education to their pupils, but what they pass on is only information on sexuality and biology. 'Information is essentially a-theoretical, there is no system of motivating or reinforcing the person who has received such information' (Hochhauser and Rothenberger 1992:107). Most AIDS prevention projects targeting young Vietnamese are in the form of preventive information. Leaflets continue to use scare tactics even if this does not work. Now there are only two methods which seem to give good results: a 'Life Skills' curriculum in school and 'peer education' out of school. Both methods are based on self-sufficiency of the young individual. The point of departure is that each young individual is a competent person with some mastery over the environment. In the case of peer education, the young become the teachers of their peers. The chief advantage of this method is that it avoids the social discomfort currently observed during interactions between teachers and pupils, or more generally between adults and adolescents. Moreover, this method can be compared to another traditional one. Historically, at school in Vietnam, when a teacher had a great many pupils, he used to ask his best pupil or perhaps the eldest in the class to help him to give lessons. These are the reasons that the peer education project was implemented in collaboration by the Australian and the Vietnamese Red Cross. It was based on the hope it could reach the objectives of a new approach to sex education in which the young people themselves are constantly involved and feel more concerned about the HIV/AIDS epidemic. Here the educators are students and the trainees are high-school boys and girls, just a few years younger than their preceptors. One objection which can be observed is that the young teachers have been recruited through the network of mass organizations like YU and Vietnamese Red Cross, and therefore are not volunteers in the absolute sense, because they are known by the People's Committee of the ward or are the children of members of the different mass organizations. Large numbers of Vietnamese people are members of at least one mass organization. In Vietnam as in most Southeast Asian countries, the association is a traditional way of life which plays an important role in managing the community and building and maintaining solidarity (Blanc 1994:22–3). Maybe it is the first step on the path to set up a new conception of sexuality in Vietnam, even if at present such a conception will reach only the middle-class. But revolutions are often begun by intellectual, middle-class people!

What we are actually seeing is that the adults are still continuing to control the activities of the young and this includes sex education. Probably the control over sex education by parents is thought to be essential because the family as a central institution of the Vietnamese society could be endangered by widespread sexual emancipation. Nowadays parents and teachers, backed up by findings of Vietnamese biologists, agree that thanks to economic development and a better diet young Vietnamese are maturing earlier than before. Puberty begins one or two years earlier. The upshot is that they begin their love life and sexual adventures earlier. A study carried out by the Department of Pharmacy at the University of Ho Chi Minh City report that more than 50 per cent of girls aged twelve are menstruating (Nguyen Thi Thuong 2000:14). The mentality of people in Vietnam is changing slowly but surely. People are willing to acquiesce to early sex in the young if there is a strong bond of love between the two partners and if marriage is planned. The well-entrenched position of adults in the society does not allow the young to create their own structures and communicate their opinion on sexuality easily. A real involvement of the young in fighting against AIDS as in many countries in the world has not yet gained ground in Vietnam. One great stumbling block is that as far as young people are concerned it seems that to be active in a social organization or a non-profit association is a characteristic of retired people and old ladies. In our survey only 18.7 percent of the young living in Ho Chi Minh City belong to a youth club or a sport association. But 61.2 per cent told us that if they had the opportunity they would like to create or participate in a club. The problem is that this kind of activity still seems to be the privilege of adulthood and old age. Despite all the obstacles seeming to impede progress, AIDS is a relevant factor in social change a factor which is inexorably contributing to the emergence of a civil society, even if in Vietnam it is a near impossibility for the civil society to operate from a mass organization.

EMERGENT CIVIL SOCIETY FACING SOCIAL AND EDUCATIONAL NEEDS IN THE CONTEXT OF THE AIDS EPIDEMIC

Since the implementation of the *Doi Moi* policy, there has been a great upsurge in the development of clubs and other associative groups in every social sector. At the moment such clubs must still inexorably belong to mass organizations. There is no law which would allow Vietnamese people to create an NGO independently of the institutional structure linked to the Party. This restrictive regulation was adopted in 1957. Even though such a regulation is considered inappropriate nowadays, it has not yet been abrogated. Another law promulgated in 1989 and again in 1990 is an explicit effort to promote the development of a non-profit sector, but it does not go far enough (Sidel 1996:300-1). The sole exception is the Vietnamese Red Cross, which has a particular status, but this organization reproduces the same structure of a mass organization, abiding by the four levels, and it benefits from some financial support from the government.

The difference between a Vietnamese NGO (VNGO) and a mass organization is that the NGO does not receive any financial support from the government. The VNGOs must find funding elsewhere and, of course, to do so turn to foreign NGOs and UN agencies. Sometimes it would be preferable to call them CBOs (Community Based Organizations) instead of VNGOs. The CBOs were created by the community (locally, in the village or in the neighbourhood) and brought together people from the community with or without skills. Foreign NGOs and UN agencies supported the idea in order to raise awareness and to launch activities thought out by the people themselves to improve sustainable development by the people for the people.

Sometimes it is wise to be cautious with some organizations which are too close to an institutional structure. Wary of a welter of bureaucratic procedures and the consequent authorizations to be sought, many foreign NGOs or other providers of potential foreign investment in charity abandon their aid programmes. Another stumbling block which irks such sources of fund is that all the aid is managed by the Ministry of Investment and Planning and the population does not receive all the benefit of the aid because of the inevitable sharing out along the vertical structure of four levels.

Undeniably, the CBOs in Vietnam do try to use every inch of the small room to manoeuvre they are allowed by the law. Since 1993 and 1994, most CBOs working on HIV/AIDS prevention have been granted an authorization by the VUSTA (Vietnamese Union of Scientists and Technicians Associations), which includes the associations of medical doctors. In the case of Hanoi, the CBOs obtain their registration at the Department of Sciences, Technologies and Environment which is part of the People's Committee. Who makes up or founds a CBOs ? Most of the founders are medical doctors, but not exclusively. When they retire the older members of the medical profession want to continue to be active in and useful to their community. Their younger colleagues create private, humanitarian clinics. This idea cuts two ways. They create their own job and in doing so they help the poor. The system they build closely resembles a mutual aid system. The richest patients are required to pay, but the poor are treated free of charge. The situation in the public health system has pushed them into acting in this way, because there are not enough jobs for young doctors in hospitals and the wages are very low. There is a ready market as STI patients prefer not to go to the public sector because of the lack of confidentiality and intimacy. A private or humanitarian STI clinic is also likely to attract those members of the population either too shy or too poor to come to consult a doctor in the ordinary way. Cogently, these kind of clinics also provide some preventive information and counselling.

In a way, the CBOs act in contravention of the law, particularly a decree from the Central Committee of the Party, which urges everybody to fight against the AIDS epidemic. However, preventive education among prostitutes or drug users was considered as illegal because the behaviour of these risk groups placed them outside the law. Members of the community, people who were not restrained by holding the position of a civil servant, could take action to organize preventive measures among people at risk and their education. Paradoxically, CBOs seem to be more developed in the North, mainly in Hanoi, than in the South. Hanoi CBOs profile themselves more openly, carrying out surveys while distributing preventive information or launching some peer education training, although there are still only a few which want to take care of the HIV patients. They often include HIV/AIDS in a broader STI care activity.

In Ho Chi Minh City, the situation is different. There are plenty of non-formal charity initiatives because of the local culture, which encourages a host of religious (Roman Catholic, Buddhist) organizations to work with compassion for the poor and the sick. Another factor is that the morbidity and mortality linked to AIDS are both more visible in the South. As a matter of principle, the authorities do not agree with the intervention of such religious organizations. Only mass organizations are granted the right to give social assistance to the population. Our observations have revealed that mass organizations are also more active in the South than the North. The reason that the former, private charitable organizations have not been encouraged is that the government has been afraid of the re-emergence of the solidarity structures which prevailed under the former southerner regime. However hard they try, mass organization structures are not effective in some poor areas or in some other places where prostitution, drug addiction and delinquency flourish. The police are usually more active in those places, but repression makes the task of prevention or education there more difficult. Before CBOs launch any activities, the police always subjects them to a thorough examination and wants to know how they plan to operate.

In the South, private charity and social workers (sometimes *assistantes sociales* and *éducateurs* in the French-style) meet together to discuss the best way to tackle urgent social problems. People who created CBOs in the South have good relationships with the foreign NGOs working in the region on the same issues. In the recent past they may well have worked as staff members of a foreign NGO or International UN agencies, like UNICEF, UNDP or WHO. Through such experience, they have acquired a good knowledge of what is involved and the skills to deal with it. In contrast, people who are involved in a National NGO in the North have often come from a mass organization. In a 1997 report, the National AIDS Committee (NAC) estimated that 'there has been about 40 local non-profit organizations that are beginning to appear in HIV/AIDS prevention and Care network in Vietnam since 1994. Some choose to define themselves as non-governmental organizations, others are clubs or associations. All require Government approval and assistance' (Chung *et al.* 1997:14). Some organizations are newly emerged or have been initiated by the NAC, but all these groups are gathered together under the umbrella of a mass organization. Most of them are associations of medical doctors at provincial or district levels. 'AIDS activists' and associations led by people living with HIV or AIDS (PLWHA) can take part to the social mobilization but only at the district level. They are primarily assigned the task of giving help or care to poor patients in hospital or at home with their families. They have insufficient means and financial support to extend their field of actions. As was just mentioned, PLWHA are restricted to working under the control of Health Department at the district level, and then only in big cities.

The Overseas Vietnamese Community plays a big part in the financial support for the CBOs in the South. The community abroad publicizes the needs of its homeland (Blanc 1994:277, 342). Of course, the activities of the CBOs could easily be construed as a covert fight for democracy in Vietnam and some of them have indeed succeeded in proving that this is possible. The Internet and the network of all the overseas Vietnamese associations around the world indubitably play an important role in the sustainability of such CBOs. In Ho Chi Minh City, for instance, the CBOs direct their activities in the field of sex education towards specific parts of the population, like high-risk groups, homeless adolescents and street children. They are more effective with poor people than are the mass organizations. They are more in touch with the population of slums and more flexible in their styles of management. In that way they present an unspoken criticism of the bureaucratic model by being able to save time and money. They can avoid meetings every day and they do not have to bother with renting an office. The people who work for them do not live far from the 'hot spots' and 'red-light' districts. Consequently they are better equipped with the practical know-how to solve the problems of the people in need because they keep their ears pricked for hints about the social needs. Also, they are more efficient because some people in them have learnt from foreign NGOs where they worked earlier. They have come from the disadvantaged sections of the population (former drug users or prostitutes and they were disoriented adolescents at the end of the war). They are re-adapting educational methods like 'peer education', applying the lessons Australian or British people taught them.

Youth clubs which are part of mass organizations like the YU are less efficient because their target is mostly young people still at school even though it cannot be denied they make huge efforts to help needy people and street children. Their usual practice is to train students to be peer educators out of school. This means that there is a social gap between the educators and the young living on the streets. This inevitably produces a communication gap which undermines the efficaciousness and efficiency of peer educational methods.

The AIDS epidemic has shown us that solidarity can re-emerge in the community, even in a society in which the State seems to be over-present at each level. In fact this issue of public health and sex education need has revealed other social and educational needs among a part of the population and these will also have to be tackled in future.

Sex education in every country is linked to two societal problems. The first one is demographic: how are the same resources to be shared with a growing population? The second one is moral (religiously based or not) and familial (particularly in a patriarchal society): how to control sexuality before marriage and ensure the continuity of the lineage. In Vietnam, STIs were never a determining factor in providing sex education. Abortion is legal and available on request. In 1992, the total abortion rate was estimated at 2.5 abortions per woman, the highest rate in Asia (IPPF 2001). This would seem to indicate that though information on contraceptive means may be widely provided, sex education which would guide people to use them remains poor.

What has the AIDS epidemic changed? The HIV/AIDS epidemic reinforced the problematical situation and prompted a greater concern about sex education among families and in the state apparatus. But so far nothing really new regarding sex education has been undertaken. Vietnam is adapting new educational methods, but cautiously and slowly.

The emergence of the civil society linked to the AIDS fight has revealed social fracture lines. Where economic, social and educational problems exact assistance for people, the CBOs have proved strongest and have been more active in giving an appropriate response. One seemingly insurmountable obstacle to this solution being embraced with arms is that the family is a strong institution in the Vietnamese society and this seriously impedes the development of CBOs. This is because in such a social structure individuals follow the rule of the family and virtually as a logical progression of this the state. Where the family is weak and poor, the CBOs and solidarity in the community tend to develop strongly and quickly. This new solidarity can probably be largely attributed to the recent economic crisis and to a development of individual awareness and self-confidence.

We know that a medical response is hard to find because of the financial costs. We are simply worried about the fact that social discrimination might push the poorest and most disadvantaged PLWHA out of the AIDS prevention and care system. The CBOs do not participate enough in the elaboration of new social or medical measures for AIDS patients. Probably this arises from a formal problem of the acknowledgement of their usefulness even though they are state-approved. This situation is one quite commonly met by AIDS activist movements all over the world (Epstein 1996). How can social workers or patients afford to find solutions instead of allowing or trusting scientists, medical doctors and the State to do this for them? At this juncture PLWHA associations are testing their citizenship. Are they still full citizens? Can they act as helpful citizens?

NOTE

1 We would like to extend our warmest thanks to Dr Nguyen Minh Thang and Dr Vu Thu Huong from POPCON (Hanoi); Dr Hong Anh from Population and Family Planning Dept. of HCM city; Mrs Nguyen Thi Thuong vice-director of the Information Center on Love, Marriage and Family at Vietnam Youth Union in HCM city and Mrs Nguyen Thu Hien who help me greatly to carry out this survey, and a special thanks to Mrs Nguyen Thi Oanh from who I learnt about social work and CBOs history in Vietnam. This survey could not have been possible without the financial support of the National Agency on AIDS Research (France) and kind advice from Dr Yves Souteyrand.

REFERENCES

Ariès, Philippe (1973) *L'enfant et la vie familiale sous l'Ancien régime.* Paris: Editions du Seuil.

Bhasin, Sanjiv Kumar and O.P. Aggarwal (1999) 'Perceptions of teachers regarding sex education in national capital territory of Delhi,' *Indian Journal of Pediatry* 66, pp. 527–31.

Blanc, Marie-Eve (1994) *La pratique associative vietnamienne: tradition et modernité.* Ph.D. dissertation, supervised by Prof. Trinh Van Thao, Aix-en-Provence: Département de Sociologie, Université de Provence, 494 pp.

Blanc, Marie-Eve (2001) 'Du modèle confucéen à la quête de l'égalité entre homme et femme,' in: Claude Bontems (éd.) Mariage-Mariages. Paris: PUF, pp. 407–42.

Chung A, Phan Huy Dung, Dang Van Khoat and Hien Bui (1997) *Joint Action and Social Mobilization for HIV/AIDS Education, Prevention and Treatment in Vietnam.* Hanoi: 34 pp.

Dawson, D.A. (1986) 'The effects of sex education on adolescent behavior,' *Family Planning Perspectives* 18, pp. 162–70.

Elia, John P. (2000) 'Democratic sexuality education: A departure from sexual ideologies and traditional schooling,' *Journal of Sex education and Therapy*, Mount Vernon: AASECT, 25 (2 & 3), pp. 122–9.

Epstein, Steven (2001) *Le virus est-il bien la cause du sida? Histoire du sida 1.* Paris: Les empêcheurs de penser en rond, 276 pp.; (1996) 1st ed., *Impure Science. Aids, Activism and the Politics of Knowledge.* Berkeley, Los Angeles: University of California Press.

Galland, Olivier (2001) 'Adolescence, post-adolescence, jeunesse,' *Revue Française de Sociologie*: Ophrys 42(4), pp. 611–40.

Hochhauser, Mark and James H. Rothenberger (1992) *AIDS education.* Dubuque: Wm. C. Brown Publishers.

International Planned Parenthood Federation (IPPF), http://www.ippf.org, http://ippfnet.ippf.org/pub/IPPF_Regions/IPPF_CountryProfile.asp?ISO Code=VN.

Jaspard, Maryse (1997) *La sexualité en France.* Paris: La Découverte, Syros, 125 p.

Khuat Thu Hong (1998) 'Study on Sexuality in Vietnam: The Known and Unknown Issues,' *South & East Asia Regional Working Papers* 11, Hanoi: Population Council, 70 pp.

Ministry of Health, Maternal and Child Health Department (1998) *Annual Report.* Hanoi.

National Committee for Population and Family Planning (1997) *Vietnam Demographic and Health Survey.* Hanoi.

Nguyen Thi Thuong (2000), 'Vi thanh nien – tuoi can duoc quan tam dac biet!,' (Adolescence. Age that need to pay a special attention!), *Phu Nu Chu Nhat* (Women Sunday) 33, August 27th, pp. 14–35.

Pedersen, Jean Elisabeth (1998) 'Something mysterious: sex education, victorian morality, and Durkheim's comparative sociology,' *Journal of the History of Behavioral Sciences* 34(2): John Wiley & Sons Inc., pp. 135–51.

Reich, Wilhem (1982) *La révolution sexuelle.* Paris: Christian Bourgois éditeur; (1936) 1st ed., Copenhague: Sexpol Verlag.

Sidel, Mark (1996) 'The Emergence of a Nonprofit Sector and Philanthropy in the Socialist Republic of Vietnam,' in: Tadeshi Yamamoto (ed.) *Emerging Civil Society in the Asia Pacific Community.* Singapore: Japan Center for International Exchange, ISEAS, pp. 293–304.

Tran Dang Kieu Minh, Hang Nga, and Ha Loan Vuong, *Giao duc gioi tinh va hanh phuc lua doi*, (Sex education and life happiness). Ho Chi Minh City : Nha Xuat Ban Tong Hop Hau Giang, 268 pp.

UNAIDS (1997) *Impact of HIV and sexual health education on the sexual behaviour of young people: a review update.* Geneva: Best Practice Collection, 64 pp.

United Nations in Vietnam (1999) *Looking ahead. A common country assessment.* Hanoi.

CHAPTER 11

SEX WORK IN TIMES OF AIDS, CAUGHT BETWEEN THE VISIBLE AND THE INVISIBLE

IVAN WOLFFERS, PAULA KELLY AND ANKE VAN DER KWAAK

In a workshop on reproductive health needs in Semarang (Indonesia) in 1987, the provincial health authorities told one of the authors (IW) that there was practically no prostitution in Central Java. Later that same evening, after we had had dinner and had driven back in the night to the hotel, the same people showed me where sex workers along the entry roads to the city were attracting their clients. Officially they denied their existence but, as men of the world, they knew where to find them. In 1988, when the English-language newspapers in Thailand started to write about the emergence of the HIV/AIDS crisis, the city authorities of Bangkok were challenged on the existence of the many massage parlours. They denied that these were places where sex work took place. It was massage and nothing else but, as it concerned adult people who had their natural needs, it was quite possible that other things might happen too. Officially the authorities denied this aspect of sex work, but they also had their private knowledge of what might happen in the rooms of the massage parlours. Now, almost fifteen years later, this attitude has changed dramatically in both Indonesia and Thailand, because it created an unworkable situation. How can HIV/AIDS prevention campaigns be developed if one of the most important ways of transmission (sexual intercourse) is denied? The HIV/AIDS epidemic has confronted countries in Asia with the ways they are dealing with sexuality.

In most societies sexuality belongs to the tacit knowledge of human beings. People know about it, have ways to communicate about it, but they hesitate to be open about it. The HIV pandemic has confronted societies with behaviours that contribute to increased risk of transmission of the virus. Sexual behaviour in particular has become the focus of attention of public health specialists and researchers. This change in attitude does not mean that all aspects of sexuality are highlighted in the same way. And it may also be expected that, in the process of making sexuality more 'visible', certain expectations of 'correct' versus 'incorrect' sexual behaviour will be introduced.

The last ten years have produced more research then ever before on sexual behaviour in Asia, though not all of it is of sufficient quality. The motivation for most research has been carried out from the perspective of health professionals looking for possibilities to educate people about Sexually Transmitted Infections and HIV/AIDS. In order to support them in their pursuit of a solution, behavioural change has been added to what had been a specific hygienists' construction of sexuality, intimate behaviour and gender relations. Such a hygienists' construction of sexual behaviour is inexorably related to a distinction between correct and incorrect behaviour, which introduces moral judgement and bias. Therefore, most of this new research has focused on specific areas of sexual behaviour. It has produced insufficient data about people's own perceptions and ignored the dynamics of sexual and gender relations in societies. However, it is a simple fact that in some societies in which twenty years ago people would not dream to discuss sexuality or consider it a topic for research, people are now forced to look more seriously at different types of sexual behaviour. This has revealed a wealth of detail about the construction of sexualities, gender relations and power positions in those societies.

Initially, in most countries, people have reacted uncomfortably to the recent attention paid to behaviour that is private and mostly hidden from others. The increased focus on sexual behaviour in combination with uneasiness about it is probably universal, though differences between societies exist. Reports on how difficult it is to discuss sexuality, even in countries with a serious AIDS threat, come from everywhere, from sub-Saharan Africa to the former Soviet Republics (Massesa 2000, Chkhatarashvili 2000). In discussions on sexual behaviour, it is sometimes claimed that Western societies are more open and direct in their communication, and thus better able to deal with the unease of discussing intimate matters. Indeed, advertisements and television spots in AIDS campaigns in the West are sometimes rather explicit, though also big differences exist between different Western countries. For instance, AIDS television spots in the South of Europe are radically different from the spots in Northern Europe.

It is often claimed that Asian societies have more problems developing AIDS campaigns because there is reluctance to be explicit about it. There seems to be a 'knee-jerk', innate response to the introduction of sex into communication: 'It is against our tradition to talk about such things.'

Cultural factors are mentioned as a reason, but as has been stated elsewhere, blaming cultural factors may be a process of denial of certain behaviour for different reasons and serving only certain groups in society (Wolffers 1997). Terms like culture and tradition have many meanings. People who use phrases in their arguments like: 'It is against our culture' or 'It is against our tradition' are not using these terms in the academic way. They use them in the popular way, in which culture is viewed as folklore and the function of the use of such arguments is to have an extra reason to maintain the status quo: do not change anything. Examples of the use of such 'cultural arguments' in Asian countries in order to manipulate power are plentiful. The best example may be the ideology of the New Order regime of Suharto in Indonesia (1965–1998). Roles of villagers, women and people with diverging opinions were defined by consciously quoting certain rules of *adat* (the set of traditions governing behaviour), which were useful tools for the ruling elites in Jakarta. We often see that such popular cultural arguments become static and an excuse for conventionalist positions.

Academic perspectives of culture are rather different. Clifford Geertz sees 'cultural interpretations' as a process of human beings continuously giving meaning to what they see and to what happens to them (Geertz 1973, 1983). And Keesing (1987) emphasizes the fact that giving meaning to certain aspects of a culture is strongly related to the world views of those who interpret and this cannot be viewed discretely from their interests and power. Assuming that certain forms of behaviour related to sexuality (for instance, the reluctance to discuss it) are normal aspects of an indirect culture, or of a 'shame culture', may prevent us from realizing the power aspect and especially from the interest that the different genders may have in not discussing it.

In this article we would like to reflect on whether uneasiness to discuss sexuality is really 'cultural' or whether other factors may be more important in the declaration in Asian societies of certain discussion topics taboo. What might the function of this tabooing be for certain sections in the population?

LET'S TALK ABOUT SEX

Over more than ten years, one of the authors (IW) has carried out workshops and trainings on HIV/AIDS awareness and education in countries like Turkey, Bangladesh, Indonesia, Malaysia, Vietnam, Cambodia, and Thailand. Among other methods, this has been done with the help of a training module, which was developed and produced at the request of WHO Europe (Wolffers 1995). Initially, there was invariably some unrest among the participants in these workshops, as they expected they would have to talk about things they would prefer to ignore. Before even starting the discussions, participants would claim that it is 'against their culture' to talk about sexuality. 'We Thais don't like to talk about it'. 'In Indonesian culture you don't discuss it'. 'Vietnamese are very shy.'

Other behaviour was easier for the participants to deal with. One of the ways to prevent talking about the relationship between HIV infection and sexual behaviour that was often used in these workshops was the claim that, in their country (e.g. Bangladesh) HIV will only disseminate through unhygienic procedures in the health care system, or that the infection is mainly seen among injecting drug users (e.g. Malaysia, Vietnam).

In the late 1990s, it became easier to discuss sexual behaviour in the light of the HIV pandemic, because an increasing number of people had grown used to talking about it. However, this is not true for the population as a whole and certainly not in all situations. Sexual behaviour remains a topic that is difficult to discuss, and in addition to this, the sexual behaviour of others is easier to talk about than one's own sexual behaviour. The rise of discussions on the place of the sex sector in Asian societies has made that rather easy (Lim 1998), because it appeared convenient to talk about the behaviour of sex workers as a specific population that was to blame.

Openness about sexuality is one of the preconditions for successful AIDS campaigns and these have now been developed in various Asian countries like Thailand, Cambodia, Indonesia, Vietnam, and China. Of course, in these countries there have always been ways to communicate about sexuality. They differ from one social group to another, from one generation to another, from how sex education is passed on in the street to how it is inculcated at an official level and from how it is different for boys/men and girls/women. Crucially, it is important to know who communicates with whom on what and how, because it gives an insight into who controls the communication and thus into who controls the construction of sexual behaviour.

As an example we would like to look at the education about sexual health of young women in Vietnam. In qualitative research that was done among an open sample (twenty) of women, active in the Youth Union, aged between eighteen and twenty-eight in Ho Chi Minh City (Van der Meer *et al.* 1998), we found how difficult it is for young women to obtain information about sexuality and that they can only talk about it with specific persons, and not with others. It makes them very dependent on certain people, which has implications for the power to decide and negotiate about sexuality. We learned that young women often have limited access to sources of sexual information. Pertinently information about sexuality that adolescents and young adults in Vietnam receive does not come from their parents. It is interesting to look at some details of the interviews that were done with young women. Because of the expectations that other Vietnamese (older people and men) have of young women, they were less exposed to sexual information. As a reaction young women would also keep themselves away from situations in which sexuality was discussed. Young Vietnamese women with only a primary-school education did not like to talk to their parents about sexuality, out of fear of rejection. 'I didn't like to talk. I felt uncomfortable when I talked. If I spoke out, I would be shouted at by my parents.' Girls were warned not to bring shame on the family and avoid indecent behaviour, but it was rarely made explicit what indecent behaviour is: 'They advised me to be careful when I went out with a boy. They taught me to be wise in every word so people don't disdain me.' Young Vietnamese women who had followed secondary and even higher education said the same things in the interviews. 'It is very uncomfortable... and I didn't know what to ask, for example, when I get married, there is a thing I can ask...' Analysing the interviews we found that young people are afraid to talk about sexuality with their parents in the first place because they fear that their parents will think badly about them. The second reason that was given was the generation gap between parents and children. The third reason mentioned was that it is simply not done in Vietnamese culture.

It does not mean that young women remain completely ignorant, but they become dependent on other, limited sources of information. Young Vietnamese women with a higher education get their information from newspapers and books. Young Vietnamese women with a lower educational standard get some information from peers, sisters and once married, from their partners. It implies that the education about how these young women should behave sexually comes either from official medical sources or from husbands and family members, often with a strongly delineated idea of the sexual role of women.

The most interesting thing we learned from the research is that in interviews with young mothers we discovered that they would like to talk about sexuality with their children once these children are a bit older, but they feel insecure. Young Vietnamese women with a higher education thought that it would be best if their daughters were to find it out for themselves. 'I think if she is a clever person, she can get a partial understanding of this matter by reading books and newspapers. If she asks me, then I will explain it to her on the basis of my own experiences.'

We can describe this as a process of passing on ignorance from one generation to another. Indisputably, sexual behaviour is hard to discuss between generations in Vietnam, as it is elsewhere. Consequently, young people are dependent on their peers. Books and newspapers are not very open about sexuality and tend to describe it from a biological perspective. As a result, sexual reality is kept invisible, or only part of it is visible.

In this example, a knowledge of Vietnamese culture is vital for understanding the importance attached to communal living and the significance accorded to group importance over individualism. The slowness to trust outsiders, which could be seen as a hesitance to speak freely about sexuality, is a matter of relationships. However, individuals will open up quickly to those who show an interest, respect, and have something to give

(Brugemann and Franklin 1996). Individuals 'come out' when they feel comfortable in the social or education setting.

All this leads to the idea that neither the 'private body' nor 'personal ownership of oneself' is seen as a person's right in Vietnam. Communal living and family ownership or husband ownership, compounded by a lack of privacy in the home, in a community without rules of confidentiality in absolutely any sphere means that 'private body' and 'right' are difficult to define by the time puberty has begun. As a result, traditional culture is often stated as the reason why sexuality cannot be addressed in Vietnam.

SEXUALITY IN A GENDER PERSPECTIVE

Gender expectations and relations are an important aspect of sexual socialization. Therefore, it is essential to use a gender perspective to look at the need in Asian cultures to keep certain aspects of sexuality invisible. The sexual worlds of men and women are clearly separated and things visible to men may be invisible to the majority of women. This is especially the case with sex work. Sex work plays a vital economic role in many Asian countries. Estimates of numbers of sex workers are hard to make, but often impressive and the sex sector caters primarily for the local market. The sex sector that targets tourists is small compared to the local sex market. The research results that have become available in the last fifteen years show how normal it is for Asian men to lose their virginity in a brothel and that a weekly night out for men will often involve a visit to a bar or a massage parlour.

We are facing two realities. One reality is that in which an official ideal for women is cherished and is one in which sexual behaviour does not seem to exist. It is not even discussed. The other reality is that of weekly brothel visits by men of all ages and recruitment among marginalized men and women to work in the sex sector. In reality both these men and women lead different lives at the same time, forced to do so by economic pressure, lack of education, gender roles, karma, sexism, misogyny and indifference (Van Kerkwijk 1995). At this juncture we will present some attempts by academics to explain the place of sex work in Asian societies.

In this context it is interesting to mention the cultural analysis by Muecke (1992) which unequivocally demonstrates how culture, gender, class, and power are intertwined. Speaking about Thai society, she argues that the beliefs the Thai laity tend to associate with Buddhism and village morality paradoxically enables the practice of prostitution in their society. She shows that while in the past mothers were food vendors, their daughters remit funds home to their families and villages of origin earned from so-called illegal prostitution, which enables them to fulfil the traditional cultural function of daughters. According to the karma laws of the Theravada Buddhism, good actions earn moral merit and wrong actions, demerit. A person can change her/his karma by purposefully making merit, for example, by giving gifts to monks and temples. In the karma stakes, men are regarded as superior to women. Sex workers rank low on merit because they are women and are from poor families. The more a sex worker suffers, the lower her karma is said to be. As Muecke states, the Buddhist way of alleviating suffering is to make merit. Women are more regularly involved in merit-making activities like providing food for monks. The work of sex workers precludes these types of merit making but does allow the merit making that involves money. Prostitutes working in massage parlours or hotels are often regarded by themselves and their families as good Buddhists, when they make merit by inviting friends for overnight excursions to stay at the village temple for the purpose of giving money to the monks. Nevertheless, overall public opinion is against the linking of sex workers and Buddhism, although they fund major temples.

Even though the media and women's organizations especially have highlighted the economic impact of the sex workers, the government has a more ambivalent attitude towards them. Under Thai law prostitution is legal when it is not advertised as such, but female sex workers are not recognized. Economic contributions by the sex sector are not mentioned, and sex workers are seen mainly as the carriers of the HIV virus. Muecke shows how in the original double standard pertaining with respect to men and women – namely Thai girls being dutiful and women loyal, while men are mischievous and irresponsible, real men need sex and good girls can control their sexuality – a new double standard emerges: between justified and unjustified sex workers. The latter are sex workers who make too little money to buy consumer goods for their parents or ensure the education of their sisters.

Another effort to explain how culture facilitated the development of commercial sex comes from Chris Lyttleton (2000). He argues that because the sanction on extramarital relationships and broken promises with regard to marriages in the Isan region in Thailand were financial, this may have prepared the ground for a materialistic view of sexual services by the villagers. This may have made it easy to take part in commercial sex, especially when it was strongly commercialized in the second half of the twentieth century.

There is another explanation possible. In Vietnam Confucianism is viewed as feudal, outdated, and not in line with the aims and objectives of the Democratic Socialist Government of Vietnam. In the past Confucianism was a system – influencing culture but not culture itself – for controlling the masses when Vietnam was ruled by China. As this system was patriarchal, it gave power to the men. In all countries men have devised systems that have perpetuated their power over women. Even in Vietnam, where the equality of men and women is a governmental aim, gender power has been divided (Connell 1991, Soucy 2000). This has enabled the power exercised by men over women to continue in the post-feudal society.

These examples are enough to demonstrate that there are many layers in the analysis of prostitution. Many aspects are involved and often it is a matter of taste or interest which particular view is adopted in scientific papers. A gender perspective, though, always seems to be essential.

To hold fast to their 'ownership' of women, men promote their sexual power preferring and promoting as 'traditional' women who are sexually appealing, i.e. submissive, naive in sexual matters, and pliable. Women thus 'act out' sexual non-verbals rather than talk about sex to men – boyfriends, lovers, and husbands.

Not only men use these binary oppositions to justify their behaviour, governments also need these labelling constructions in order to realize their 'female sex worker as a disease vector' approach – they are to be blamed and banned, as we will see below for the case of Vietnam. In using terminology such as good and bad women, direct and indirect sex workers, the traditional static view of women being 'good wives and mothers' or 'bad sex workers' and nothing else is maintained. In order to create more openness in the discussion on sexuality and HIV/AIDS, an essential point of departure is by looking at the different identities of the women and men involved. In this context, Eric Ratcliff (1999) shows how many women working in Philippine go-go bars disassociate themselves from the sex worker representation, and transform some of their clients into more acceptable 'boyfriends' and by doing so avoid viewing themselves as sex workers in their relationships with these men. Ratcliff shows that the women and men in the bar move in and out of these identities as they see fit, thereby creating personalized practices and identities. These are certainly overlooked by any collective approach to the problem of AIDS.

Here it is important to realize that women and men are actors with multiple shifting identities, even in cultural settings in which it seems appropriate to distinguish only among public/open and private/covert culture. Besides the incapacity and inability to negotiate safe sex or the fact that a higher degree of familiarity with certain sexual partners may withhold women from using condoms, covert romantic feelings and expectations may also play a role in sexual practices. These are matters which are often not being addressed by interventions or campaigns.

We believe that it is inexpressibly important to move away from the cultural moral distinctions used to define sexual behaviour and practices, and instead to use a social and gender-sensitive analysis of the context of sexual decision making in which men and women are not stripped of their origins of gender, power, and class relations. This implies a different approach and moves away from more traditional research methods.

THE BATTLE AGAINST SOCIAL EVILS

Control of a society can be effectuated by a number of means – one is to enforce a specific morality. In Vietnam, this is what is currently happening under the concept of 'social evils'. Social evils are written about, talked about, and hence have become common knowledge. They include any form of bad social conduct and are not necessarily written down in laws. Prostitution and drug addiction are two of these, but when the festive season is on, the government also warns about the social evil of gambling. Also AIDS is associated with social evils: the section called 'Fight Against Social Evils and AIDS' in the Social and Economic Development Strategy for 2001–2 (documented in the *Vietnam News*), mentions among such evils, traffic accidents, AIDS and concomitantly prevention of AIDS by adopting a healthy way of life (i.e. not visiting prostitutes), and addiction.

Prostitution is against the law, i.e. its procurement, organizing, and facilitating is illegal. A sex worker is seen, in the law, as a victim and not as the perpetrator of social evils. However, it is she (usually a woman) who is 'punished' via re-education to return her to her 'true nature of womanhood', rarely the client. Prostitution in Vietnam (and as a matter of fact everywhere in Asia) is in fact widespread and part of the culture regardless of the rhetoric. Men state 'when you eat rice you want bread' (Brugemann 1996, Beesey 1998). Men are said to be 'forced' into situations with their workmates and bosses which require them to drink regularly at a *bia-om* (a room or space in an establishment where women serve beer and encourage its consumption, many submitting themselves to sexual harassment through physical sexual acts). From the *bia-om*, men are 'forced' by peer pressure to solicit a prostitute. The nature of a man is such, it is believed, that men cannot say 'no' when presented with this situation (Beesey 1998).

Vietnamese society has always had a mechanism which has allowed men to enjoy more than one sexual partner. Though there is a law of monogamy now, concubines and second wives still exist and are socially (not legally) approved of, especially if the union with the legal wife does not produce a son. Second wives and concubines are not sex workers, but their existence is illustrative of the position of women in Vietnam. For men who are not able to have second wives and concubines, there are more convenient and cheaper ways of having sexual contacts with women other than their official wives. The sexual pleasures of men have been provided for in the increase in sex available on a commercial basis as well as in the second wife phenomenon. The advantage of the former is that it allows men to have more than one partner without the emotional and financial commitment and responsibilities that come with the second wife. It also allows for sexual experimentation without procreation, thus pleasure without responsibility.

Women must submit to sexual demands in marriage or in partnerships, or else husbands will take another wife or frequent prostitutes. They must also present themselves as being as sexually appealing as their 'competition', otherwise they will be 'blamed' for failing to make their husband 'happy'.

What is seen in many societies is the paradoxical combination of sexual attitudes. There is the sex sector in which many different services are offered, which is accessible to men from all layers of society. At the same time, women are supposed to be not aware of this side of sexuality and are expected to display diametrically opposed behaviour. During a workshop in Cambodia organized by one of the authors, the male participants were very explicit in their expectations about their own wives, sisters, mothers, and daughters. Simultaneously, they frankly said that they were forced to go to sex workers to enjoy sex properly; because these sex workers would do things their wives would never consent to perform. The question of whether it would not be more convenient were their wives to do to them what sex workers usually do, evoked shocked responses, because that was the sort of behaviour a decent woman would not indulge in.

What we see is a mixture of moral views that are protected by the 'official culture', meaning the popular culture, sometimes even reinforced by the authorities through legislation, with secrecy that protects the space that men need to satisfy their sexual needs.

THE REALITY OF MEN

Most Asian countries have a flourishing sex sector. In some Asian countries it has developed into a thriving economic sector on which many marginalized women and men have become dependent (Lim 1998). The number of sex workers in Thailand is estimated to be between 400,000 and 900,000, depending on what definitions are used. In Indonesia the number of sex workers is estimated to be 400,000. In Malaysia the estimated number of sex workers is 150,000.

The gender aspect is extremely important with regard to communication and education about sexuality. In societies where the highest ideal for girls is to marry as virgins, but where men make frequent visits to sex services, we are not only dealing with different realities, but with the shifting identities of people.

It is dubious whether all sexual transactions between people who are not bound by marriage can be classified as sex work. Epidemiologists may define these exchanges of sexual favours for economic benefits as sex work, but the persons involved in these transactions will never define it in these terms. In Asian countries there is a wide variety of sex transactions and, depending on one's point of view, these can be defined as sex work or not. How should one classify small sexual favours to older men or 'sugar daddies' who help younger women with the cost of living? Are women who go to the discotheque once a week and leave with a man who also gives them some money sex workers? In what instances is a woman a sex worker and not a girlfriend, second wife or a one-night-stand? Does money paid directly after the sexual act make it prostitution, whilst long-term financial support or gifts do not?

If we look again at the situation in Vietnam, we see that prostitution pervades every district of the country. The government is concerned and instructs families to 'stamp out this social evil', blamed on the sexuality of women, not the sexual desire of men. Men are believed to be constitutionally unable to refuse the advances of women (Franklin 1993). Simultaneously, families are known to sell daughters to middle agents for prostitution (Kelly and Le 1999). Yet, families are also expected to be the moral educators of children. As units of production within the new economy (generally referred to as *Doi Moi* – renewal), they may feel they have little choice – the demand for such services is there, and the return for providing the supply will help feed the family.

Some aspects of this can be viewed primarily as 'cultural', like the need for girls to submit to the father, and like the compelling of children to show eternal gratitude to their parents, including acceptance and obedience (Le Thi 1995, Kelly and Le 1999, Jamieson 1995). In point of fact, these 'ideals' simply facilitate the power of men over women. Prostitution is an economic activity (in every country), which is male-driven; it is no different in Vietnam. It is simply only the facilitation of this which differs according to the culture.

There is a whole range of possible interactions that may involve some kind of sexual transaction. A distinction is made between direct and indirect sex work, but that does not really solve the problem of definition and the fact that a moral judgement is involved in it. Whatever we call it, a system in which men can obtain sexual services (ranging from kissing, touching, to sexual intercourse), which is not visible to most of the women from their own social class, but in which a lot of men and women are working, simply has to be based on hypocrisy and double standards. There is some kind of cultural agreement that these two realities never mingle. An Indonesian expression says: *'Pura-pura, tidak mau'*. This translates best as 'always pretend that you don't want something'. If you go into a shop and want to buy something, do not show an interest in the product you really want to purchase, because if you do the vendor may increase the price. If people offer you something to eat or drink, it is impolite and greedy to accept it immediately. *Ergo*, though a man is attracted to the many and easy ways of buying sexual services, he has to pretend not to be interested. It does simply not exist officially.

In most countries, dominant groups will define prostitution as a negative phenomenon (Wolffers 1997), and this will add to the importance of a separation between these two realities. In a study we carried out in 1996 and 1997 we tried to understand the impact of the separation of these two realities on the women working in the sex sector (Wolffers *et al.* 1999). We could distinguish self-defined identity and the identity as defined by others. In addition, women who identify themselves as being sex workers will see certain relationships as sex work, while others that are also based on an exchange of sexual favours for economic benefits are not seen as sex work.

A negative conception of prostitution is expressed in the Indonesian word for sex worker. This is *'perampuan tuna susila'*, meaning woman without morals or *'pelacur'*, meaning a person displaying incorrect sexual behaviour. Officially prostitution is not allowed in Indonesia and sex workers caught soliciting can be sent to a rehabilitation camp, but in some areas of the big cities, brothels are tolerated and often run by army and police personnel. The societal disapproval of prostitution creates an extra reason for sex workers to keep their identities well separated from each other.

A similar situation is seen in other Asian countries. Sex work has a negative image and is often illegal, even though simultaneously it is in high demand and those working in the sector move in and out from one identity to another. In Vietnam we see something similar.

THE NEW ROLE OF SEX WORK

There is a relationship between sexuality, gender, and sex work which is based on the power of men to control women and it functions thanks to the invisibility of sexual reality. The recent focus on sex work in the light of the HIV pandemic has changed this slightly, but by only focusing on the sex workers and not on their clients or on other forms of sexual behaviour, it continues the same functions. Were people initially to deny that sex work was widespread in their country, in the later stages of the epidemic they reluctantly acknowledged it, but simultaneously it has provided the opportunity to distinguish between sex workers and others, between the good and the bad.

Sex workers have become the scapegoats who are responsible for the HIV pandemic and are seen as a different category. The existence of sex workers that was denied in most countries was suddenly accepted, because it functioned as an excuse and explanation for the HIV pandemic. 'They', 'the others', the 'sex workers' display risky behaviour, but the 'normal' Thais, the 'normal' Indonesians, the 'normal' Vietnamese were not like that. Like Gilmore and Somerville (1994:1339) argue: 'Despite the great discoveries and advances of science and medicine, primitive reactions to being confronted with disease continue to divide people, and communities into them and us. This is particularly evident in reactions to epidemics of dread diseases, which have long been associated with stigmatisation, scapegoating and discrimination. Sadly with AIDS is no exception.'

These authors show the three functions of stigmatization, namely that it can be a response to a risk, threat, or adverse situation. Second, it can be a means of strengthening a community and its values by purging the community of undesirable traits. In doing so, it adds to social cohesion. Thirdly it can be a means of social control of both the persons stigmatized and those who are not, by marginalizing and excluding the former (Gilmore and Somerville 1994).

One of these stigmatizing strategies is indeed to make a difference between 'normal' Thai, Malaysian, Indonesian, or Vietnamese behaviour and 'deviant' behaviour, and by doing so falling back on the popular cultural argument. In this way people are able to ban everything that does not fit their middle-class ideology. They simply say that it is 'non-Thai' or 'non-Malaysian' or 'very un-Vietnamese'. Another rather similar strategy is to make the distinction between the original indigenous culture and imported habits, as if they (from their class perspective) had the right to decide about what is real and what is fake Thai, Malaysian, Indonesian, or Vietnamese. It is clear that culturalist stigmatizing strategies as described here are all exercises of power. And those in power fear that if one de-stigmatizes sex workers, by for instance stating openly that Thai sex workers are good mothers and devout Buddhists, this would do too little to secure social structuring.

This new role and acceptance of sex work in Asian societies leads to a stronger distinction between what has been called 'direct sex work' and 'indirect sex work'. The process of stigmatization and limiting their opportunities may lead to activism against the stigma. Stigmatization may stimulate self-empowerment and mobilization (Gilmore and Somerville 1994). The so-called direct sex workers have accepted the identity of sex worker. They can make use of the new possibilities, like sex workers' organizations and they are in a much better position to advocate the rights of sex workers. Sex workers who do not identify themselves as sex workers have become more dependent on keeping their different identities separated. This often leads to denial of their sex work and it makes it more difficult to create the openness that is needed to discuss reproductive health and the consequences of different sorts of behaviour.

CONCLUSIONS: HIDDEN SEXUALITY BENEFITS MEN

The majority of sex workers are marginalized women who have few other options in their struggle for survival. Simultaneously, there are many people involved in the organization of the sex sector: those who recruit men and women, buy them, sell them, find clients, and provide protection against police and aggressive clients. Many others are also involved, ranging from rickshaw and taxi drivers to former sex workers who work as recruiting agents, hotel owners, tour operators, corrupt police officers and so on and so forth. This implies that it is also a power issue.

Connell (1991) and Soucy (2000) categorize these gender divisions as labour, power, and cathexis (emotional relations), however better terms would be labour, patriarchy i.e. 'natural order', and sexuality. Men hold power over women to a greater or lesser degree in all societies in these three areas. It is not a matter of 'culture'. It is a matter of the 'construction of maleness'. In Vietnam, the government is working hard to minimize the male power over labour and patriarchy in the family but, while these power holds are declining, the holding power of sexuality has increased (Soucy 2000). Vietnamese women are forced, if they want any credibility, to present themselves as sexualized people, predominantly downplaying their intellectual, cultural, entrepreneurial and other such characteristics in order to win social acceptance. This is the exemplification of the presentation and downplay of dominant patriarchal ideology that both men and women support. This is not cultural but structural, and it is the result of Vietnamese male response to losing power in other areas.

This submission by women to sexuality as their essential female character advantages men. It may be one of the reasons why HIV/AIDS is rapidly spreading in Vietnam. Women must be fragile, submissive, shy and the like (sometimes said to be 'traditional') in sexual matters and men must be the opposite – such power in the hands of men enhances the chances of HIV spread.

Such domination is covert and manifested publicly as 'indirectness' and hidden behind a veil termed 'culture' – it is not culture specific but it is more prevalent in the world where women as yet have not been sufficiently empowered or educated to a level of awareness of their predicament. For many women, including women in Vietnam, it is easier to accept and have power in other ways – labour, family, control of home, money and so on.

It is time to stop claiming that cultural and religious factors are the main constraints to being more open about sexuality in HIV/AIDS campaigns. What can be said, written and shown is at the moment a battlefield for different interest groups in Asian societies. The most positive outcome of the epidemic is that the oppositions have become clearer than ever: men against women; sex workers against 'regular housewives'; rich against poor; self-identified sex workers against not self-identified sex workers; health workers against sex workers and their clients. And because these oppositions have become clearer than ever, the battle for what is considered to be the popular national culture has become more visible than ever before.

REFERENCES

Beesey, Allan (1998) *The Crossroads of Risk and Responsibility – Truck Drivers and HIV/AIDS in Central Vietnam.* Vietnam: World Vision International – Vietnam and AusAID.

Brugemann, Ilonka and Barbara Franklin (1996) *Love and the Risk of AIDS for Women in Vietnam.* Vietnam: CARE, Vrije Universiteit, Unicef.

Chkatarashvili, K. (2000) *How to Improve Adolescents' Sexual and Reproductive Health in Georgia.* Thesis at the 36th International Course in Health Development. Amsterdam: Royal Tropical Institute.

Connell, Robert (1991) *Gender and Power: Society, the Person and Sexual Politics.* Cambridge: Polity Press.

Department of Social Evils Prevention (1998) *Report to Radda Barnen of Survey on Trafficking of Women and Children for Prostitution* (unpublished, on file).

Efroymson, Debra and P.N. Thanh Vu (1995) *Nha Trang Youth Speak Out.* Hanoi: Ham Long Street.

Franklin, Barbara (1993) *The Risk of AIDS in Vietnam.* Vietnam: CARE International in Vietnam.

Gammeltoft, Tina (1999) *Women's Bodies, Women's Worries.* U.K.: Curzon/Nordic Institute of Asian Studies.

Geertz, Clifford (1973) *The Interpretation of Cultures.* New York: Basic Books.

– (1983) *Local Knowledge: Further Essays on Interpretative Anthropology.* New York: Basic Books.

Gilmore, Norbert and Margaret A. Somerville (1994) 'Stigmatization, Scapegoating and Discrimination in Sexually Transmitted Disease: Overcoming "Them" and "Us",' *Social Science & Medicine*, 39(9), pp. 1339–58.

Jamieson, Neil (1995) *Understanding Vietnam*. University of California Press.

Keesing, R.M. (1987) 'Anthropology as Interpretative Quest,' *Current Anthropology* 28, pp. 161–76.

Kelly, Paula and Duong Bach Le (1999) *Trafficking in Humans From and Within Vietnam*. Hanoi: ILO, Radda Barnen SCF (UK) and Unicef.

Le, Thi (ed.) (1995) *Vietnam Family: Responsibilities and Resources in the Changing of the Country*. International Year of the Family 1994. Hanoi: Social Science Publishing House.

Lim, L.L. (1998) *The Sex Sector. The Economic and Social Bases of Prostitution in Southeast Asia*. Geneva: International Labour Office.

Massesa E.O. (2000) *Improving Sexual and Reproductive Health Needs among Adolescents in Tanzania: A Neglected Group*. Thesis at the 36th International Course in health Development. Amsterdam: Royal Tropical Institute.

Muecke, Marjorie A. (1992) 'Mother Sold Food, Daughter Sells Her Body: The Cultural Continuity of Prostitution,' *Social Science & Medicine* 35(7), pp. 891–901.

Lyttleton Chris (2000) *Endangered Relations. Negotiating Sex and AIDS in Thailand*. Amsterdam: Harvard Academic Publishers.

Ratliff, Eric (1999) 'Women as "Sex Workers", Men as "Boy Friends": Shifting Identities in Philippine Go-go Bars and their Significance to STD/AIDS Control,' *Anthropology & Medicine* 6(1), pp. 79–101.

Soucy, Alexander (2000) *Masculinity and Reproductive Health: The Imperative and Integrated Approach to Gender*. Paper presented at the Gender Donor Group Meeting, Hanoi (unpublished).

Thuc, D. *et al.* (1996) 'Family Under Siege'. *Saigon Times Weekly,* 224.

Tjiong, Dewi and Reiner Groeneveld (2001) *HIV/AIDS, A Foreigners' Disease? A Study on Tourists and the Sex Industry in Vietnam*. Ho Chi Minh City: MRSC.

Van Kerkwijk, Carla (1995) 'The Dynamics of Condom Use in Thai Sex Work with Farang Clients,' in: Han ten Brummelhuis and Gilbert Herdt (eds) *Culture and Sexual Risk. Anthropological Perspectives on AIDS*. Canada: Gordon and Breach Publishers, pp. 115–43.

Van der Meer, Maaike, Marieke Verhoeven, Nguyen Nguyen Nhu Trang, Paula Kelly, Anke van der Kwaak and Ivan Wolffers (1998) *The Knowledge of Body, Sex, Sexuality & Risky Behaviour of Young Adults in Vietnam*. Ho Chi Minh City: Care International.

Vietnamese Studies (1993) *The Traditional Family in Transitional Period.* Hanoi: Vietnam Studies 3 Xuhasaba.

Wolffers, Ivan (1995) *HIV/AIDS and the Mass Media. Capacity Building Module for Journalists, Broadcasters and Other Media Representatives.* Copenhagen: WHO.

– (1997) 'Culture, Media and HIV/AIDS in Asia,' *Lancet,* 349, pp. 52–4.

Wolffers Ivan, Rika S. Triyoga, Endang Basuki, Didik Yudhi, Walter Devillé and Rachmat Hargono (1999) 'Pacar and Tamu: Indonesian Women Sex Workers' Relationships with Men,' *Culture, Health & Sexuality* 1, pp. 39–53.

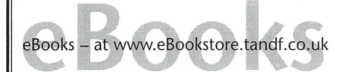
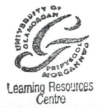

Learning Resources
Centre